Nursing Ethics

Nursing Ethics

Normative Foundations, Advanced Concepts, and Emerging Issues

Edited by

MICHAEL J. DEEM AND JENNIFER H. LINGLER

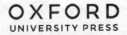

OXFORD
UNIVERSITY PRESS

OXFORD
UNIVERSITY PRESS

Oxford University Press is a department of the University of Oxford. It furthers
the University's objective of excellence in research, scholarship, and education
by publishing worldwide. Oxford is a registered trade mark of Oxford University
Press in the UK and certain other countries.

Published in the United States of America by Oxford University Press
198 Madison Avenue, New York, NY 10016, United States of America.

Library of Congress Cataloging-in-Publication Data
Names: Deem, Michael J., editor. | Lingler, Jennifer H., editor.
Title: Nursing ethics: normative foundations, advanced concepts, and emerging issues /
[edited by Michael J. Deem and Jennifer H. Lingler].
Description: New York, NY : Oxford University Press, [2024] |
Includes bibliographical references and index. |
Identifiers: LCCN 2024024880 | ISBN 9780190063559 (pb) |
ISBN 9780190063580 (epub) | ISBN 9780190063573 (ebook) |
ISBN 9780190063566 (ebook)
Subjects: LCSH: Nursing ethics.
Classification: LCC RT85 .N8795 2024 | DDC 174.2/9073—dc23/eng/20240621
LC record available at https://lccn.loc.gov/2024024880

DOI: 10.1093/med/9780190063559.001.0001

Printed by Marquis Book Printing, Canada

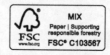

Contents

PART II. EMERGING ETHICAL ISSUES IN CLINICAL PRACTICE

Preface

Nursing ethics is no fledgling field. For roughly a century and a half, nurses have been publishing books and articles on ethical issues—from the esoteric to the mundane—that arise in clinical practice. The profession of nursing has had a formal code of ethics in place since at least 1950 and, over the past three decades in particular, nursing ethics has established itself as a significant field of ethical inquiry and research. Despite this storied history, there is wide recognition that the broader field of bioethics has been slow to consider ethical perspectives peculiar to nursing practice. During the formation of bioethics as both an academic and clinical field from the late 1940s through the late 1970s, concerns regarding ethical conduct of clinical research and the ethical and practical challenges arising from the *physician*-patient relationship dominated much of bioethical inquiry. It wasn't until the early 1980s that bioethics as a whole began to show interest, albeit limited, in the unique ethical challenges and insights arising from nursing practice, the particular duties that stem from nurses' professional and moral identities, and the ethical and policy implications of interprofessional and organizational structures in healthcare. One of the first publications to address these issues from both philosophical and nursing perspectives, and to help to establish nursing ethics as a recognized subfield in bioethics, was published by this very press: Martin Benjamin and Joy Curtis, *Ethics in Nursing: Cases, Principles, and Reasoning* (1981).

Since that time, introductory texts in nursing ethics have proliferated. Most of these volumes share a common approach and scope; that is, providing a comprehensive and accessible introduction to a broad array of ethical issues in nursing. While such texts have a vitally important role in undergraduate nursing education, they rarely feature the sort of original and rigorous analyses that might distinguish nursing ethics as a distinct subfield of bioethics. Instead, this latter, more advanced and rigorous work tends typically to appear in peer-reviewed journals in nursing, nursing ethics, or general bioethics.

The present volume was born out of a twofold concern. As faculty teaching ethics courses to students in both baccalaureate and graduate nursing programs, as well as to students across a range of other health professions, we wished to gather between two covers a set of original essays that would enable students in the health professions to engage in high-level discussions of central and emerging issues in nursing ethics, exposing them to the work of ethicists from multiple disciplines whose work is of particular relevance to nurses, including advanced practice nurses and nurse researchers. In addition to this pedagogical concern, we saw the need for a single volume comprising essays by an interdisciplinary group of scholars as an important step toward securing a recognized place among other subfields within bioethics, broadly construed. In other words, we envisioned a volume that shows the importance of nursing ethics not just to nurses, but also to other clinicians and bioethicists. At the same time, we wished to show the relevance of philosophical, legal, and *broadly* clinical inquiry to the ethical and practical issues that nurses face. While related fields, such as medical ethics and public health ethics, are replete with advanced, interdisciplinary, and scholarly volumes of this kind, the same is not yet true of nursing ethics.

To these ends, we sought to gather new essays from a wide range of academic and clinical perspectives that provide extended, rigorous examination of the normative foundations, advanced concepts, and new directions in nursing ethics. The resulting volume, to be sure, is not an introduction to nursing ethics, nor does it purport to be a comprehensive overview of the field. Rather, this volume gathers essays that provide both conceptual, normative analyses and practical reflections that push discourse and debate in nursing ethics beyond what one might find in an introductory book or an initial nursing or healthcare ethics course. While the volume is a suitable complement to basic volumes introducing the field, it will be of particular utility to ethics courses in advanced practice nursing programs (e.g., MSN, DNP, PhD), whose students increasingly have had prior exposure to fundamental topics and issues in ethics. Most importantly and more ambitiously, we hope the volume makes a contribution to scholarly bioethical discourse, well beyond the academic and professional boundaries of nursing.

The volume is divided into two parts. Part I focuses on foundational normative issues in nursing ethics, including questions about its independence as a field of inquiry among other subfields in bioethics, its methods, and its potential contribution to forming ethical environments for healthcare professionals. Several chapters address questions surrounding the scope, reliability, and limit of nurses' ethical knowledge and expertise, and the moral and practical identities that nurses take on *qua* nurses. These chapters are marked by rigor and a plurality of approaches to these issues, including conceptual analysis, narrative explorations, and feminist ethics.

Part II focuses on emerging issues in clinical practice and nursing education. This wide-ranging set of essays includes contributions from academic and clinical ethicists from nursing, medicine, philosophy, and law. Current and anticipated ethical challenges in the care of persons, families, and communities impacted by both physical and mental health conditions are addressed. Several chapters aim to proactively identify ethical concerns posed by new developments in areas such as biotechnology, health policy, and cultural shifts. Essays focusing on education feature novel analyses of the conditions under which explicit con-sent is required of participants in the education of nurses, including consent to care by clinical trainees and consent to the use of photographic images of per-sons in texts and lectures on tragic historical events in clinical practice or re-search. Like Part I, the essays in Part II reflect the diversity of approaches found in the published literature on nursing ethics, including policy analysis, empirical research, case studies, and relational ethics analysis.

This is an exciting period in nursing ethics. It is our hope that this volume will serve as a single, advanced resource that will contribute to the reinforcement of the field as a distinct and important subfield of both academic bioethics and clinical ethics. Collectively, the essays contained within this volume hold the po-tential to propel a flourishing area of scholarship toward the continued pursuit of high-quality, in-depth ethical inquiry and analysis. On a practical level, these essays should appeal to academic bioethicists, healthcare professionals, clinical ethicists, professional nurses and advanced practice nurses working in clinical and research contexts, and healthcare institutions seeking to establish more prominent roles for nurses in clinical ethics and ethics education.

We are grateful to the scholars and clinicians who contributed essays to this volume. We warmly remember Robert Veatch, who passed away before comple-tion of the volume. He provided encouragement early in the process of devel-oping the project and graciously contributed one of his last essays to it. He is missed.

Acknowledgments

This project benefited from the generosity of several individuals and institutions. We thank the Phillip H. Wimmer and Betty L. Wimmer Family Foundation for its financial support.

We are grateful to Heidi Funke, Jeremy Garrett, and Claire Horner, who served as expert reviewers of early drafts of the chapters in this volume and provided helpful feedback to contributors. Rebekah Cheng, Melissa Knox, Caroline Ronsivalle, and Lisa Tamres provided valuable editorial assistance in the later stages of production.

The 2018 and 2020 Carol Carfang Conference for Nursing and Health Care Ethics, organized by the Duquesne University School of Nursing, provided a welcome opportunity for connecting with many of the contributors to the volume and for discussing ideas for chapters.

Our thanks to Oxford University Press's editorial team, whose professionalism and patience enabled the volume to remain on a smooth track through its development and publication. Hannah Doyle and Brent Matheny provided valuable assistance on contractual and editorial matters. Suriya Narayanan led the copy-editing effort and ensured timely production of the volume. We especially express our gratitude to Lucy Randall, our OUP editor, who championed the project from the start, provided continuous feedback and support through its development, and ensured that the volume met the press's standards and expectations.

Finally, we are grateful to our nursing students, whom we have had the privilege to teach over the past two decades at CUNY College of Staten Island, Duquesne University, and the University of Pittsburgh. Their insightful, pressing, and challenging ethical and social questions were a significant inspiration behind this project.

Contributors

Jalayne J. Arias, JD, MA
Associate Professor, Department of Health
Policy & Behavioral Sciences
School of Public Health
Georgia State University
Atlanta, GA, USA

**Jennifer L. Bartlett, PhD, RN-BC,
CNE, CHSE**
Associate Professor, Georgia Baptist
College of Nursing
Mercer University
Macon, GA, USA

Katherine Brown-Saltzman, MA, RN
Co-Founder and former Co-Director,
UCLA Health Ethics Center
Los Angeles, CA, USA
Ethics Instructor, School of Nursing
University of California, Los Angeles
Los Angeles, CA, USA

Angel C. Carter, DNP, APRN, NNP-BC
Nurse Practitioner, Neonatal/Perinatal
Medicine
Children's Mercy Kansas City
Kansas City, MI, USA

Brian S. Carter, MD, FAAP
Marjorie and William Sirridge Endowed
Professor
Department of Medical Humanities and
Bioethics, School of Medicine
University of Missouri–Kansas City
Kansas City, MI, USA
Interim Director, Bioethics Center
Children's Mercy Kansas City
Kansas City, MI, USA

Helen Yue-lai Chan, RN, PhD
Professor, The Nethersole School of
Nursing
The Chinese University of Hong Kong
Shatin, N.T., Hong Kong

**Helen Stanton Chapple, PhD, RN,
MA, MSN**
Professor, School of Medicine
Creighton University
Omaha, NE, USA

Ho-yu Cheng, RN, PhD
Assistant Professor, The Nethersole
School of Nursing
The Chinese University of Hong Kong
Shatin, N.T., Hong Kong

Wai-tong Chien, RMN, PhD
Director and Professor, The Nethersole
School of Nursing
The Chinese University of Hong Kong
Shatin, N.T., Hong Kong

Connie Yuen-yu Chong, RN, PhD
Assistant Professor, The Nethersole
School of Nursing
The Chinese University of Hong Kong
Shatin, N.T., Hong Kong

Michael J. Deem, PhD
Associate Professor, Department of
Human Genetics, School of
Public Health
Core Faculty, Center for Bioethics &
Health Law
University of Pittsburgh
Pittsburgh, PA, USA

Judith A. Erlen, PhD, RN, FAAN
Professor Emeritus, Department of Health
& Community Systems
School of Nursing
University of Pittsburgh
Pittsburgh, PA, USA

Heather Fitzgerald, DBe, MS,
RN, HEC-C
Interim Director, Office of Professional
Fulfillment, and Resilience Clinical
Ethicist
Stanford Medicine Children's Health
Palo Alto, CA, USA

Megan Gillen, RN
Director of Nursing, Hospice Caris
Healthcare
Charleston, SC, USA

Pamela J. Grace, PhD, RN, FAAN, HEC-C
Associate Professor Emerita, William
F. Connell School of Nursing
Boston College
Chestnut Hill, MA, USA

Laura K. Guidry-Grimes, PhD, HEC-C
Associate Staff Bioethicist, Center for
Bioethics
Cleveland Clinic
Clinical Assistant Professor of Medicine,
Cleveland Clinic Lerner College of
Medicine
Clinical Assistant Professor of Bioethics,
Case Western Reserve University School
of Medicine
Cleveland, OH, USA

Christa M. Johnson, PhD
Associate Professor of Teaching
The Ohio State University
Columbus, OH, USA

Richard Kim, PhD
Associate Professor, Department of
Philosophy
Loyola University Chicago
Chicago, IL, USA

Emily A. Largent, PhD, JD, RN
Emanuel & Robert Hart Assistant
Professor of Medical Ethics and
Health Policy
Department of Medical Ethics &
Health Policy
Perelman School of Medicine
University of Pennsylvania
Philadelphia, PA, USA

Philip J. Larkin, PhD, MSc
Chair of Palliative Care, Nursing Palliative
and Supportive Care Service
Institute of Higher Education and Research
Healthcare Lausanne University Hospital
University of Lausanne
Lausanne, Switzerland

Doris Yin-ping Leung, PhD
Associate Professor, School of Nursing
The Hong Kong Polytechnic University
Hung Hom, Hong Kong

Joan Liaschenko, PhD, MA, MS, RN,
HEC-C, FAAN
Professor Emerita, Center for Bioethics
and School of Nursing
University of Minnesota
Minneapolis, MI, USA

Jennifer H. Lingler, PhD, MA,
CRNP, FAAN
Professor and Vice Chair for Research,
Department of Health & Community Systems
School of Nursing Faculty, Center for
Bioethics & Health Law
University of Pittsburgh
Pittsburgh, PA, USA

Elizabeth Peter, PhD, RN, FAAN
Professor, Lawrence S. Bloomberg Faculty
of Nursing
Member, Joint Centre for Bioethics
University of Toronto
Chair, Ethics Review Board Public Health
Ontario
Toronto, Ontario, Canada

Cynda Hylton Rushton, PhD, RN, FAAN
Anne and George L. Bunting Professor
of Clinical Ethics, Berman Institute of
Bioethics
Professor, School of Nursing
Professor, Department of Pediatrics,
School of Medicine
Johns Hopkins University
Baltimore, MD, USA

Erica K. Salter, PhD, HEC-C
Associate Professor, Albert Gnaegi Center
for Health Care Ethics
Associate Professor, Department of Pediatrics
Saint Louis University
St. Louis, MI, USA

Liz Stokes, PhD, JD, RN
Director, Center for Ethics and
Human Rights
American Nurses Association
Silver Spring, MD, USA

Carol Taylor, PhD, RN, FAAN
Senior Clinical Scholar, Kennedy Institute
of Ethics
Professor, Department of Nursing and
Medicine, School of Nursing
Georgetown University
Washington, DC, USA

Robert M. Veatch, PhD
Senior Research Scholar, Kennedy
Institute for Ethics
Professor Emeritus, Department of
Philosophy
Georgetown University
Washington, DC, USA

Eric Vogelstein, PhD
Associate Professor, School of Nursing &
Department of Philosophy
Duquesne University
Pittsburgh, PA, USA

Jamie Carlin Watson, PhD, HEC-C
Associate Staff Bioethicist, Center for
Bioethics
Cleveland Clinic
Cleveland, OH, USA

Daniel A. Wilkenfeld, PhD
Associate Professor, Department of Acute
& Tertiary Care, School of Nursing
University of Pittsburgh
Pittsburgh, PA, USA

PART I
CONCEPTS, KNOWLEDGE, AND PRACTICAL IDENTITY

1

An Argument for the Distinct Nature of Nursing Ethics

Pamela J. Grace

In this chapter, I argue that *nursing ethics* is rightfully viewed as a distinct field of critical inquiry relevant to the nursing profession and its purposes. While there are areas of overlap and mutual interests with bioethics, medical ethics, and the ethics of other disciplines, nursing ethics is concerned with the particular purposes and perspectives of the profession and problems faced in trying to achieve its goals. Nursing ethics, as a field of inquiry, has to do with the purposes of the profession, the scope and limits of practice, expectations of nurse clinicians, educators, and scholars, and the future direction of disciplinary knowledge development. Nursing ethics, like other professional ethics, is informed by insights from centuries of moral philosophizing, the conceptualization of nurse scholars and researchers about the distinct nature of the profession, and the experiences of frontline nurses. It is an *applied, professional* ethics.

I use philosophical argumentation, prior research, personal practice experiences, and the contemporary sociopolitical context of healthcare to support the argument that nursing ethics is its own entity with its own sphere of inquiry. Finally, I advance a definition of nursing ethics, comparing and contrasting it with those of bioethics, medical ethics, and the ethics of other healthcare professions. Importantly, the contemporary move to propose that bioethics be the parent discipline under which all healthcare professional and sociopolitical issues can be subsumed is challenged. Bioethics to date has shown that as a field of inquiry it is ill-equipped to provide ethical guidance for healthcare professional practice in the absence of insights from everyday clinician experiences and concerns. These types of concerns have been called "microethics" by Truog and colleagues (2015) and "everyday ethics" by others. Issues affecting daily nursing practice, whether these are inpatient-, institution-, or community-oriented, are rarely addressed in bioethics conferences and literature. The problems of daily professional practice often remain invisible to the "bioethics lens" unless highlighted by the nurses and other healthcare professionals who experience them. Moreover, the often intimate and prolonged encounters that accompany bedside and primary care nursing work render visible patient and family vulnerabilities stemming from their contexts and how they are affected by sociopolitical conditions. This is not to argue that all nurses are experts at addressing unjust social policies; many are quite obviously not. But nurses do see firsthand the sequelae, and for the most part in a more sustained way, of ill health stemming from poverty, inadequate access, premature hospital discharges, poor nutrition, and toxic living and working environments. Expectations that nurses will act to address unjust policies (unit, institutional, and societal) exist nationally and internationally (American Nurses Association, 2015; International Council of Nursing, 2012). The level at which nurses act thusly will, of course, differ according to the ethical awareness of nurses related to the ethics of everyday practice and the origins of obstacles to practicing well (Milliken et al., 2018), the role assumed, and education level. Curricula content at the baccalaureate, master's, and doctoral levels generally includes policy content, and professional organizations, such as the American Nurses Association, American Academy of Nursing, and those in other countries, all have policy arms.

For nurses, guided by the profession's raison d'être or historically developed goals (Fowler, 2016; Grace & Willis, 2012), an understanding of one's ethical responsibilities is not solely the purview of scholars and academics but of every nurse. Thus, nursing ethics is not about esoteric moral theories—although certainly insights from such theories can provide clarity about what one ought to do in certain difficult circumstances—but rather about how one can practice well on a daily basis, and how to address obstacles to good practice. Further, nurses do have responsibilities to join or collaborate with others in identifying and addressing social injustices that give rise to poor health. Not to do so is equivalent to treating a patient for an infection such as the parasite *Giardia* from a community, but not doing anything to cause community awareness of the problem so that changes can be affected. The root cause of the problem is left unaddressed and thus the problem recurs or is perpetuated.

The field of inquiry that is nursing ethics has given rise to ethical guidelines such as codes of ethics (ANA, 2015; ICN, 2012) and social policy statements (ANA, 2010). So, codes of ethics and the historically determined goals and perspectives of the profession outline both a nurse's obligations related to everyday practice and, in concert with others, to address the roots of ill health in societal conditions (Grace, 2001; Grace & Willis, 2012). Finally, distinguishing nursing ethics, other professional ethics, and bioethics, rather than being problematic, broadens the areas of potential knowledge development by highlighting how each can inform the others and provide added value to the enterprise of promoting the "good" of health for individuals and the society.

Background

Before detailing the facets of my argument for accepting nursing ethics as a separate area of inquiry distinct from that of either medical ethics or bioethics, I provide some history of how I came to this realization. Varied and lengthy nursing experiences in both the United Kingdom and the United States, in critical care and later as a nurse practitioner, along with doctoral studies in philosophy, were all influential. It might seem odd, as it does to some of my faculty colleagues, that I chose to pursue a philosophy rather than a nursing PhD. How that came about is serendipitous. During my master's level nursing studies, I had the opportunity to enroll in a graduate-level bioethics course offered as an elective to nursing students. This course, taught by philosopher Mark Wicclair, was enlightening. I realized that the critical thinking and analytic skills developed during the class were just what I needed to help me understand in more depth the nuances of the countless practice problems I had faced in my career and thus their likely resolution. Eventually, on the advice of Mark, I enrolled in the University of Tennessee-Knoxville's (UTK) philosophy program. This program was particularly suited to my goals of developing ethical decision-making abilities, since it had an additional concentration in medical ethics. I was also fortunate to secure a part-time faculty position in the UTK College of Nursing, where I taught undergraduate and graduate nursing students both adult health content and nursing theory.

Learning to Be a Philosopher

It must have been obvious to my philosophy professors and peers from the beginning that I had difficulty separating my nursing role from that of philosophy scholar. I was often the recipient of the reminder, "take off your nursing hat and put on your philosophy hat," when I gave clinical examples related to a philosophical argument. While I tried desperately to do this, in awe of their intellectual skills and so hoping that this would enable my development as a true philosophy scholar with sharply honed skills of critical and ethical analysis, I found that I could not. I was constantly frustrated in this desire; no matter how hard I tried, I was not able to isolate "me the philosophy student" from "me the experienced nurse." Even during deep dives into the writings of various philosophers to understand what they were doing, I would question, "Why was X compelled to explore this?" The voices of various patients would rise to my consciousness, asking, "How will your knowing this help me?"

Steeped in nursing work since the age of 18 (I was 39 years old when I started doctoral studies), I had intimate contact with people facing the extremes of life's boundaries. These experiences inevitably dispel naivete about life and its travails. Patients expect and have to trust that they will receive help in navigating the physical and existential difficulties that bring them to a healthcare setting (Grace, 2001; Sellman, 2006). They are not necessarily aware of the various obstacles that nurses and other clinicians face in striving to meet their needs.

Because of our close and sustained contact with patients and their families, nurses often become the repositories and auditors of their stories and hopes. I vividly remember Carol, one of my first patients. She was a young woman with an extruding abdominal cancer that she had hidden until it was no longer curable. The daily extensive wound dressings and the foul odor emanating from the wound caused her severe psychological and physical distress that could only be lessened but not eliminated by compassionate care, which she did not always receive. Among the collage of other strong memories was that of the nameless homeless man found unconscious on the street, whose undershirt had to be gently peeled off from the chest hair that had grown through it before we could delouse him. There was Hari, the 9-month-old abandoned baby with a brain injury, whose pitiful cries could not be pacified even though I held and rocked him while pacing the ward floor to monitor others in my charge. These and other indelible memories contaminated my ability to engage in philosophical studies from a neutral stance. Indeed, they were what led to my desire to improve my analytic skills and to learn how to better understand and articulate the nuances of both complex and daily practice problems. Often, my colleagues and I faced obstacles to what we saw as good patient care. For example, inadequate staffing was an ongoing issue. Sometimes there was a lack of support from supervisors and the institution, whose priorities seemed to differ from ours. There were hierarchical issues where nurses' perspectives on the patient's needs and preferences were either not heard or dismissed. At other times, it would be hard to access a physician for a needed order change or to validate our assessment of a patient's deterioration and intervene in a timely manner. Resources to resolve these sorts of problems were rare. For most of my career, clinical ethics resources were not readily available.

Even in more recent times, when many hospitals have an ethics resource or consultant, available services tend to be aimed toward the resolution of dilemmatic crises rather than the everyday issues with which point-of-care nurses often struggle. Yet the ability to engage in "preventive ethics"—that is, recognizing and addressing emerging ethical issues expediently and bringing them to the attention of the team—is an important aspect of ethical nursing practice. Preventive actions are in alignment with the ethical principle of nonmaleficence, particularly in terms of minimizing potential harms.

Preventive ethics is a relatively new term proposed by Forrow and colleagues (1993), capturing the idea that some ethical issues can be anticipated and addressed before they escalate to dilemmas. As Epstein summarizes (2012), "preventive ethics proposes that ethical conflict is largely predictable and can be avoided with proactive interventions aimed at the organization, unit, and individual levels" (p. 217). As an example, a nurse notices that a comatose patient's family is confused about the severity of his condition based on information they have been given by different members of the team. Taking actions to ensure the family is given consistent messages by the team can prevent the situation from becoming conflictual in a way that undermines the family's trust in the team. For these reasons, it is important that nurses are prepared to recognize and address ethical issues in practice and beyond. The development of nurses who are confident in their ethical decision-making skills is a task for the field of nursing ethics, as I argue below. While non-nurses may be involved in the ethics education of nurses, the appropriate ethics education of nurses is a task for the field of nursing ethics to determine.

So, two related conditions prevented me from assuming a purely philosophical stance in my PhD studies. The first had to do with the fact that I saw myself as a *nurse*, and this had become relatively inseparable from my identity. The second was, as described above, the difficulties in practicing well in the face of multiple confounding influences and derived from the reason I was pursuing this course of study in the first place.

Subjectively a Nurse First

These experiences of caring for people at their most vulnerable as well as most resilient moments were the very reason for my pursuing a high-level degree in philosophy. I came to understand that, infused as I was by practice experiences, taking a purely objective stance was no longer either possible, necessary, or desirable. My motivation for engaging in philosophy studies was to gain the skills and tools to empower myself as both an educator and clinician, and to develop nurses' moral agency on behalf of good patient care. I wanted to be able to use these skills to help nursing students and practicing nurses understand the extent of their professional responsibilities to patients and society, develop their confidence in ethical decision-making, and build their moral agency. For nursing purposes, and in alignment with James Rest's four-component model of moral action (1982, 1983), moral agency means that the nurse understands his or her professional responsibilities as *ethical* in nature, can engage in ethical decision-making (alone or in a team setting), has an understanding of ethical precepts and their relationship to nursing goals and perspectives, and is motivated to act to resolve actual or potential ethical problems.

Developing Skills: Remaining Concerned With
Everyday Nursing Problems

Besides exposure to ideas of philosophers ranging from ancient to contemporary times, during the philosophy studies part of the degree, there were courses on logic, moral philosophy, and value theory. The medical ethics concentration also involved a clinical ethics practicum. However, I discovered that the emphasis on medical and bioethics-type problems involving ethical conflicts and dilemmas did not accommodate my concern with issues of everyday nursing practice, which had led me to philosophy studies in the first place. Those everyday problems, for the most part, did not float up to the attention of clinical ethicists or ethics committees, yet they often underlay the later development of conflicts. Thus, I saw that it was up to me to make the applications of my learning to the work of nurses.

As noted above, daily ethical issues for nurses include such things as not having enough staff to provide optimal care, difficulties transmitting knowledge of patient preferences to those making treatment decisions, family members pressuring patients to accept treatments that they do not want, patients not understanding what was being proposed, and getting patients adequate pain control, among innumerable other problems. Unless nurses effectively articulate how such issues affect patient care, and why it is in the interests of everyone that they are addressed, they are unlikely to be heard and the root causes of problems remain uncovered. I have a vivid memory of an ethics practicum experience where I was in a hospital ethics committee meeting. The discussion was about an elderly patient from a nursing home. She had suffered aspiration pneumonia, and the question was whether it was permissible to insert a gastrostomy feeding tube even though she had "passed a swallow test." Serendipitously, I had been supervising student nurses doing their clinical practice in the same nursing home as part of my faculty role in the college of nursing. I had noted how there was only one nurse's aide to feed those patients who could not feed themselves. A given aide had up to four patients to feed on any particular day and had to rush from one patient to another. The situation was ripe for patients to aspirate stomach contents into their lungs. Thus, the primary ethical question should not have been about the permissibility of placing a gastronomy tube, but rather why were there inadequate staff in the nursing home to safely feed patients. This was not the sort of question that could be answered in the absence of understanding the context of care in the particular nursing home (or perhaps in nursing homes in general). Yet, who was looking at these recurring problems, the root causes of which lay in the larger sociopolitical environment?

As Garrett (2015) critiques, the individual "duty of rescue" perspective that pervades bioethical deliberations tends to neglect the reality that bioethical dilemmas, for the most part, are not solely isolated problems to be resolved in the moment. To provide a more enduring good, it is necessary to explore the sociocultural patterns from which the makings of dilemmas spring and which often require agents from different disciplines, as well as the public, to bring about needed sociopolitical change.

The Critical Nature of a Nurse's Observations

From incidents such as that of the nursing home patient described above, I realized four important things. First, the perspective of knowledgeable nurses at the immediate bedside is critical when it comes to good inpatient care. The intimate contact they have with patients, families, and the caregiving environment makes them privy to factors that would not appear even within the peripheral vision of others whose interactions are more fleeting. Second, many of the problems that later develop into ethical crises could be identified and intercepted earlier if the voices of nurses were heard and their perspective on the patient's needs accounted for. Third, some problems that arise in practice have their roots in sociopolitical conditions that disadvantage the most vulnerable, and nurses are often well positioned to recognize this (Grace, 2001). Finally, my experiences as a nurse, along with the privilege of education in philosophy and philosophical analysis, put me in a unique position to see these gaps and attempt to bridge them. Thus, it would be up to me to make the application of my growing philosophical skills and knowledge to these seemingly more mundane nursing problems that were not easily visible in the clinical ethics enterprise. Moreover, it solidified my understanding that "nursing ethics" is a venture that is largely distinct from medical or biomedical ethics, although these fields of study have areas of overlapping and reciprocal interests related to individual and societal goods. How a nurse responds to his or her inability to provide optimal care for patients when assigned too many to adequately meet the needs of any one of them is a problem for nurse scholars to explore. It would be virtually impossible for a physician or ethicist to grasp the contextual nuances of such a situation without being informed by the perspective of the nurse.

As evidenced from the literature, each of the disciplines came into being because of a particular type of human need that was not otherwise being met. Each went through a process of knowledge development unique to the particular field. That is, the focus of the lens through which a problem is perceived is directed by the professional role (or disciplinary role, in the case of ethicists who do not belong to a healthcare profession). For example, a review of several decades of nursing literature revealed a focus on humanizing the healthcare environment and viewing the person's healthcare needs within the larger contexts of their lives (Willis et al., 2008). Historically, nurses have also been concerned with sociopolitical conditions that impair the health of the least well off (Fowler, 2017).

In part, the focus of the ethical enterprise for each healthcare profession depends on the goals and perspectives of the given profession as developed and articulated over time in response to societal need for particular services. Healthcare professions have disciplinary (academic and knowledge development) arms and practice arms which are, ideally, mutually informative (Adam, 1985; Bayles, 1981; Donaldson & Crowley, 1978; Meleis, 2018). Both the nursing and medical professions have clearly articulated goals conceptualized by disciplinary scholars as foci for practice, educational, and research endeavors toward the provision of a human good. However, the goals of bioethics and bioethicists are not yet articulated in a cohesive way that could provide a strong, unified foundation for knowledge development, decision-making, and agency.

Moreover, it is doubtful that there can be unifying goals due to the varied nature of the bioethics enterprise. One reason for this may be the considerable extent to which bioethics is shaped by moral philosophy. The focus of moral philosophy is on theorizing about whether there is or can be a human good to which all humans strive. Ideas derived from moral philosophy and resulting moral theories when applied in practice are applied ethics. Clearly, applied ethics for professional practice focuses on what is needed to realize the specified goals of the profession, including the appropriate development, roles, and responsibilities of its members. Not so clear are the distinct and specific goals of bioethics, as will be discussed shortly. While there is now a code of ethics for clinical ethics consultants in the United States (American Society for Bioethics and the Humanities, 2014), it is specific to the role, rather than to the broader discipline. These reasons are the basis for my argument below that bioethics cannot serve as the parent discipline for the healthcare professions generally, or the nursing profession specifically. Bioethics is an adjunct discipline. As Kopelman argues, bioethics is rooted in many professions, disciplines, and fields and is best understood as a second-order discipline. A second-order discipline is one where members have a broad perspective and "include many perspectives and areas of expertise" (Kopelman, 2009, p. 263). The issues they explore are complex and impinge on many disciplines. Finally, there is reliance upon the primary "field(s) to set their educational or other standards of competency" (Kopelman, 2009, p. 263). A brief look at the development of bioethics as a discipline in comparison to that of the healthcare professions is illustrative of Kopelman's points.

Bioethics, Medical Ethics, and Nursing Ethics

There are areas both of distinction and overlap among these entities. Some have advocated that bioethics be considered the parent discipline for the healthcare professions, but this is not a logical proposition as argued in what follows.

Bioethics: Parent, Offspring, or Other?

Albert Jonsen (1998), one of the pioneers of bioethics as a field of inquiry, traces its development from its beginning in the 1960s up to the publication date of his book, *The Birth of Bioethics*. During and after World War II (1939–1945), the development of biological and technological innovations related to human trauma, disease, and incapacity was rapid and exponential compared to such developments in earlier years. Applications in the context of healthcare gave rise to new sorts of quandaries that were beyond the ability of the medical community to resolve on its own. Medical education and expertise were clinical in nature, and its applications were largely in the care of individual patients. Medical ethics, as discussed in more detail later, was concerned with the proper education and conduct of physicians in relation to their patients or practice area. As Pellegrino and Thomasma (2004) note, it stems from "a philosophy of medicine in which the good of the patient determines the obligations and virtues of the health professional" (p. 17). Medical ethics as a field of inquiry considered not just disease and ill health, but also the responsibilities of physicians to patients. Physicians were, generally, not skilled in evaluating philosophical, social, or moral questions. Yet, the unprecedented development of biotechnology and its applications to human disease and incapacity were posing just such sorts of problems. The complexity of such problems warranted the analyses of those skilled in unpacking complex problems. Clarity was needed about not only what best served the needs of patients and prospective patients individually, but also what was in the interests of society more generally. Additionally, the question of just application of scarce resources for healthcare purposes became a problem that required scrutiny beyond that of individual-physician interactions.

For example, in 1960 a patient in kidney failure received the first arteriovenous shunt permitting him to receive hemodialysis from a specially designed machine. Initially, however, there were more people in line for these machines than available machines, presenting a true moral dilemma (Jonsen, 1998). A true moral dilemma is a particular type of ethical problem where a person is forced to choose between two undesirable alternatives. The term "dilemma" comes from the Greek *di*, meaning "two," and *lemma*, meaning "premise" or "assumption" (Brown, 1993). The term as used in contemporary healthcare settings does not always denote a true or pure dilemma. Many so-called dilemmas would actually be resolvable or have a preferable choice of action or actions given more information, or access to resources. However, the issue of allocating a scarce resource—dialysis machines—was not purely one requiring medical judgment; rather, it was a social one requiring a value judgment. A broader ethical analysis was required, necessitating the use of different tools than those of clinical decision-making, to promote a just solution. Thus, the knowledge, skills, and input of other humanities and social sciences disciplines were sought. This is not to say that medicine abrogated its professional goals, but rather that help was needed from philosophers and social scientists in discerning how to meet those goals when complex human and sociopolitical questions arose related to the use and management of biotechnological advances.

Two Conceptions of Bioethics as a Discipline

Hence, the discipline of bioethics was born in the 1960s. Bioethics, according to *The Encyclopedia of Bioethics* (Reich, 1995) is "the study of the moral dimensions—including moral vision, decisions, conduct and policies—of the life sciences and health care, employing a variety of ethical methodologies in an interdisciplinary setting" (p. xxi). On this perspective, bioethics is essentially a multidisciplinary field that takes into account the goals of a profession in decision-making about individual and social good, but it does not develop or refine these goals. Indeed, a bioethicist, unless he or she were also a member of the given profession, would generally not understand the profession well enough to be capable of influencing the profession's goals. *The Encyclopedia of Bioethics'* perspective is the wider-ranging of the two definitions of bioethics available in the literature. It has been criticized as being too broad to be meaningful (Benatar, 2006). A central disciplinary focus or reason for being, as well as unified goals are missing. Moreover, few bioethicists are bioethicists first and foremost; most have a primary discipline and, related to their interests in bioethical issues and dilemmas, bioethics as a secondary interest (Kopelman, 2006). Allied to the question of disciplinary goals, the question could be raised, "Under which conditions would a physician bioethicist follow the goals of medicine and under which bioethical goals?" (assuming such goals exist or are discernible). The answer would have to be that it depends upon the role being assumed at the time of questioning.

There are a few institutions that currently offer doctoral and master-level degrees in bioethics and which do not also presume experience in either a professional or academic discipline. However, an informal survey of a sample of these programs fails to uncover a unifying focus, purpose, or practice area. Indeed, it is unclear in what sense pure bioethicists—those who do not have a prior practice profession—can be considered either professionals or practitioners. This is not to argue against the usefulness of bioethics education in problem-solving dilemmas and ethically complex issues, but rather to point out its inadequacy as a discipline for prescribing or overseeing the ethical actions of practice professionals. This task is the emic purview of the disciplinary arm of a profession, informed by the input of its members.

Benatar (2006) argues that a narrower view of bioethics is preferable: "On the narrower construal, bioethics, although it may draw on these other disciplines, is itself only an area of philosophical inquiry. More specifically, bioethics is one branch of practical (or applied) ethics, which is one branch of ethics, which in turn is one branch of philosophy" (p. 17). Viewing bioethics this way avoids the problem of "disciplinary slip" (p. 18). "Disciplinary slip" is the problem of assuming expertise to resolve a problem in a practice area for which one has not been trained. Regardless of which view of bioethics one holds, neither can subsume the ethics of the various professions for reasons given above and supported below.

Bioethics as an Overarching Discipline

Some commentators have argued quite strongly that bioethics should be understood as the overarching discipline for all areas of healthcare, including human subjects research, and the ethics of the healthcare professions. For example, Ruth Faden (2011), a humanities, bioethics, and public health scholar, when accepting a lifetime achievement award from the American Society of Bioethics and Humanities, argued that bioethics should be accepted as the parent term for all healthcare-associated ethics, including the ethics of the professions. Her point was that having bioethics as the overarching discipline gives a conceptual, strategic, and methodological advantage by consolidating power to influence change in the healthcare environment. She noted:

> At this point, some might respond that I am working with a stipulative definition of bioethics that by its very structure makes my conceptual point. If bioethics is defined broadly enough, as something like the ethics of health care, the ethics of the health of populations, and the ethics of biomedical science then of course it would subsume narrower areas like nursing ethics, neuroethics and so on. (Faden, 2011, p. 2)

This perspective misses the critical point that healthcare professions need to be self-reflective about their practices and attendant ethical obligations and such inquiries are the specific domain of the given profession. Certainly for nurses, concerns are likely to continue to remain hidden or dismissed as unimportant if subsumed under the rubrics of bioethics. Earlier in this chapter, I highlighted some of the problems I experienced as a bedside nurse. Other examples—to name just a few—include inadequate staffing for the acuity level of patients, which changes a nurse's emphasis from providing good care to minimizing risks of harm, orders for a patient from one specialist that conflict with orders from another specialist, and orders to discharge a patient who has no one at home capable of attending to his needs. In each of these cases, nurses are responsible for doing their best to resolve the immediate problem and address the underlying conditions that gave rise to the problem.

Clearly, these are not the sorts of problems with which the discipline of bioethics is typically concerned. So, rather than strengthening a power base for sociopolitical change, accepting bioethics as the discipline covering professional ethics both weakens the power of the individual healthcare professions to determine the details of their practice and adds to the vulnerability of those with less powerful voices (patients and professionals). Certainly, we can add to the bioethics discourse and benefit from bioethics-type assistance without subsuming our professional identities and associated responsibilities.

The Distinct Nature of Professions and Professional Ethics

The experiences and perspectives of healthcare professionals are important to the health and well-being of both individuals and society. Such perspectives cannot adequately be imagined by those who have not been educated in and/or lack experience in the given professional role. As Bayles (1981) notes, while there are no well-defined criteria for what constitutes a profession, "three necessary features have been singled out by almost all authors who have characterized professions" (p. 7). These are a prolonged education period, the accumulation of extensive knowledge related to the proposed services, and the provision of an important service to society. Further, professions have a certain amount of autonomy over the scope and boundaries of their practice (Grace, 1998). Healthcare professions are critical service professions (Windt, 1989). They have a "grinding life or death importance" (Windt, 1989, p. 7) in the lives of individuals and for the flourishing of society. Thus, they have focused goals related to human well-being, and those goals are necessarily ethical goals. That is, the profession's goals are to provide a human good, and they can be criticized to the extent that they do or do not further that good (Grace, 2001). Their fields of ethical inquiries are geared to exploring such questions as: Why does the profession exist? What needs does it serve? What characteristics are expected of the profession's members? What knowledge, experiences, and skills are needed to practice well? How are obstacles to good practice to be anticipated and overcome?

My argument in this chapter is that nursing ethics is rightly seen as a distinct field of inquiry not only from bioethics, but also from the ethical inquiries of other healthcare professions. There are, of course, areas of overlap. Nurses work with physicians and other professionals and encounter situations that cannot be resolved without the input of all concerned. Moreover, biotechnological advances are pervasive in the environment and in healthcare. Problems arising from their use are ubiquitous and frequently require disparate disciplines for their explication and resolution. Thus, my argument for nursing ethics to be understood as a separate field of inquiry is confined to exploring the historical development of the profession, the reason for its existence as a profession, and the proper development of its members and their ethical responsibilities related both to the care of individuals and to society more generally.

In the past, nursing ethics inquiries would have been subsumed under medical ethics or the ethics of the medical profession. Indeed, even in many schools of nursing where there is a mandated course in ethics, content is often taught under the rubric of "medical ethics" or "bioethics." While such courses are helpful in supplying the language and tools associated with ethical analysis of dilemmatic situations, in the absence of a concerted effort to make applications of such content to nursing work, these courses fail to prepare nurses for the everyday issues they will face in practice (Jurchak et al., 2017; Milliken & Grace, 2017). Truog and colleagues (2015) have highlighted a similar problem in medical education and practice. They note that everyday issues faced by physicians are not always viewed as *ethics* problems, yet there are ethical implications related to a physician's professional obligations. One example they use involves informed consent and anesthesia. As Truog et al. (2015) point out, "Anesthesiologists regularly obtain informed consent from otherwise healthy patients for routine low-risk anesthesia. Although the informed consent document typically lists 'death' as a potential complication of anesthesia, few patients actually read the form, and anesthesiologists vary widely" (p. 11) in their opinions about how this should be addressed. This is a question for medical ethics to resolve. Medicine and nursing generally have different microethics issues to resolve based on role, perspectives on how the role should play out, and associated responsibilities, but they also have shared concerns as well. As noted earlier, I discovered this during the medical ethics concentration of my philosophy doctoral studies, which stimulated my dissertation work analyzing the role responsibilities of medicine, nursing, law, and clinical ethics related to advocacy.

Medical Ethics as a Distinct Field of Inquiry

The medical profession internationally has a lengthy history of inquiry into the ethics of its practice and the conduct and the responsibilities of its members (Pellegrino & Thomasma, 2004). Philosophers, historians, and physicians have all undertaken such analyses. This philosophical field of inquiry is properly termed "medical ethics" and is a professional ethics. Allert and colleagues (1996) document an initiative to (re)conceptualize the goals of medicine. Led by project director Daniel Callahan, groups of physicians and other interested parties from 14 countries, after discussions over a four-year period, achieved consensus on four goals of medicine. These are: "The prevention of disease and injury and promotion and maintenance of health. The relief of pain and suffering caused by maladies. The care and cure of those with a malady, and the care of those who cannot be cured. The avoidance of premature death and the pursuit of a peaceful death." (Allert et al., 1996, para. 3). Medical ethics, then, is a field of inquiry about what is needed to develop physicians who can meet the profession's goals. Conflicts related to the impact of biological and technological advances inevitably impact how physicians go about meeting these goals. In such instances, bioethicists and clinical ethicists may be needed to assist in problem-solving. However, as noted earlier, it is unlikely that there can be unified goals for the discipline of bioethics, for the simple reason that it is not a practice profession per se. While there is an applied branch of bioethics in the United States, that of healthcare ethics consultants, for which goals have been proposed and documented, these are not directive. The goals of ethics consultation are asserted as being responsive "to questions from patients, families, surrogates, healthcare professionals, or other involved parties who seek to resolve uncertainty or conflict regarding value-laden concerns that emerge in health care" (American Society for Bioethics and Humanities, 2011, p. 2). Siegler (2019) argues, in essence, that the professionalization of clinical ethics consultants is premature. The goals, as articulated, are inadequate because they are not focused on patient good, and the recent certification process for clinical ethicists is premature in the absence of more empirical data (Siegler, 2019).

Nursing Ethics as a Distinct Field of Inquiry

The argument so far, augmented by several decades of literature documenting nursing's development into a distinct profession (Grace, 1998, 2001), supports the claim that nursing ethics is its own field of inquiry into the boundaries of practice, the appropriate knowledge base for that practice, and apt characteristics of members (Fowler, 2017; Fry, 2002; Grace, 2018). Elsewhere, I have proposed that the term *nursing ethics* can viewed be in two ways (Grace, 2018): first, as a field of inquiry; and second, as appraisal of nurses' actions to the extent that they are focused on furthering nursing goals in practice, education, and/or research. For example, a nurse is distracted by an illness in his family and lacks the energy and focus to interact with patients; instead, he performs tasks in a perfunctory manner. Nursing ethics as a critique of actions (the second sense of nursing ethics) would determine that the nurse failed to focus on upholding the goals of nursing. Nursing goals are defined as "the protection, promotion, and restoration of health and well-being; the prevention of illness and injury; and the alleviation of suffering, in the care of individuals, families, groups, communities and populations (ANA, 2015, Preface). While the goals of medicine, nursing, and the other healthcare professions tend to mutual interests, the perspective of nursing about how those goals are to be met is distinct and is based on the contexts and nature of nursing practice. Colleagues and I (Willis et al., 2008) explored several decades of nursing scholarship to uncover what, if any, were common perspectival themes. This culminated in our articulation of a *Central Unifying Focus for the Discipline*. Basically, our disciplinary efforts over the past six decades have been concerned with: "facilitating humanization, meaning, choice, quality of life, and healing in living and dying" (Willis et al., 2008, E28). Thus, the goals of nursing and perspectives on how those goals can be furthered, along with the prescriptions of nursing codes of ethics, are all features that distinguish nursing ethics from the fields of inquiry of other disciplines, while acknowledging that there are shared interests related to promoting individual and social good.

Nursing ethics, then, as a field of inquiry, is a professional applied ethics, like medical ethics. It is specific to the nature of nursing, nursing perspectives, and the scope and boundaries of nursing work as developed over time by nursing's philosophers, theorists, and researchers (Fowler, 2016) and informed by practicing clinicians. One result of this back-and-forth between nursing scholars, whose intellectual work and associated research almost always derived from practice experiences, and contemporary practitioners is the formulation of theories about the scope and boundaries of nursing practice. Determinations of the scope and boundaries of practice for a critical human service profession highlight the obligations of the profession. These obligations are in a sense "promises" (Grace, 1998, 2001) made to those served about what can be expected in the form of goods (services). In this sense they are the result of an ongoing process of ethical reasoning about what services are needed and what actions are permissible, obligatory, and prohibited.

Codes of ethics are only the tentative end results of professional deliberations about what is owed to society (Grace 1998, 2001). These codes are fluid in the sense that they must be revised as societal contexts and the needs for services change. As Marsha Fowler (2017), a nurse philosopher and historian, describes, the nursing profession has a long history of fighting for improved social conditions. Starting with Florence Nightingale, "an ardent social reformer" (Fowler, 2016, p. S9), and the later establishment of national nursing societies in various countries, nursing started to establish itself as a professional body with the need to determine the scope and obligations of its work. In 1893, the American Nurses Association was formed and there was early recognition that a code of ethics was needed (Fowler, 2016). In 1926, a "suggested code" was formulated; however, it was not until 1950 that a formal code of ethics was published. The latest *American Nurses Association (ANA) Code of Ethics for Nurses with Interpretive Statements* was published in 2015 and includes four provisions that speak to responsibilities toward individuals, families, and groups; one provision that speaks to the nurse's responsibilities to her- or himself; and four provisions that are focused on influencing broader professional, social, and healthcare contexts. In contrast, the American Medical Association (AMA)'s *Code of Medical Ethics* (2001) is focused predominantly on medical goals and medical practice with some, but much less, emphasis on responsibilities for remedying social inequities.

A code of ethics lays out guidelines for good practice and the expectations of members. Provisions of codes of ethics have to be practicable in order to meet the philosophical principle "ought implies can." That is, in order to avoid mandating that nurses do what they cannot because of intractable obstacles, codes of ethics have to reflect contemporary environments and provide guidance for the members should it become impossible to adhere to the provisions of the code. In American medicine, for example, there have been concerns that medical practice is more and more guided by what insurers will pay, rather than clinical judgment (Reich, 2012).

Most developed countries have published country-specific nursing codes of ethics. These tend to be similar in nature, although somewhat refined in line with the development of the profession in the particular country. The International Council of Nurses, a federation of more than 130 national nursing organizations, also has a code of ethics informed by those of its member states.

I suspect that some will object to my claim that nursing has its own field of inquiry related to ethical practice. One objection I have heard, which is founded on a misunderstanding of modern nursing, is that since nursing exists to support medical practice, and nurses' actions are largely dependent upon physician orders, medical ethics is the proper field of inquiry for good nursing practice. This objection mistakes the contemporary environment of nursing practice. It is true that some nursing actions support medical practice and are dependent on medical orders. However, even in these cases (e.g., dispensing medication) the nurse must use his or her judgment to decide if what is ordered is actually in the patient's interests, and he or she is accountable for questioning the order if it is not. Among the many independent nursing actions are responsibilities to evaluate a patient's physical and psychosocial status in a given setting and to address identified needs. Nurses make judgments about what resources are needed and how to access them. They evaluate what is being proposed for their patients and help them understand the meaning of interventions. Nurses are both legally and ethically accountable for the many independent judgments made daily in the interests of good patient care. Moreover, the nurse is accountable for questioning physician orders that do not align with their own clinical judgments.

Arguably, the nursing profession has been more reflective about its work than has medicine. This is in part because of the recent maturing of what was a vocation or occupation into a profession, partly because the problems associated with nursing practice have remained beneath the vision of philosophers, and partly because nursing has and continues to be a majority female endeavor. The discipline's scholars, informed by its practicing members, have clarified the goals of the profession and how those goals can be met. Nursing ethics inquiries, philosophical and empirical, have been ongoing and are aimed at understanding the characteristics of ethical nurses, good practice, identification of obstacles to good practice, and the responsibilities of nurses for individual and social well-being.

Conclusion

Nursing ethics is its own area of inquiry. It cannot realistically be considered under an umbrella concept such as bioethics, healthcare ethics, or medical ethics. None of these fields of inquiry is concerned with why nursing exists as a profession, what nurses' ethical responsibilities are, how nurses should act, or what nurses should do to identify and overcome obstacles to good practice that occur on a daily basis. While more attention has been paid recently to everyday practice issues from the bioethics and medical ethics community, this attention still tends to focus on problems of medical than nursing practice (Komesaroff, 1995; Truog et al., 2015). The nursing ethics literature, however, is much more developed than the medical ethics and bioethics literature in its attention to the problems that nurses and the healthcare team face in an increasingly complex healthcare system (Jurchak et al., 2017). There are many reasons for this, but perhaps the most compelling is that nurses spend the most time with patients, for the most part are exposed to the contextual aspects of person's lives, and often work within systems that hinder in various ways their ability to practice well. Additionally, their storied interactions with patients facilitate the profession's ability to question the root causes of problems, as these lie within sociopolitical contexts and give broader ethical responsibilities than to the patient alone.

References

Adam, E. (1985). Toward more clarity in terminology: Framework, theories and models. *Journal of Nursing Education*, 24(4), 151–155.

Allert, G., Blasszauer, B., Boyd, K., & Callahan, D. (1996). The goals of medicine: Setting new priorities, executive summary. *The Hasting Center Report*, 26(6), S1–S27.

American Medical Association. (2001). *AMA code of medical ethics*. American Medical Association. June 17–18.

American Nurses Association. (2010). *Nursing's social policy statement: The essence of the profession*. Nursesbooks.org.

American Nurses Association. (2015). *Code of ethics for nurses with interpretive statements*. https://www.nursingworld.org/practice-policy/nursing-excellence/ethics/code-of-ethics-for-nurses/.

American Society for Bioethics and Humanities. (2011). *Core competencies for healthcare ethics consultation* (2nd ed.). Author.

American Society for Bioethics and Humanities. (2014). Code of ethics and professional responsibilities for healthcare ethics consultants. Author. https://asbh.org/uploads/publications/ASBH%20Code%20of%20Ethics.pdf

Bayles, M. D. (1981). *Professional ethics*. Wadsworth.

Benatar, D. (2006). Bioethics and health and human rights: A critical view. *Journal of Medical Ethics*, 32(1), 17–20.

Brown, L. (Ed.) (1993). *The new shorter Oxford English Dictionary*. Oxford University Press.

Donaldson, S. K., & Crowley, D. M. (1978). The discipline of nursing. *Nursing Outlook*, 26(2), 113.

Epstein, E. G. (2012). Preventive ethics in the intensive care unit. *AACN Advanced Critical Care*, 23(2), 217–224.

Faden, R. (2011, Oct. 26). *The boundaries of bioethics*. [Talk] ASBH Annual Conference. Minneapolis, MN. Retrieved August 4, 2019, from http://bioethicsbulletin.org/wp-content/uploads/2011/10/asbh-ruth-final.pdf.

Forrow, L., Arnold, R. M., & Parker, L. S. (1993). Preventive ethics: Expanding the horizons of clinical ethics. *Journal of Clinical Ethics*, 4(4), 287–294.

Fowler, M. D. (2016). Nursing's code of ethics, social ethics, and social policy. *Hastings Center Report*, 46, S9–S12.

Fowler, M. D. (2017). Why the history of nursing ethics matters. *Nursing Ethics*, 24(3), 292–304.

Fry, S. (2002). Guest editorial: Defining nurses ethical practices in the 21st Century. *International Nursing Review*, 49(1), 1–3.

Garrett, J. R. (2015). Collectivizing rescue obligations in bioethics. *The American Journal of Bioethics*, 15(2), 3–11.

Grace, P. J. (1998) *A philosophical analysis of the concept 'advocacy': Implications for professional–patient relationships*. University of Tennessee-Knoxville, Hodges Library Thesis 986.G73. Proquest order no. 9923287.

Grace, P. J. (2001). Professional advocacy: Widening the scope of accountability. *Nursing Philosophy*, 2(2), 151–162.

Grace, P. J. (2018). *Nursing ethics and professional responsibility in advanced practice* (3rd ed.). Jones & Bartlett Learning.

Grace, P. J., & Willis, D. G. (2012). Nursing responsibilities and social justice: An analysis in support of disciplinary goals. *Nursing Outlook*, 60(4), 198–207.

International Council of Nurses. (2012). The ICN code of ethics for nurses. Geneva, Switzerland. Retrieved November 14, 2020, from https://www.icn.ch/sites/default/files/inline-files/2012_ICN_Codeofethicsfornurses_%20eng.pdf.

Jonsen, A. R. (1998). *The birth of bioethics*. Oxford University Press.

Jurchak, M., Grace, P. J., Lee, S. M., Willis, D. G., Zollfrank, A. A., & Robinson, E. M. (2017). Developing abilities to navigate through the grey zones in complex environments: Nurses' reasons for applying to a clinical ethics residency for nurses. *Journal of Nursing Scholarship, 49*(4), 445–455.

Komesaroff, P. A. (1995). *Troubled bodies: Critical perspectives on postmodernism, medical ethics, and the body.* Duke University Press.

Kopelman, L. M. (2006). Bioethics as a second-order discipline: Who is not a bioethicist? *The Journal of Medicine and Philosophy, 31*(6), 601–628.

Kopelman, L. M. (2009). Bioethics as public discourse and second-order discipline. *Journal of Medicine and Philosophy, 34*(3), 261–273.

Meleis, A. I. (2018). *Theoretical nursing: Development and progress* (6th Ed.). Wolters Kluwer.

Milliken, A. & Grace, P. J. (2017) Nurse ethical awareness: Understanding the nature of everyday practice. *Nursing Ethics, 24* (5), 517–524.

Milliken, A., Ludlow, L., DeSanto-Madeya, S., & Grace, P. (2018). The development and psychometric validation of the ethical awareness scale. *Journal of Advanced Nursing, 74*(8), 2005–2016.

Pellegrino, E. D., & Thomasma, D. C. (2004). The good of patients and the good of society: striking a moral balance. In M. Boylan (Ed.), *Public health policy and ethics* (pp. 17–37). Springer.

Reich, A. (2012). Disciplined doctors: The electronic medical record and physicians' changing relationship to medical knowledge. *Social Science and Medicine, 74*(7), 1021–1028.

Reich, W. T. (1995). Introduction. In W. T. Reich (Ed.), *The encyclopedia of bioethics* (pp. xix–xxxii). Simon & Schuster.

Rest, J. (1982). A psychologist looks at the teaching of ethics. *Hastings Center Report, 12*(1), 29–36.

Rest, J. (1983). The major components of morality. In P. Mussen (Ed.), *Manual of child psychology* (Vol. *Cognitive development*, pp. 556–629). Wiley.

Sellman, D. (2006). The importance of being trustworthy. *Nursing Ethics, 13*(2), 105–115.

Siegler, M. (2019). Clinical medical ethics: Its history and contributions to American medicine. *The Journal of Clinical Ethics, 30*(1), 17–26.

Truog, R. D., Brown, S. D., Browning, D., Hundert, E. M., Rider, E. A., Bell, S. K., & Meyer, E. C. (2015). Microethics: The ethics of everyday clinical practice. *Hastings Center Report, 45*(1), 11–17.

Willis, D. G., Grace, P. J., & Roy, C. (2008). A central unifying focus for the discipline: Facilitating humanization, meaning, choice, quality of life, and healing in living and dying. *Advances in Nursing Science, 31*(1): E28–E40.

Windt, P. Y. (1989). Introductory essay. In P. Y. Windt, P. C. Appleby, M. P Battin, L. P. Francis, & B. M. Landesman (Eds.), *Ethical issues in the professions* (pp. 1–24). Prentice Hall.

2

Nursing Ethics as an Independent Subfield of Healthcare Ethics

Eric Vogelstein

In any academic field in which we apply ethics to real-world cases, policies, and practices, both empirical investigation and normative analysis will play key roles.[1] Empirical inquiry is necessary because we cannot draw *relevant* ethical conclusions about real-world issues, or even ask the right ethical questions, unless we know all the morally relevant facts, and many of those facts might be known only through empirical investigation. That said, empirical inquiry *by itself* will not allow us to draw any ethical conclusions—this is simply an instance of Hume's dictum that one cannot derive an "ought" from an "is"—and thus empirical investigation cannot qualify as *ethics* unless it is combined with some form of normative ethical analysis, such as the sort of inquiry undertaken in the field of philosophical ethics. To put it simply: if we're doing applied ethics, empirical inquiry without normative analysis is incomplete, and normative analysis without empirical inquiry is blind (cf. Vogelstein & Colbert, 2020).

The field of nursing ethics is, as I take it, an applied ethical field: it aims to determine what is right and wrong, good and bad, virtuous and vicious, just and unjust, within the practice of nursing. Thus, the field must involve a marriage of normative and empirical approaches. There is some room for leeway here: empirical investigation about facts that have normative import, even if one refrains from incorporating any significant normative analysis into one's work, might rightfully be included within the field of nursing ethics. After all, the discovery of facts that are clearly relevant to the ethical practice of nursing, or facts that have potential ethical import (perhaps depending on the right normative analysis), will directly *aid* in drawing ethical conclusions. Thus, if empirically knowable facts are investigated with their application to ethical conclusions squarely in mind, we might rightly call such inquiry a form of *ethical investigation*. And, of

---

[1] The term "normative" refers to anything involving *deontic* or *evaluative* facts, judgments, etc. Deontic norms are rule-based, and are described by such terms as *ought, ought not, required, right, wrong, permissible*, and *impermissible*. Evaluative norms are value-based, and are described by such terms as *good, bad, better, worse, virtuous*, and *vicious*. Ethical or moral facts and judgments are, by their nature, normative (Dancy, 2000).

course, normative analysis that *incorporates* empirical research can be sufficient for drawing ethical conclusions that are relevant to nursing practice, even if one does not *conduct* any such research.[2] This is the way in which I shall understand the broad outline of nursing ethics as an academic field: as being inclusive of both empirical and non-empirical (viz. normative or philosophical) methods, while at the same time being focused *primarily* on the ethical conclusions one's work entails, regardless of whether that work involves empirical science, normative/philosophical analysis, or a combination of those approaches.

The aim of this chapter is to delineate more precisely the contours and boundaries of the field of nursing ethics. The way to approach this chapter's main aim is to describe how nursing ethics differs from healthcare ethics in general, and from the ethics of the other healthcare professions. By distinguishing nursing ethics in those ways, the prospect for a unique academic field and a set of norms particular to nursing emerge. The task, then, will be to explicate clearly the *grounds* for thinking that ethics for nurses differs substantively from ethics for other clinicians. To the extent to which such grounds exist, nursing ethics can be justified as an important field of inquiry—one to which considerable scholarly resources should be devoted. But there remains a question about whether that is the case. Some authors question the significance of nursing ethics as an independent academic field, separate from more general healthcare ethics; and there exists additional debate among those who believe nursing ethics should be considered a separate field about just what that involves, and the *degree* to which nursing ethics stands to be an important and robust area of inquiry (Gallagher, 1995; Kuhse, 1997; Melia, 1994; Volker, 2003). In this chapter, I shall provide some tentative answers to these questions, although the more precise details of nursing ethics, that is, specifically what ethical problems and issues it confronts and just how robust the field stands to be (based on the volume and importance of the field's content), will be left somewhat open. Instead, I shall focus on the more general question of *where to look* for such problems and issues (i.e., the general *shape* of the field of nursing ethics). That said, I shall suggest that there is indeed a significant body of moral problems and questions that apply to nursing per se, and I provide examples of the sorts of issues that plausibly provide key content to the field. What will emerge is a view on which nursing ethics has significant contributions to make, but perhaps for different reasons, and in a more attenuated fashion, than the field's most ardent supporters would claim.

---

[2] My views on the relationship between empirical and normative inquiry in bioethical fields specifically and applied ethics generally are broadly consistent with the more detailed discussion in McMillan (2018).

Outline of Unique Ethical Issues for Nursing

A large core of the ethical obligations that apply to nurses' professional lives also apply to other healthcare professions, especially physicians. The "canon" of clinical ethics (Wear, 2005)—the set of standard, widely accepted, and institutionalized ethical norms that apply in clinical practice, such as those related to confidentiality (and its exceptions), informed consent, the right to refuse treatment, decisional capacity and surrogate decision-making, parental autonomy (and its limits), and so on—is no less valid for nurses than for other clinical professionals. But these general norms in healthcare ethics are not part of *nursing* ethics, as we should understand it, because those norms do not apply to nursing per se. If we wish to find genuine nursing ethics, we must look beyond the clinical ethical canon to specific moral problems and issues that nurses face *qua* nurses. That is not to say either that *all* nurses face those issues, or that *only* nurses do so—rather, it is to say that the prevalence with which nurses confront the issues in question is significantly *disproportionate*: if an issue is one in nursing ethics, then significantly *more* nurses should face the issue in question, and *most* of those who indeed confront the issue (or a large plurality) should be nurses, compared with other healthcare professionals. Only under those conditions is the issue in question one *for nurses* (by and large), as opposed to one *for healthcare professionals*; and that is what would justify delineating a realm of *nursing* ethics.[3]

So, what is the general form of an issue that would apply disproportionately to nurses? There seem to be two possible types: (1) issues that fall directly out of the essential nature of nursing, and are therefore intrinsic to nursing practice; and (2) issues that happen to disproportionately affect nurses, as a matter of circumstance or contingency, and are in that way extrinsic to nursing practice.

Two prominent examples of the *basis* for putative *intrinsic* ethical issues in nursing are the propositions (a) that nurses, and only nurses, are responsible for the *care* of patients (while physicians, e.g., focus only on *cure* or the "medical model"), and (b) that nurses have a special role as the patient's *advocate*. These are sometimes thought to be unique and essential professional aims of nursing; if that is correct, then, perhaps, the moral norms that apply to nurses based on

---

[3] Must an issue be faced by a *sufficient* proportion of nurses in order to count as an issue in nursing ethics? We should think not. Even if an issue is rarely faced, and even if only a small proportion of nurses ever face it, if that issue is nevertheless disproportionately faced by nurses (the limiting case being that *only* nurses face that issue), then it is an issue in nursing ethics. In general, the *absolute* prevalence of an ethical issue for nurses is not relevant to determining whether it is a nursing ethics issue—rather, the *relative* prevalence (i.e., disproportion), compared with other healthcare professions, is what matters. That is how nursing ethics is plausibly distinguished from a field of healthcare ethics that applies across clinical professions.

those aims are themselves unique and thus form the basis for genuine nursing ethics.

An important example of the basis for putative *extrinsic* ethical issues in nursing is the particular type of *inter-professional* relations that exists between nurses and other providers, especially physicians, and the power imbalance that derives from the kind of institutional authority physicians (and others) have and nurses lack. That relative difference in power creates unique moral problems for nurses in navigating their position within the relevant hierarchy. This is, at least *prima facie*, fertile soil for nursing ethics, but these issues are not intrinsic to the nature of nursing (nothing about *being a nurse* implies anything about the degree of clinical authority nurses have within the domain of their expertise)— they are a consequence of contingent logistical facts and institutional structures that exist in modern healthcare.

These issues shall be explored in more detail below. I shall suggest that ethical issues intrinsic to nursing are far more difficult to justify than are extrinsic ethical issues—but that does not negate the latter's status as issues that rightly fall under the category of nursing ethics.

Nurses' Professional-Role Obligations

A natural place to look for nursing ethics properly conceived is in the special obligations that nurses may incur in virtue of their *professional role*, since that is what distinguishes nursing from other clinical professions. That role plausibly grounds moral obligations because it involves tacit or explicit *promises* or *commitments* to professional aims, and because the aims themselves are morally good. It goes without saying that nurses have such obligations (Cooper, 1988). The question for purposes here, however, is whether those are *special* obligations (i.e., obligations for nurses per se).

Now, there is a trivial sense in which any two professions have professional ethical obligations that apply to each uniquely. That is because distinct professions are committed to different aims (or else the professions would not be distinct) which manifest via differing professional *actions*, and therefore we can correctly say that different professions have distinct moral obligations to carry out their respective professional aims via such actions. Nurses are morally obligated to engage in nursing-actions, and physicians in physician-actions, because they have committed themselves to doing so, and because those actions are morally good. But a genuine nursing ethics should involve more than the existence of this trivial sort of ethical fact, even if such facts apply uniquely to nurses—it should involve *contestable* ethical judgments (i.e., morally controversial issues), or at least the potential for the discovery of *new and interesting* ethical norms.

These are the pillars of ethics as a worthwhile and significant discipline: the existence of reasonably disputable moral claims, or (otherwise) the possibility of discovering novel moral facts (even if they are not reasonably disputable). Only then would there be propositions that, collectively, we *don't know*, within the domain in question, which then justifies *inquiry* within that domain.

One sort of attempt to explain the uniqueness of nursing ethics is based on the idea that different *moral principles or values* apply to nursing than to other healthcare professions. This is one way of understanding the claim, made by some nursing ethicists, that an *ethics of care* is the appropriate moral-theoretical framework for nursing (Fry, 1989a, 1989b; Grace, 2018; Tschudin, 2003; Twomey, 1989). On this view, nursing, unlike other healthcare professions, is grounded (at least in part) on a *principle of care*, we might say, which entails ethical obligations unique to nursing, and which can be discovered and discussed from within that framework. Another moral principle or value that is sometimes considered unique to nursing is one of *patient advocacy* (i.e., the principle that nurses ought to advocate for their patients); the claim at issue, then, would be that this is a unique obligation for nurses (Grace, 2001, 2018). On this general paradigm, we have the possibility both for the discovery of new ethical facts, as well as debatable issues, based on different possible ways in which we might understand the caring or advocacy roles being implemented in practice (both in general and in individual cases). Thus, if it is borne out, this would indeed be a basis for genuine nursing ethics.

The challenge for the sort of view in question is to explain why these moral principles and values, which are on their face quite general, wouldn't apply to any healthcare professional regardless of their particular role in healthcare provision. Physicians, for example, should indeed be concerned with *caring* for their patients. The claim to the contrary—the idea of a sharp contrast between the *caring* role of the nurse and the *curing* role of the physician—is simply not borne out by reflection on what we should want out of a good physician, or the actual practice of medicine. It is clear that the aim of such practice is not merely to cure, or to heal, or to preserve life, or any simply identifiable technical aim. There are doctors who do none of those things (e.g., cosmetic surgeons), and there are physician-acts that seem to run *contrary* to them (e.g., withdrawing life-support). Moreover, physicians are, and ought to be, concerned with the general well-being of their patients, just as nurses are—in that way, their role is indeed one that includes caring (Gallagher, 1995; Kuhse, 1997; Melia, 1994; Volker, 2003). Finally, nurses routinely perform curative acts, both independently (e.g., as advance practice nurses), as well as under physicians' orders. To be sure, the caring role is emphasized—and perhaps should be emphasized—more in nursing than it is in medical practice. That is something that shall be explored in more detail below. The point here is that it is implausible that a *fundamentally* different moral orientation applies to nursing compared with the practice of medicine, based on a strict care/cure dichotomy. Such a dichotomy might exist as a matter of emphasis or focus, but not as a matter of principle.

Similar issues arise regarding patient advocacy. The notion of advocacy is grounded on the idea that certain forces within the healthcare system (people, policies, procedures, etc.) might stand to *wrong* patients in some fashion—the *advocate*, then, is the patient's defender against such wrongs. The view in question is that advocacy is the special obligation of nurses. But it is hard to see why that would be the case. All healthcare professionals should be advocates for their patients—all should be concerned with the welfare and autonomy of their patients such that they protect patients from any relevant moral violations (Melia, 1994; Volker, 2003). That said, due to logistical contingencies of nursing practice, nurses might be *better positioned* to advocate for patients than physicians (more on this below)—but that is different from the claim that a principle of patient advocacy is unique or inherent to nursing.

Ethics and the Nurse's Professional Role

Let us return to the care/cure dichotomy, and the claim that care is a unique obligation within nursing practice. I have suggested that such a dichotomy is not implied by any fundamental distinction between nursing and other healthcare professions—but there might be a more indirect way in which the "nurses care, physicians cure" maxim is correct, and which generates distinct ethical obligations for nurses that ground a robust nursing ethics. The basis for this thought is the particular division of labor that currently exists between nurses and other clinicians—the nature of nurses' work *as it presently manifests* means that the frequency, duration, and type of interactions nurses have with patients will be significantly different from those that other clinicians have with patients. The idea is that nursing ethics falls out of this arrangement because those differences give rise to special ethical obligations of care that are far more *feasible and necessary* in the nursing role than in the roles of other clinicians—given the type of relationship with patients that nursing work currently involves, nurses are better *able* to care for patients, and the caring role is more *needed* for patients coming from those who interact with patients in the way nurses do. Nurses, simply put, are poised to care for patients *differently* and *better* than are other clinicians—not as a matter of necessity, but as a matter of fact.

For instance, patients might feel more comfortable talking with nurses than other clinicians about sensitive issues related to their treatment options—in that case, nurses would stand to play a unique role in the informed consent process, which might generate moral obligations to do so. Indeed, merely spending more time with patients could provide nurses with insights into the kind of information patients desire before making a treatment decision, or reveal pertinent aspects or implications of their treatment options that a patient does not fully understand—thus an obligation to be especially sensitive to those aspects of the informed consent process might exist for nurses although it doesn't exist for other clinicians (even physicians, who are usually in charge of obtaining informed consent). Or, patients might be more open to emotional support from nurses than from other clinicians, based on the sort of comfort that develops with the relevant time spent and nursing tasks performed. Associated moral obligations to provide such support might follow. These kinds of obligations—discussing sensitive information about treatment, being sensitive to patients understanding their treatment options, and providing emotional support—plausibly fall under the category of "care."

Relatedly, because nurses spend more time with patients and may engage with them in more intimate ways, nurses may be in a special position to advocate for their patients—nurses stand to know the patients' desires and various facets of their well-being more intimately than would clinicians with whom patients spend less time, and with whom patients may be less forthcoming. Nurses may therefore be more readily aware of when violations of autonomy or harm to patients occur—they will thus have both greater ability and greater standing to advocate for patients than will other clinicians, which might give rise to a special moral obligation of patient advocacy.

At this point, it is also worth considering just what it means to *care* for patients. Indeed, debate about the meaning of "care" in this context may be one *within* nursing ethics; and reasonable definitions of "care" and "caring" give rise to additional nursing ethics issues. For example, it is plausible that caring involves (at least primarily) *being sensitive to patient needs and providing for those needs.* Such needs might include, for example, additional information about one's diagnosis, prognosis, or treatment, reassurance or other sorts of emotional support, and discussion about treatment choices. Caring, in this sense, requires *empathy*; but it might also require having caring emotions oneself, such as compassion or warmth toward patients. Note that empathy, in this sense, is not itself an emotion—rather, it is the ability to feel, or understand, what others feel. Empathy is the reflective mirroring of others' emotional states (either viscerally or intellectually).[4] Thus, two controversial issues emerge: (1) whether the obligation to care for patients requires *emotional* empathy (feeling what others feel), as opposed merely to *intellectual* empathy (understanding what others

---

[4] This is a common stipulation regarding how "empathy" is to be defined, and the one I adopt here, although some researchers use "empathy" to refer to *sympathy* or *compassion*, i.e., the emotion characterized by concern for others' well-being, especially as it manifests as aversion to others' suffering. For an excellent overview of the concept of empathy and related research, see Stueber (2019).

feel); and (2) whether or not the obligation to care for patients requires having *caring feelings* toward patients (e.g., sympathy or compassion). The common issue in dispute in (1) and (2) is whether nurses (or any healthcare professional, for that matter) are morally required to have certain *feelings* or *emotions*, as opposed merely to perform certain *actions* (e.g., by fully assessing patient needs and acting accordingly). Given that nurses have a special obligation to care for patients, either in kind or in degree, these issues are nursing ethics issues.

As it stands, the framework thus described would be an *extrinsic* basis for nursing ethics, since it would be based on contingencies of the division of labor between nurses and other clinicians.[5] In order for the framework to be *intrinsic* to the nurse's professional role, we would need the additional claim that what it *is* to be a nurse is to have a professional role based on the sort of divided labor at issue (i.e., that much of what we have thus far classified as *contingent* elements of nurses' work is, in fact, essential to nursing per se). Such a claim will be contentious, and indeed it is in tension with the various sorts of advanced practice nursing positions that exist in modern healthcare, such as nurse practitioners and nurse anesthetists. Furthermore, we might imagine hypothetical situations (or worlds) in which the technical clinical expertise of nurses is in such high relative demand that they do *not* have time to develop the sort of relationships with patients at issue—they simply move from patient to patient too quickly to do so.[6] In that world, perhaps, *physicians* are better positioned, logistically and institutionally, to develop with patients what are in today's world the types of relationships that are more common with nurses. Such a situation would not make the nurses in that world *not really nurses*, nor would they be *bad* nurses, especially if we assume that physicians (with their comparatively abundant time to spend with patients) are better able to develop the relevant sorts of relationships and thus provide care and advocacy to patients. The upshot is that special moral obligations of care and advocacy, if they exist for nurses, appear to do so because of various contingencies (clinical, logistical, institutional, and historical), that is, the way the world happens to be, rather than due to the intrinsic nature of nursing. However, that does not make these issues any less important or any less a part of nursing ethics.[7]

[5] It should be noted that the division of labor between nurses and physicians will have both essential and contingent elements. The claim under consideration here is that the ethical obligations unique to nurses do not derive from the essential elements of their profession that differentiate them from other professionals, but rather from how those essential elements interact with the context of contemporary nursing practice, which in turn gives rise to contingent features of nurses' work that have ethical implications for practice.

[6] Some would argue that we live in a world close to this today, and they would no doubt be correct when it comes to certain clinical settings.

[7] One might object that the contingencies I have been discussing are indeed part of the nature of nursing because professions can *take on* contingent roles and *thereby* be defined accordingly. The idea, in other words, is that the profession of nursing has *incorporated* certain contingent elements, and thus any profession that does not possess them would not be *nursing* (it would be a

Furthermore, it is important to note that the case I have presented for care-based and advocacy-based obligations is meant to be neither definitive nor exhaustive—it is merely intended to describe some plausible areas in which special moral obligations might derive from the practical conditions of nursing practice. Indeed, debate about whether these aspects of nursing practice ground special obligations would itself fall within the field of nursing ethics. For example, it could be argued that adopting the bulk of care or advocacy duties will have deleterious consequences, such as consecrating institutional roles that may be unjustified or harmful, and thus that we should question or reject the relevant division of labor (Kuhse, 1997; Pinch, 1996). Nevertheless, generally speaking, it is at least plausible that there exists an independent domain of nursing ethics grounded on the structure of current nursing practice, even if it is not based on the notion that the values in question (e.g., care or patient advocacy) are unique to nursing practice or are intrinsic to the nurse's professional role.

Power, Authority, and Ethics

There is an additional and important extrinsic basis for nursing ethics, based on the sort of power and authority that nurses have in relation to physicians. Insofar as the concept and authority of the "physician order" remains intact, nurses will remain in an institutionally and clinically subordinate position that will generate ethical problems in cases of conflict and disagreement between physicians and nurses (Redman & Fry, 2000; Yarling & McElmurry, 1986).

More specifically, ethical problems emerge from conflicts in which the *domains of knowledge* of nurses and physicians *overlap*, and thus when there is a legitimate question about who is correct, and whose position warrants deference from others, when a nurse and physician disagree—questions that cannot simply be settled by appeals to greater expertise. Such disagreements might be either *clinical* or *ethical* in nature. A clinical disagreement is one in which parties disagree about some clinical (medical, biological, scientific, etc.) fact that bears on the patient's case, while an ethical disagreement is only about the morality of a certain course of action *given* agreement about the more "factual" clinical aspects of the case (Vogelstein, 2019). Nurses might have greater knowledge than a physician in either domain—clinically due to the fact that a nurse may have more *experience* or *specialization* in an area than a particular physician, or because the physician happens to be making a mistake within an area of clinical

nursing-adjacent profession). It is not clear how much of ethical import turns on this point, since it concerns merely how we *classify* the source of the obligations in question (i.e., whether they are considered intrinsic or extrinsic to nursing), and not the *basis* for those obligations (the contingent elements themselves). In any case, whether this view is correct depends on our reaction to the sorts of hypotheticals and purported counterexamples mentioned above (regarding nurses for whom the contingencies at issues do not apply) that I have suggested count against the view in question.

practice about which a nurse has sufficient knowledge to identify the error; ethically simply because nurses have no less knowledge about ethics or ability to make morally sound decisions than do physicians.

When a physician's authority outstrips his or her knowledge (clinically or ethically) and a collaborative solution is not forthcoming (because the physician chooses to exercise his or her authority rather than attempt collaboration), a nurse's *moral* obligation might conflict with his or her *organizational* or even *legal* obligation. This often gives rise to *moral distress*—the sort of emotional distress that results from knowing the right course of action but being institutionally constrained from carrying it out (Epstein & Delgado, 2010; Jameton, 1984). And this stands to be a disproportionate (although not unique) problem for nurses given their relatively subordinate position in organizational hierarchies, as well as their potential for (often unacknowledged) *equal* or *superior* knowledge clinically or ethically.

Thus, special issues of nursing ethics emerge, especially ones based on how to navigate the conflicts at issue. For instance, we might ask what general rules or framework might be developed for handling such conflicts, for example, principles for deciding when to question or "disobey" physician orders, and when to carry out orders with which one disagrees (Benjamin & Curtis, 2010; Vogelstein, 2019). Likewise, given that moral distress can lead to burnout and turnover (Karakachian & Colbert, 2019; Rushton et al., 2015), which can significantly affect the welfare of patients, there might be various moral obligations surrounding the reduction of moral distress or increasing nurse-autonomy. Even the topic of how much focus these issues warrant might be a matter of debate (Bishop & Scudder, 1987). These are questions that fall squarely within nursing ethics properly conceived.

Skepticism About Nursing Ethics

The sort of position I have sketched here runs contrary to the views of some writers who believe that nursing ethics lacks the essential resources to define itself separately, in a significant way, from medical ethics or healthcare ethics (Gallagher, 1995; Kuhse, 1997; Melia, 1994; Veatch, 1981; Volker, 2003). One prominent line of reasoning that can be gleaned, in one form or another, from such authors is that because there is a large degree of overlap between the *aims* or *goals* of the healthcare professions (put simply, we might say that those goals are the health-related well-being and autonomy of patients), there is likewise significant overlap among the *roles* of such professions. Therefore, on this argument, any role-based distinction between nursing *ethics* and the ethics of other clinical professions—which would be the only potential basis for distinguishing the ethics of those professions—will be minor, at best.

These authors are correct that the professional goals, and thus the professional ethical obligations that nurses have, largely overlap with those of physicians and other providers—that is reflected in the fact that the clinical ethics canon is generalizable and universally applicable in the ways I have noted. That is to say, they are correct that the *fundamental* role-based moral principles that apply to nursing will not be different from those of healthcare providers in general, since the overall aims (patient well-being, respect for patient autonomy, etc.) remain the same for all clinicians. And they are correct that in some form or another the professional roles of nurses and other clinicians must explain (even if partially or indirectly) any difference in their respective professional ethics. What they fail to appreciate, however, is that the unique position of nurses—in particular, their status in relevant power hierarchies and the time spent and activities undertaken with patients (even if those are merely *contingent* aspects of nursing practice, and thus [we might say] represent nurses' *extrinsic* professional roles)—might give rise to unique, common, and significant moral obligations and ethical challenges for nurses per se. To be sure, the authors in question discuss these areas of nursing and acknowledge that they might be ethically relevant—but these facets of nursing practice are given short shrift when it comes to providing a basis for a significant nursing ethics. The authors appear to imply that the ground for such a field must come from special moral obligations *intrinsic* to nursing practice, that is, moral norms that would be based on, and would be unique to, the essential professional role of nurses (which, as we have seen, are difficult to justify). They fail to recognize that there can be extrinsic yet special nursing ethical obligations—those that do not derive from the nature of the profession itself, but rather obligations that nurses have contingently, yet uniquely—that might provide just as important and fertile a ground for a robust field of nursing ethics.

Nursing Ethics and Healthcare Ethics

Given what has been said thus far, where ought we to situate nursing ethics within, or alongside, related fields such as bioethics, healthcare ethics, and medical ethics? To be sure, these terms have no strict definitions, and may be used differently by different people. Here is how I conceive of the fields. *Bioethics* is the academic discipline in which we address moral problems in healthcare and the biological sciences—it is a subfield of the broader normative field of *applied ethics* or *practical ethics*. Within bioethics we have *healthcare ethics*.[8] This may or may not be coextensive with *medical ethics*, depending on how "medical" is used: the term might mean something like *pertaining to the science and practice of healthcare*, or it might

---

[8]   Also within bioethics are the non-health-related ethical issues that arise vis-à-vis the biological sciences. The ethics of cloning and genetic enhancement (as opposed to genetic therapy or disease prevention) are prominent examples of topics within that area of bioethics; sometimes environmental ethics and animal ethics are grouped within bioethics, as well.

Table 2.1 Divisions of Bioethics

Bioethics		
Healthcare Ethics		Non-Health-Focused Biological Science Ethics
General Healthcare Ethics	Professional Healthcare Ethics	
Examples of topics	*Examples*	*Examples*
• Confidentiality • Informed consent • Surrogate decision-making and advance directives. • Assisted dying • The right to healthcare	• Nursing ethics • Physician ethics • Pharmacy ethics	• Animal ethics • Environmental ethics • Ethics of genetic manipulation (e.g., cloning, genetic enhancement)

simply refer to what *physicians* do.[9] Given the former sense, "medical ethics" is synonymous with "healthcare ethics"; given the latter, it is synonymous with "physician ethics." In any case, within healthcare ethics, we have the ethics of the specific healthcare professions (nursing ethics, physician ethics, pharmacy ethics, etc.), determined, in one way or another, by the professions' respective roles.

The sense of "healthcare ethics" I have thus described differs from another sense of the term, according to which "healthcare ethics" denotes a field that addresses only the ethical problems relevant to *all* healthcare professions (such as those that pertain to the clinical ethics canon). The definition implied thus far, on the other hand, includes the professional ethical fields (which address ethical issues relevant only to particular healthcare professions) *within* the broader category of healthcare ethics. The idea here is, simply, that because these are *healthcare* professions, the ethical fields in question may be categorized under *healthcare ethics*, in one sense of the term. That said, the other sense of "healthcare ethics," which would not include the ethics of specific healthcare professions but instead only ethical issues that apply to all such professions, itself describes an important area of study, and thus deserves its own label. We might call this *general healthcare ethics*—that category would then be a subfield of *healthcare ethics*, alongside the various professional ethical fields which we can group under *professional healthcare ethics*. Thus, we have the academic division in Table 2.1.[10]

---

[9] Veatch (1981), e.g., uses it in the former sense—thus *nursing ethics*, in his view, is a subfield of medical ethics (as is *physician ethics*).

[10] This division should not be controversial even to those who believe that nursing ethics is a field with content that makes it entirely distinct from healthcare ethics per se (e.g., Grace, 2018; Fowler,

Conclusion

This chapter has sketched a basic outline of the field of nursing ethics as an independent subfield of healthcare ethics. The specific issues that nursing ethics should grapple with are plausibly determined by the ways in which the type of interaction nurses disproportionately have with patients (frequency, duration, and clinical activities) differs from those of other clinicians. The following questions represent some of those issues.

- Do nursing roles give rise to special moral obligations of care or patient advocacy on the part of nurses? If so, are those roles part of the inherent nature of nursing practice, or are they merely contingent aspects of the way nursing practice currently works? If the latter, is the relevant division of labor between nurses and other clinicians one that ought to be supported? Are there other nursing obligations that arise out of either intrinsic or extrinsic aspects of the nurse's professional role?
- What, specifically, do nurses' obligations of care and advocacy entail? For instance, does appropriate care require caring attitudes (feelings, emotions, etc.) or merely caring behaviors or actions? Does it require emotional empathy, or is intellectual empathy sufficient? How might care-based obligations introduce or augment clinical responsibilities, for example vis-à-vis informed consent or emotional support? How, precisely, should nurses advocate for patients, and how do obligations of advocacy interact with issues related to patient autonomy and physician authority?
- What are the ways in which nurses should navigate disagreements, clinical and ethical, with clinicians who have (in various ways and to varying degrees) greater organizational or clinical authority? For example, what sort of principles should nurses use to decide when, and how, to expressly question or refuse to implement physician orders? What sorts of institutional reforms might mitigate harms, to nurses and their patients, that are associated with conflicts between nurses and physicians?

2017). That is just to say that nursing ethics is distinct from general healthcare ethics, a view with which I agree (the content of nursing ethics is not subsumed by that field, nor can it be derived from it). But because nursing is a healthcare profession, nursing ethics is a *kind* of professional healthcare ethics, by definition. This is a mere categorization, not an expression of the particular content of the field.

This is only a sample of the issues that fall within the field of nursing ethics—but even so, it is obvious, given the relevance and importance of the issues thus described, that the field of nursing ethics contains robust content and involves inquiry vital to the practice of nursing.

References

Benjamin, M., & Curtis, J. (2010). *Ethics in nursing: Cases, principles, and reasoning* (4th ed.). Oxford University Press.

Bishop, A. H., & Scudder, J. R., Jr. (1987). Nursing ethics in an age of controversy. *Advances in Nursing Science, 9*(3), 34–43.

Cooper, M. C. (1988). Covenantal relationships: Grounding for the nursing ethic. *Advances in Nursing Science, 10*(4), 48–59.

Dancy, J. (Ed). (2000). *Normativity*. Blackwell.

Epstein, E. G., & Delgado, S. (2010). Understanding and addressing moral distress. *The Online Journal of Issues in Nursing, 15*(3).

Fry, S. T. (1989a). The role of caring in a theory of nursing ethics. *Hypatia, 4*(2), 87–103.

Fry, S. T. (1989b). Toward a theory of nursing ethics. *Advances in Nursing Science, 11*(4), 9–22.

Fowler, M. (2017). Why the history of nursing ethics matters. *Nursing Ethics, 24*(3) 292–304.

Gallagher, A. (1995). Medical and nursing ethics: Never the twain? *Nursing Ethics, 2*(2), 95–101.

Grace, P. (2001). Professional advocacy: Widening the scope of accountability. *Nursing Philosophy, 2*(2), 151–162.

Grace, P. (2018). *Nursing ethics and professional responsibility in advanced practice*. Jones & Bartlett.

Jameton, A. (1984). *Nursing practice: The ethical issues*. Prentice-Hall.

Karakachian, A., & Colbert, A. (2019). Nurses' moral distress, burnout, and intentions to leave: An integrated review. *Journal of Forensic Nursing, 15*(3), 133–142.

Kuhse, H. (1997). *Caring: Nurses, women, and ethics*. Wiley-Blackwell.

McMillin, J. (2018). *The methods of bioethics: An essay in meta-bioethics*. Oxford University Press.

Melia, K. M. (1994). The task of nursing ethics. *Journal of Medical Ethics, 20*(1), 7–11.

Pinch, W. J. (1996). Is caring a moral trap? *Nursing Outlook, 2*(44), 84–88.

Redman, B. K., & Fry, S. T. (2000). Nurses' ethical conflicts: What is really known about them? *Nursing Ethics, 7*(4), 360–366.

Rushton, C. H., Batcheller, J., Schroeder, K., & Donohue, P. (2015). Burnout and resilience among nurses practicing in high-intensity settings. *American Journal of Critical Care, 24*(5), 412–420.

Stueber, K. (2019). Empathy. In *Stanford encyclopedia of philosophy*. Retrieved February 2021 from https://plato.stanford.edu/entries/empathy.

Tschudin, V. (2003). *Ethics in nursing: The caring relationship* (3rd ed). Butterworth-Heineman.

Twomey, J. G., Jr. (1989). Analysis of the claim to distinct nursing ethics: Normative and nonnormative approaches. *Advances in Nursing Science, 11*(3), 25–32.

Veatch, R. M. (1981). Nursing ethics, physician ethics, and medical ethics. *Journal of Law, Medicine, and Ethics, 9*(6), 17–19.

Vogelstein, E. (2019). Questioning orders: A bioethical framework. *Nursing, 49*(1), 14–16.

Vogelstein, E., & Colbert, A. (2020). Normative nursing ethics: A literature review and recommendations for expansion. *Nursing Ethics, 27*(1), 7–15.

Volker, D. L. (2003). Is there a unique nursing ethic? *Nursing Science Quarterly, 16*(3), 207–211.

Wear, S. (2005). Ethical expertise in the clinical setting. In: L. Rasmussen (Ed.), *Ethics expertise: History, contemporary perspectives, and application* (pp. 243–258). Springer.

Yarling, R. R., & McElmurry, B. J. (1986). The moral foundation of nursing. *Advances in Nursing Science, 8*(2), 63–73.

3

The Relevance of Feminist
Ethics for Moral Communities
in Healthcare Work

Joan Liaschenko and Elizabeth Peter

Fundamentally, ethics is about who is in *the* group and who is not. To be in *the* group is to be worthy of moral consideration; *the* group is the moral community. A central concern of moral philosophy throughout its history has been who or what is worthy of moral consideration and thus worthy of membership in the moral community (Gunkel, 2014). To be worthy of moral consideration and a member of a moral community means that members must consider the impact of their actions on the welfare of others. Membership in the moral community "is the foundation for understanding how we should treat the entities we encounter in the world" (Neely, 2014, p. 97). One could say that the history of ethics has been the history of the expansion of the moral community to include those previously excluded. As Gunkel (2014) claims, "Although initially limited to 'other men,' the practice of ethics has developed in such a way that it continually challenges its own restrictions and comes to encompass what had been previously excluded individuals and groups—foreigners, women, animals, and even the environment" (Gunkel, 2014, p. 113). And as Neely (2014, p. 97) notes:

> Over time, our notion of this community has expanded; those we take as nonmembers have changed and the criteria used to make that distinction have also altered. Historically . . . criteria such as intellect and rationality were used to separate white men from women and non-whites. Taken to be governed primarily by emotion rather than rationality, these people were seen as moral inferiors, deserving of lesser or no moral consideration.

The work of feminist scholars and feminist political activists throughout history has been driven by the goal of full inclusion of women and other excluded groups in the moral community. This can be said of any group previously excluded on the basis of race, class, sexual orientation, ethnicity, religion, and the seemingly innumerable ways that humans have of denying others access to the material and social goods of a way of life. Through membership in a moral community, people account to each other in fulfilling their responsibilities. In return, they have protections in that others are obligated to not harm them and to help them if possible. Human communities also have culture, customs, and values which "determine the use of resources and the functions performed in the social division of labor" (Aroskar, 1995, p. 135). Communities overlap and must jointly accept responsibilities and work together. Aroskar (1995) is noteworthy in her mention that although communities are generally viewed in a positive light, they have a "darker side" in that they can be "authoritarian and oppressive" (p. 135) and not look with compassion on the struggles of their members. At the same time, members must be accountable to each other.

It would seem that "moral community," then, is important to understanding morality itself. The ongoing expansion of inclusiveness can be seen in animal ethics, where there is an argument for the inclusion of (at least certain) animals in the moral community. Work in the ethics of artificial intelligence and robotics is, likewise, aimed at developing arguments for including some machines in the moral community. The call from nurses to be recognized as full members in the moral community of healthcare has been a major focus in nursing ethics whether or not the term "moral community" was explicitly used.

We take for granted the significance of moral communities, even their necessity as a condition of morality in the first place. Although it is a central concept in moral philosophy, as far as we are aware, the idea of a moral community appeared only a few decades ago in healthcare ethics literature. Pellegrino first addressed it in medicine in 1990 and Aroskar in nursing in 1995. Recently, however, "moral community" has appeared more often in the nursing ethics literature. There has been a call to recognize healthcare work environments as moral communities and to acknowledge how doing so provides a new ethics resource for coping with the ethical concerns encountered by all healthcare workers in challenging and very complex work environments (Austin, 2007; Epstein et al., 2020; Hardingham, 2004; Liaschenko & Peter, 2016; Pavlish et al., 2014; Traudt et al., 2016; Wocial, 2018).

Our goal in this chapter is modest. We seek to make a case for why feminist ethics is best suited to represent actual moral communities and, therefore, is able to serve as a resource for the challenges they face in contemporary healthcare workplaces. First, we describe the history of the use of the concept of moral community in the healthcare ethics literature and review some of the ethics literature that calls attention to the importance of moral communities. We then cull the characteristics of moral communities delineated in the more current literature that calls attention to the importance of moral communities to see how they square with the theoretical representation of morality in feminist ethics. We examine in detail the general feminist concept of the "situated knower," or the subjectivity of the knower, and what that means for moral communities.

The History of the Concept of Moral Community in Healthcare

The idea that moral communities are present in healthcare was first made by physician Edmund Pellegrino (1990) over 30 years ago when he argued that medicine was a moral community. Five years later, Mila Aroskar (1995) made the same argument for nursing. Both of these scholars highlighted the importance of relationships in healthcare to the idea of a moral community. Pellegrino (1990) argued that physicians had ethical responsibilities beyond the physician/patient dyad. In focusing only on the dyad, he claimed they "neglected the obligations of the profession as a moral community" (p. 221). For Pellegrino (1990), physicians as members of a moral community meant that they had collective responsibilities to society beyond the care of the sick, for example, "the just distribution of health care" (p. 225).

Like Pellegrino (1990), Mila Aroskar (1995) acknowledged the need to focus ethical attention on relationships beyond the patient-caregiver relationship. Whereas, Pellegrino (1990) focused on medicine's collective responsibility to society, Aroskar (1995) drew attention to the relationships necessary to deliver care in ever more complex environments. In particular, she noted the dearth of attention to other working relationships important in nursing practice, specifically, nursing colleagues and other nursing caregivers. This was a key contribution by Aroskar (1995) because in so doing, she emphasizes the interrelatedness of all those providing care. In this way, she introduces a decidedly feminist way of understanding moral agency. She even referred to moral communities as a kind of "moral ecology" (p. 135), noting that the actions of individual moral agents affect the welfare of both their colleagues and their patients. In her analysis, a moral community is a kind of human community, that is, a place where needs are met; in this case, for both patients and nurses. She declared that "nurses and others who contribute to delivery of nursing care *should* identify themselves as citizens of a moral community" (p. 134, emphasis is ours) and that as members they "must be accountable for their working relationships" (p. 134).

Aroskar (1995) introduces a decidedly feminist outlook in three ways. First, she emphasizes the interrelatedness of all those providing care. Second, in calling moral communities a kind of "moral ecology," she acknowledges moral agents as embedded in social structures that both determine the use of resources and assign responsibilities through the division of labor. She stresses both the necessity of accounting to each other for our responsibilities and the importance of the need to work collaboratively. Third, she notes the damage done to moral agents by authoritative and oppressive communities.

Although Wendy Austin (2007) does not reference Aroskar (1995), she, nonetheless, extends her work by making explicit the feminist connections, which Aroskar made implicitly. Like Aroskar, Austin stresses the importance of work relationships and, in particular, interdisciplinary relationships and the role of the social environment in shaping the ethical behavior of moral agents. Austin (2007) appeals directly to the work of feminist moral philosopher Margaret Urban Walker (1997, 1998), whose work addresses many of the concepts that Aroskar used to describe nurses' working relationships and moral community.

In providing a feminist description of the kinds of ethical issues that are most common in healthcare, Austin (2007) also contributed to the feminist analysis of healthcare ethics, albeit in a roundabout way. She critiqued bioethical theory's focus on the hot issues of medicine to the detriment of what physician and nonfeminist author (Komesaroff, 1995) called "microethics," or the ethics of the everyday healthcare issues. These issues rarely achieve "the status of the serious" in bioethics (Warren, 1989, p. 78). Because nursing work is the work of the everyday in healthcare (Davis, 2005), the focus on the hot issues means that the ethical concerns of nurses remain invisible. Yet, the limits of bioethical theory and the ordinariness of most healthcare issues were first noted several years earlier, in 1989, by feminist philosopher Virginia Warren—she called the everyday issues "housekeeping issues," in contrast to the hot or "crisis issues" of medicine.

There are also numerous empirical studies that identify the ethical concerns of nurses which clearly show how they arise from the work of nursing. Here we specifically mention the research of Traudt et al. (2016), who studied intensive care unit (ICU) nurses, and Pavlish et al. (2014), who studied the ethical concerns of ICU and oncology nurses. Both teams of researchers argued that many of these tensions could be prevented within a moral community. Traudt et al. showed how highly experienced nurses manage these difficult situations by enacting their moral agency, exercising moral imagination, and sustaining and utilizing their moral community. It is now well documented that mismanaged end-of-life situations can lead to moral distress. The Traudt et al. study was not examining moral distress, but rather the communication of experienced ICU nurses with families and physicians to achieve consensus on withdrawing aggressive treatment and transitioning to comfort care. What they noticed, however, was that the nurses in their study did not experience moral distress. In their analysis, Traudt and her colleagues found that moral agency, moral imagination, and moral community were the resources that enabled these highly experienced and skilled nurses to communicate in such a way that facilitated the achievement of consensus regarding the transition to comfort care, thereby allowing the patient to die. By so doing, they were able to avoid the experience of moral distress.

In the Pavlish et al. study, we see how the social positioning of nursing in a healthcare hierarchy dictated by the values of the dominant profession of medicine shapes how nurses identify and experience their ethical concerns. These nurses experienced tensions in their work between the general goals they worked to achieve: "relieving patient suffering, being honest with patients, and contributing meaningfully to patient improvement and stated goals" and other work challenges: "administering treatments that cause suffering, being honest without removing hope, and considering the risks of speaking up, that often thwarted the goals of care" (Pavlish et al., 2014, p. 130). In working with these tensions, nurses frequently found themselves in conflict with other providers and families, that is, when the goals of the latter foiled the attainment of the nurses' goals. These are not crisis issues but housekeeping issues, and few in bioethics outside of nurses see them as worthy of academic attention; we still largely continue to teach the standard bioethical principles and framework to students and other providers. If we heed the advice of Austin (2007), Traudt et al. (2016), and Pavlish et al. (2014), healthcare ethics academics would be teaching about moral communities.

For Austin (2007), Traudt et al. (2016), Pavlish et al. (2014), and Hardingham (2004), an ethics which makes the moral community central would be more helpful in resolving the most frequently experienced ethical concerns. For Austin (2007), such an ethic requires "attentiveness to action" (p. 85) and "perpetual responsiveness to others" (p. 86). These qualities in an ethics would: (1) allow all voices to be heard; (2) facilitate the raising of challenges and uncertainties; (3) improve understanding of moral reasoning by understanding contexts; (4) allow shared meanings to be created and knowledge critical to the opening and sustaining of genuine dialogue to be acquired; and (5) move attention to practices and the institutional processes involved in making healthcare environments morally habitable places (p. 86), all of which are aspects of feminist ethics. These qualities imply the necessity of community members' willingness to engage in conversations about differing moral perspectives that touch on one's identity, responsibilities, and values. Likewise, Hardingham (2004) believes that members of a moral community should openly share their ethical concerns, bringing them to light in a way that creates mutual respect and understanding, because without these, integrity cannot be preserved in situations of compromise.

Pavish et al. (2014) explicitly note that a moral community provides two things: first, "processes for timely, honest, planned communication" in the context of "open, respectful team relationships" (p. 135); and second, leadership that is responsive to the needs and values of its staff, manifested in leadership's acknowledgment that the institution's success depends on downstream labor. Most important to the participants in their study was "timely, respectful dialogue about moral perspectives and responsibilities" (p. 137). For Pavlish and her colleagues, epistemic humility, dialogue, and collaboration make for quality relationships given that these "comprise the landscape of moral communities" (p. 137). Similarly, Traudt et al. (2016) described the importance of healthcare professionals having a caring engagement with their work, a primary commitment to patients, and a willingness to challenge hierarchies as foundational to enacting their moral agency. Importantly, their participants accepted accountability for their moral perspectives, actions, and skills, which enabled them to work through any internal or external constraints to their agency (p. 204).

While moral communities transcend personal interest, Wocial (2018) argues that they cannot exclude the interest of self-care. While we think that the term "self-care" is not the most useful, we recognize that Wocial is calling attention to the fact that moral communities have the obligation not only to not harm their members, but also to nurture and support them. Aroskar (1995) noted that human communities could be authoritative and oppressive, failing to show their members compassion, and for Wocial, this is crucial. In fact, Wocial maintains that moral communities show compassion for their members even when they make mistakes because they can be devasting not only for patients, but also for professionals. It is also critical for Epstein and her colleagues (2020), who are primarily concerned with burnout in healthcare workers as a result of moral distress and secondary traumatic stress experienced in their workplaces—workplaces with failed moral communities. They argue that moral communities, with their fundamental responsibilities to their members, are the starting point for change to happen in a meaningful way.

Previously, we have argued that moral communities can foster positive identities, repair damaged identities, and support moral agency (Liaschenko & Peter, 2016). As noted in all the above literature, this work depends on communication. In our 2016 paper, we described moral communities as "places, both literally and figuratively, that keep moral space open, where moral language can flourish in conversations about our identities as moral agents, our understandings of mutual responsibilities, and the values and beliefs we hold as members of a particular community" (p. S20). These are not easy conversations to have, and healthcare institutions are not used to having them and may not even understand their purpose or value. They are, nonetheless, essential to resolving conflicts of differing moral perspectives or conflicts that damage identities.

Moral communities offer a space to repair damaged identities through the creation of counterstories (Liaschenko & Peter, 2016). Counterstories challenge grand narratives by offering a new way to see and by being open to learn about the identities of others from their perspectives. Moral communities can challenge grand narratives of nurses as being unknowledgeable and unskilled. They can begin to question and, at least, voice resistance to the grand narrative of corporatism that marginalizes caring practices. "Moral spaces are necessary for an institution to understand the needs of all of its members, including both patients and paid care providers, because *all* people require care" (Liaschenko & Peter, 2016, S20, emphasis in original).

Summary of Themes in the Literature

Several common themes, including *characteristics of moral communities, what is needed to sustain them,* and *why they are important,* have been identified in the literature we examined.

Characteristics of Moral Communities

The characteristics include two primary aspects: relationships and moral communicative work. Moral communities necessitate intra- and interdisciplinary relationships that are based on trust, mutual respect, and a willingness to explore one's own and each other's moral understandings of responsibilities, identities, and values. Furthermore, a moral community is characterized by members' willingness to readjust these moral understandings if need be. Perhaps, most importantly, a moral community is one in which moral communicative work can take place. Moral communicative work is the work of attending to, responding to, participating in, or initiating "the verbal and nonverbal social interaction that enhances one another's understanding of the moral situations they are in and informs moral decision making and action" (Traudt et al., 2016, p. 209). Moral communicative work is necessary to both manage and repair relationships damaged when mutual accountability fails, that is, when members of the community cannot answer to each other for their respective positions and cannot readjust their moral understandings.

What Is Needed to Sustain Moral Communities

Institutional and structural support is necessary to sustain moral communities. At its most basic, this support is a recognition by both the institution and individual members that the building and maintenance of moral communities takes work at all levels, as well as a willingness to do the work.

Why Moral Communities Are Important

First, they nurture the development and enactment of moral agency. Second, they are necessary to the repair of damaged identities and to the resolution of conflicts among members with differing moral perspectives. Third, they facilitate members' recognition of the importance of narratives in the formation of moral identity and the enactment of moral agency.

A Feminist Interpretation of Moral Community

> Morality is not only about what is thought but about what is perceived, felt, and acted out; and not only what is perceived and felt and enacted by individual persons but what is constructed and reproduced *between them.*
>
> —Walker (1998, p. 8, emphasis in original)

Moral communities in healthcare are not the product of abstract theorizing by professional philosophers. They exist in the social lifeworld and are constituted by embodied beings in the constellation of myriad relationships necessary to the work of the particular community. In return, they contribute to the formation and maintenance of those relationships. Responsiveness to particular others in concrete, actual circumstances has been an argument against the universalism of traditional moral epistemology. These relationships bring together many moral actors; for example, the moral community of an ICU will consist of numerous nurses and physicians, as well as, to a much more limited extent, respiratory therapists, social workers, dieticians, physical and occupational therapists, care coordinators, unit managers, and possibly, clinical ethics consultants. Each of these has an identity or identities that are tied to their roles in the work of the particular community and to the responsibilities attached to those roles. Because these relationships unite moral actors in a common endeavor and because they involve one's identity, responsibilities, and values, they require moral communicative work to share the moral understandings of its members. For this reason, they can and should bear more scrutiny than do those relationships in which people are not united in a common goal, broadly understood as the good of the patient.

Knowledge of the respective roles of members of the community is critical because it is foundational to trust in the possibility of coordinated action. Members of a healthcare community must know what each moral agent is minimally expected to perform. Such knowledge allows for trust between members, where trust is understood both as competence and goodwill (Baier, 1986). Such knowledge allows for coordinated action to be routine in response to a variety of circumstances. For example, when a patient codes or a trauma patient is brought into an emergency department, staff know what to do. Consider, however, the knowledge that is necessary to respond to conflict in moral perspectives between members of the community or the knowledge necessary to repair damaged identities. Such knowledge is not abstract theoretical or scientific in the sense of being able to be stated propositionally (i.e., S knows that p). Rather, it is practical knowledge requiring a set of skills like the nurses in Traudt et al.'s study (2016) who demonstrated: "skill in establishing rapport, preparing for conversations, asking questions, active listening, giving reflective feedback, being clear, and knowing when not to speak" (p. 209). These skills are grounded in a sensitivity to "attentiveness to action" (Austin, 2007, p. 85) and "perpetual responsiveness to others" (Austin, 2007, p. 86).

The kind of knowledge necessary to respond to and work toward resolving different moral perspectives so that goals and coordinated action can move forward requires several things. First, it begins with the knowledge already mentioned, that is, members of the moral community must know what each moral agent is minimally expected to perform. This usually involves basic, task-oriented actions that are visible and taken for granted. For example, bedside nurses administer medications, change dressings, bathe patients, and so forth. Respiratory therapists assist with intubation and monitor intubated patients and ventilators. Physicians diagnose disease, direct the therapeutic regimen, and perform certain kinds of procedures. It could be said that this knowledge is the lowest common denominator for people in a given culture to have in order to say they understand what a given professional does. Knowing only this, however, will get one nowhere in navigating moral differences, unless they are resolved by power. Before discussing how knowledge only of minimal role expectations limits moral understandings, it is important to make a brief mention of power.

One way to move beyond such differences is to impose a course of action through the use of power, understood as power over, that is, power used to compel others to act in a certain way. Power "is a relation of domination," in which the power relation "is unjust and illegitimate" (Allen 2016, section 3). There is a large literature in nursing that points to the harms done to nurses in "relation[s] of domination," including moral distress and loss of integrity.

Second, while the knowledge of minimal role expectations is essential, it is not sufficient. Importantly, it is necessary to understand others' understandings of their values, responsibilities, and identity if the goal is to resolve differences in moral perspectives not settled by power over. Knowledge only of role excludes the rich and highly important knowledge of the invisible work of a practice (Bjorklund, 2004), what feminist epistemologists might call an "epistemology of everyday life" (Code, 1993, p. 16). It is in this knowledge that members of a moral community will often find a fellow member's commitments to values and understandings of their responsibilities and identities in how they fulfill those responsibilities. It will reveal "what we care about, what our responsibilities are, what our commitments and relationships mean" (Walker, 1992, p. 32). For example, ICU nurses generally believe it is a moral imperative for them to help patients have a good death, that is, as physically and psychologically comfortable as possible and ideally with family and loved ones present. These goals can be thwarted, however, when others have goals that support continued aggressive treatment. Given this, it is not surprising that end-of-life issues are at the top of the list for issues causing moral distress among nurses.

Third, self-knowledge, which Traudt et al. (2016) referred to as self-awareness, is critical to resolving differences in moral perspectives within a moral community. Indeed, self-knowledge helps us evaluate a moral community and whether or not we can live in it. Stanley Cavell, quoted in Walker (1992, p. 32) states: "The point of moral assessment, argument, or deliberation is not simply to determine what to do but 'to determine *what* position you are taking, that is to say, *what position you are taking responsibility for*—and whether it is one I can respect . . . whether, or to what extent, we are to live in the same moral universe'" (1992, p. 32, quoting Stanley Cavell, *The Claim of Reason*, 1979, p. 268, emphasis is Cavell's). For Cavell, what makes a moral argument rational is not that we will find the one thing that can be known and that should be done. Neither is it that we will always come to agreement about what ought to be done. Rather, it is, "following the methods which lead to a knowledge of our own position, of where we stand; in short, to a knowledge and definition of ourselves" (Cavell, 1979, p. 312, quoted in Walker, 1992, p. 32) There is much that could be said about self-knowledge, but in the interests of time, we move on to knowledge of others.

Knowing others' understandings of their identity, relationships, responsibilities, and values, all of which are essential for resolving differences in moral perspectives that are encountered in healthcare work, requires "taking subjectivity into account" (Code, 1993, p. 15). To take subjectivity into account is to attend to the social location of the knower because this "affects what and how she knows" (Anderson, 2020, n.p.). What she knows is situated knowledge: "knowledge that reflects the particular perspectives of the knower" (Anderson, 2020, n.p.) and it is the central concept in feminist epistemology and feminist moral epistemology. "Feminist philosophers explore how gender situates knowing subjects" (Anderson, 2020, n.p.). It is useful to quote feminist epistemologist, Elizabeth Anderson (2020, n.p.) at some length.

Individuals' social locations consist of their ascribed social identities (gender, race, sexual orientation, caste, class, kinship status, trans/cis etc.) and social relations, roles, and role-given interests, which are affected by these identities.

Individuals are subject to different norms that prescribe different virtues, habits, emotions, and skills thought to be appropriate for their roles. They also have different subjective identities—identities incorporated into their self-understandings—, and attitudes toward their ascribed identities, such as affirmation, rejection, pride, and shame" (Anderson, 2020, n.p.).

From their earliest challenges to mainstream epistemology and ethics, feminists have sought to highlight the importance of the knower in claims to knowledge. The idea of situated knowledge is the feminist response to the universalism and individualism of standard analytic theories of knowledge, which takes the form "S knows that p," where "S" in the subject or knower and "p" is some observable aspect of the world. This is "propositional knowledge: knowledge that such-and-such is the case" (Steup, 2006, n.p.). It can be shown to be true or false based on some observables and is the model for scientific knowledge. In these theories, the observer is, in Lorraine Code's words, "infinitely replicable" (Code, 2014, p. 150). Infinitely replicable means that any contextual differences between knowers, such as gender, class, race, work roles, able-bodiedness, education, and so forth, must be stripped away to preserve the objectivity in knowledge.

Of course, this is not how it works in complex, clinical environments: clinicians are not interchangeable with those within their own discipline, those from other disciplines, or management. From a feminist moral perspective, what to do in a given situation of moral concern cannot be determined by "correct" moral theorizing without doing violence to a feminist understanding of morality itself and to certain moral actors. Standard ethical theories represent moral agents as peers operating to maximize autonomy and self-interests. They are disembodied, independent, isolated, self-sufficient, and purely rational (Lindemann, 2006). Such an agent is not a situated knower, as they are not bound by particulars or contingencies of life that would prevent a purely impartial view, what professional philosophers refer to as "the view from nowhere" or "the moral point of view." Impartiality is believed to lead to the apprehension of pure, moral knowledge by using one's autonomous reason that can be action-guiding for "us." Feminist ethicists challenge the representation of "us": they believe "us" are the situated knowers that authored the theory but are represented as the universal "us." As feminist epistemologist, Lorraine Code, describes their position, "If one cannot take up this 'view from nowhere,' this 'moral point of view' then one cannot know anything (or at least anything worth knowing)" (1993, p. 16). But in the actual world, "differently placed people know different things" (Walker, 1998, p. 6), and it is a point of great significance. Many in the moral community are thus dismissed, ignored, or even denigrated either because others with more power and influence claim authority to set the terms of any discussion, or individual members of the community believe they don't have anything to say worth knowing. Walker (1998) warns us: "What some people know hides or obscures what is known by others, and differences between people in what they can get away with claiming they know are among the most important differences in moral and social places" (p. 6).

Moral Communicative Work

Communication is essential to a moral community. For Walker, morality is a social achievement and not a matter of theoretical knowledge that an individual moral agent works out cognitively in their own head. Morality is communicative and requires narrative understandings (Walker, 1989, 1998). Communication is the only way to access members' moral understandings of a situation and to negotiate responsibilities in ways that do not do violence to members' identities, values, and relationships. Moral communicative work is "the verbal and non-verbal social interaction that enhances one another's understanding of the moral situations they are in and informs moral decision making and action" (Traudt et al., 2016, p. 209). In Traudt et al.'s research, the nurses' goal was to facilitate a good death for patients, which, obviously, necessitated that physicians share the goal. In those cases when they did not, nurses took the responsibility to approach their colleagues and initiate discussions in which they shared their moral reasoning for altering the plan of care from aggressive treatment to end-of-life care.

We believe that this study also highlighted the moral significance of relationships, stated so well by ecofeminist Karen Warren (2015). "For ecofeminist ethicists, *relationships themselves*, and not just the moral status of the *relators* in those relationships, have moral value and are subject to moral critique. This means that *how* humans are in relationship to others (including nature) matters morally" (Warren, 2015, n.p., emphasis in original). In this study, nurses had strong interprofessional relationships that allowed for questioning and tolerated the expression of uncertainty; importantly, these relationships could withstand and manage the frequently strong affect that accompanied discussions (Traudt et al., 2016, p. 210). Nurses were able to and took responsibility for initiating necessary conversations, often telling physicians directly that they needed to address prognosis and treatment with patients and families. It is worth noting, because generally it is rare in today's healthcare environments, that these nurses worked for an average of 17 years on the same unit. Nurses' ability to initiate and sustain interprofessional relationships, often in contested situations about what course of action to pursue in a patient's care, was at least partly due to the time they spent together. Time is important because it allows trust to be built between members, but we will return to the issue later. For now, we might ask, trust in what?

Trust also involves goodwill and competence (Baier, 1986). We would also place trust in the goodwill and competence of colleagues, both those within one's discipline and those in other disciplines, as a minimal expectation in healthcare moral communities. Trust at this level is necessary if the work is to proceed at all. It is only if there is reason to suspect the competence and goodwill of a colleague or a demonstration of failure to meet the most basic expectations of the role that trust is questioned, if not suspended, giving way to distrust. Trust in relationships is also highly significant to a moral community in healthcare because it is necessary to do a different kind of work, that is, the moral work of resolving differences in perspective and goals when the resolution is necessary to good patient care and the viability of the moral community itself. Trust in relationships enables members to weather the inevitable threats to identities, responsibilities, values, and to relationships themselves when moral perspectives between community members are not aligned regarding the course of a patient's treatment. Further, we believe that trust in relationships is necessary if they are to withstand the risks that often must be taken in resolving conflicting moral perspectives. This is a complicated subject that extends beyond the scope of this chapter, but it is nonetheless necessary to make a few brief comments.

Resolving disputes stemming from differences in moral perspective often involves risk-taking by members. Precisely because speaking from the place of a "situated knower" can reveal "what position you are taking responsibility for" (Cavell, 1979, quoted in Walker, 1992, p. 32, emphasis in original), speaking out can be a threat to one's identity, responsibilities, values, and relationships, as well as those of others. In our view, this is more likely to occur when two conditions occur: first, when there is unequal social power among members, which not infrequently translates to unequal moral status among members; second, when those lower in the social hierarchy speak as situated knowers while those higher up speak not as situated knowers but as if they have some impartial insight to a universal truth. In such a situation, it is the latter who claim knowledge. These practices silence members from speaking to their own responsibilities and values, as well as asking fellow members to speak to theirs.

If the group is one in which power over is the dominant means of handling differences, people can be at risk for a range of consequences, from having their concerns dismissed to facing censorship and punishment. In such a group, a genuine, honest exchange of perspectives and exploration of the meaning of various options to members' responsibilities, relationships, identities, and values will be severely curtailed. In contrast, a moral community is one in which these risks to members are low. It is not that power is absent in a moral community. On the contrary, "morality 'itself' is a disposition of powers through an arrangement of responsibilities" (Walker, 2003, p. 106, emphasis in original). But in a moral community when differences are present and must be resolved, members are able to undertake communicative work in a way that helps both themselves and others to speak to their individual and collective understandings of their responsibilities. This sharing of knowledge and exploration of meaning subjects power to moral critique. As Walker states, "a moral inquiry that reflects on practices of responsibility for an actual social life will not talk about morality instead of power but, rather, will explore the moral authority of some powers and the arbitrariness, cruelty, or wastefulness of others" (Walker, 2003, p. 114).

We now return briefly to the issue of the length of time members are in relationship to their colleagues. The nurses in Traudt et al.'s study (2016) worked together in the same ICU for an average of 17 years each. This is extraordinary and certainly not routine in healthcare today. We think this history was helpful because nurses trusted each other and their physician colleagues. Furthermore, they learned to do the communicative work that situated themselves as knowers, allowed and encouraged others to do so as well, and communicated in a way that tolerated questioning, uncertainty, and the expression of affect. We do not mean to suggest, however, that moral communities in healthcare cannot be formed or work well in the absence of relationships built over such a long period—not at all. Because relationships are essential and most work environments do not have the luxury of a long-shared history between members, all members must be open to new members and the contributions they can make to the work of the moral community. We believe that seasoned members of the community have a responsibility to teach by role-modeling, particularly if the new members are also new to their profession.

Conclusion

That feminist ethics is relevant to nursing is certainly not a new claim, as the nursing literature is replete with references to feminist ethics frameworks for nearly 30 years. What we have tried to do, however, is focus specifically on its relevance for moral communities in healthcare. We have argued that feminist ethics is the most relevant and, therefore, applicable ethical framework for moral communities in healthcare in general. While a physician was the first, as far as we can determine, to call the discipline of medicine a moral community, in our view, it has been nurses who have moved the conversation forward. They have done so in four ways. First, they are aware of the significance of the fact that healthcare happens in moral communities (or failed moral communities); second, they have been writing about moral communities explicitly since 1995, calling attention to some of the characteristics of a moral community in healthcare; third, they have been using concepts from feminist ethics, in some cases without explicitly identifying them as such; and fourth, nurses do a considerable amount of the communicative work necessary to the establishment and maintenance of moral communities. We maintain our position that nurses be taught ethics from a feminist perspective so that they recognize that their work environments are more than the physical location of their work, but moral communities.

Acknowledgments

The authors thank the two anonymous reviewers for their helpful comments and, especially, Dr. Anastasia Fisher for her thoughtful review of previous drafts of this manuscript.

References

Allen, A. (2016). Feminist perspectives on power. In E. N. Zalta (Ed.), *The Stanford encyclopedia of philosophy.* https://plato.stanford.edu/archives/fall2016/entries/feminist-power/.

Anderson, E. (2020). Feminist epistemology and philosophy of science. In E. N. Zalta (Ed.), *The Stanford encyclopedia of philosophy.* https://plato.stanford.edu/archives/spr2020/entries/feminism-epistemology/.

Aroskar, M. A. (1995). Envisioning nursing as a moral community. *Nursing Outlook, 43*(3), 134–138.

Austin, W. (2007). The ethics of everyday practice: Healthcare environments as moral communities. *Advances in Nursing Science, 30*(1), 81–88.

Baier, A. (1986). Trust and antitrust. *Ethics, 96*(2), 231–260.

Bjorklund, P. (2004). Invisibility, moral knowledge and nursing work in the writings of Joan Liaschenko and Patricia Rodney. *Nursing Ethics, 11*(2), 110–121.

Cavell, S. (1979). *The claim of reason.* Oxford University Press.

Code, L. (1993). Taking subjectivity into account. In L. Alcoff & E. Potter (Eds.), *Feminist epistemologies* (pp. 15–48). Routledge.

Code, L. (2014). Ignorance, injustice and the politics of knowledge: Feminist epistemology now. *Australian Feminist Studies, 29*(80), 148–160.

Davis, R. L. (2005). The practice of the everyday in the literature of nursing. *Journal of Medical Humanities, 26*(1), 7–21.

Epstein, E. G., Haizlip, J., Liaschenko, J., Zhao, D., Bennett, R., & Marshall, M. F. (2020). Moral distress, mattering, and secondary traumatic stress in provider burnout: A call for moral community. *AACN Advanced Critical Care, 31*(2), 146–157.

Gunkel, D. J. (2014). A vindication of the rights of machines. *Philosophy & Technology, 27*(1), 113–132.

Hardingham, L. B. (2004). Integrity and moral residue: Nurses as participants in a moral community. *Nursing Philosophy, 5*(2), 127–134.

Komesaroff, P. A. (1995). From bioethics to microethics: Ethical debate and clinical medicine. In P. A. Komesroff (Ed.), *Troubled bodies* (pp. 62–86). Duke University Press.

Liaschenko, J., & Peter, E. (2016). Fostering nurses' moral agency and moral identity: The importance of moral communities. *Hastings Center Report, 46*(5), S18–S21.

Lindemann, H. (2006). *An invitation to feminist ethics* (1st ed.). McGraw-Hill.

Neely, E. L. (2014). Machines and the moral community. *Philosophy & Technology, 27*(1), 97–111.

Pavlish, C., Brown-Saltzman, K., Jakel, P., & Fine, A. (2014). The nature of ethical conflicts and the meaning of moral community in oncology practice. *Oncology Nursing Forum, 41*(2), 130–140.

Pellegrino, E. D. (1990). The medical profession as a moral community. *Bulletin of the New York Academy of Medicine, 66*(3), 221.

Steup, M. (2006). The analysis of knowledge. In E. N. Zalta (Ed.), *The Stanford encyclopedia of philosophy*, https://plato.stanford.edu/archIves/spr2010/entrIes/knowledge-analysis/

Traudt, T., Liaschenko, J., & Peden-McAlpine, C. (2016). Moral agency, moral imagination, and moral community: Antidotes to moral distress. *The Journal of Clinical Ethics, 27*(3), 201–213.

Walker, M. U. (1989). Moral understandings: Alternative "epistemology" for a feminist ethics. *Hypatia, 4*(2), 15–28.

Walker, M. U. (1992). Feminism, ethics, and the question of theory. *Hypatia, 7*(3), 23–38.

Walker, M. U. (1997). Geographies of responsibility. *Hastings Center Report, 27*(1), 38–44.

Walker, M. U. (1998). *Moral understandings: A feminist study in ethics.* Routledge.

Walker, M. U. (2003). *Moral contexts.* Rowman & Littlefield.

Warren, K. J. (2015) Feminist environmental philosophy. In E. N. Zalta (Ed.) *The Stanford encyclopedia of philosophy* (Summer 2015 ed.). https://plato.stanford.edu/archives/sum2015/entries/feminism-environmental/.

Warren, V. L. (1989). Feminist directions in medical ethics. *Hypatia, 4*(2), 73–86.

Wocial, L. D. (2018). In search of a moral community. *The Online Journal of Issues in Nursing, 23*(1), Manuscript 2.

4

Moral Expertise and Epistemic Peerhood

Implications for Nursing Practice

Jamie Carlin Watson

Nurses' Standing in the Medical Team: Moral and Epistemic

The practice of nursing, perhaps even more than medicine generally, emerged from a motive to care for others. While some early physicians were more interested in studying disease than helping patients, nurses have always been focused on the patient (Theofanidis & Sapountzi-Krepia, 2015; Turgut, 2011). Because of this fundamental orientation to care, Andrew Jameton described nursing as "the morally central health care profession" (1984, p. xiv). But even if nursing has always been morally central to healthcare, nurses themselves have not always been in a position to help facilitate the morally best care for a patient. Jameton notes that "nurses have struggled to find their rightful place in health care for over a century" and that early nursing textbooks, like that of Isabel Hampton Robb (1900), largely "accepted the traditional subservience of nurses" (1984, p. xiv).

Happily, times have changed, and nursing is now largely viewed as part of a "collaborative profession" alongside medicine, rather than "subordinate to" it (Volbrecht, 2002, p. 3). Nurses are better respected as professionals with important insights for patient care and, thereby, as partners in decision-making (Dubler & Liebman, 2011, p. 39).[1] Nurses can work to:

- Protect the autonomy and rights of patients
- Promote advocacy
- Open interdisciplinary lines of communication
- Create an ethical environment in which other nurses can advocate for patients and families (Wlody, 1999, p. 513).

---

[1] In a 2006 survey of 4,036 working nurses, "more than half of the nurses rated as positive the quality of communication and collaboration among nurses and physicians in their work units" (Benjamin & Curtis, 2010, p. 104; the survey is Ulrich et al., 2006).

And the nursing profession expects nurses to fulfill these roles. The American Nursing Association (ANA)'s 2015 *Code of Ethics for Nurses with Interpretive Statements* states that nurses are "responsible for contributing to a moral environment," which includes:

- Respectful interactions among colleagues
- Mutual peer support
- Open identification of difficult issues
- Obtaining ongoing professional development in the area of ethical problem-solving
- Assuring that employees are treated fairly and justly
- Being involved in decisions related to their practice and working conditions (p. 13).

Further, many nursing educators and bioethicists emphasize that nurses have duties, not only to patients, families, and the ethical environment, but also to themselves. In other words, as moral subjects who are also vulnerable to moral harms, they have a responsibility to protect themselves and their patients from the negative implications of harms like compassion fatigue and moral distress (Hamric & Blackhall, 2007; Perregrini, 2019).

What is less widely discussed is *how* nurses achieve this moral standing, that is, how they (or anyone on the clinical team, for that matter) acquire the ability to speak or advise authoritatively on moral matters, especially on behalf of others. The "how" question matters because the issue of moral authority in nursing is partly an *epistemic* issue—that is, an issue of how *beliefs* and *attitudes* are *interpreted* and *justified*. In the case of ethics, these beliefs and attitudes are about what's good or bad, better or worse, fair or unfair, for providers, patients, family members, or communities. Thus, a nurse's epistemic competence with moral matters helps determine the degree to which they can speak authoritatively on those matters.[2] I'm using "competence" here in a broad sense to include both knowledge *that* something is true and knowledge of *how* to do something. Thus, those with a strong epistemic position in ethics have a *prima facie* right to be taken seriously when they address ethical issues.[3] So if we expect nurses to have a morally authoritative voice, we should have a good idea of how we expect them to acquire it. But what does it mean to acquire a strong epistemic position

---

[2] Epistemic competence is not the only factor that determines whether someone is authoritative. Certainly, issues of motivation and character matter as well, such as intent, trustworthiness, and interest in facilitating moral decision-making.

[3] That is, if the only relevant issue is epistemic competence. Someone can easily abrogate their right to be taken seriously if they have proved themselves untrustworthy or indifferent to the issue for which their competence is needed.

in ethics? And how does anyone go about it? As we will see, good common sense and experience at the bedside is not enough.

In the next section, I briefly review the history of ethics education in nursing, highlighting its impact on the moral expectations of nurses and on the prospects for developing moral expertise.[4] In the subsequent section, I review some foundational concepts about epistemic placement in a domain of practice, including what it means to have an epistemic advantage, to be an epistemic peer, and to be an expert. With these concepts in hand, in "The Trouble With Moral Expertise," I review prominent arguments against the idea that someone could have an epistemic advantage over others about ethical matters, that is, arguments against moral expertise. In the final section, I show that these arguments are unsuccessful and summarize recent empirical findings that suggest how nurses can improve judgment in complex environments, like health care. These findings suggest that working collaboratively with others on moral problems in specialized environments can help nurses not only to improve moral decision-making, but also to establish themselves as moral authorities among medical staff.

Ethics Education in Nursing

Every nursing textbook emphasizes that nurses have a moral responsibility to care selflessly for patients. The technical part of that responsibility is straightforward—it comes through extensive training and practice doing the clinical things that nurses do. And when nurses need to learn more about those things, there are clear standards and experts to whom they can turn. But not all aspects of nursing are technical. When patients refuse interventions, when they face tough decisions about whether to continue a painful treatment or transition to comfort care, when a surrogate decision-maker asks for things that a capacitated patient refuses, or when caregivers pressure family members into accepting treatments they aren't comfortable with, nurses face an ethical challenge. And this challenge is not resolved by, for example, learning more about pharmaceuticals or managing a Foley catheter. When nurses need to learn more about ethical issues, to whom can they turn? And can turning to someone help them improve their ability to handle such challenges in the future?

Nursing curricula today vary widely in attempts to equip nurses to address ethical challenges. Most nursing programs now include ethics as a component of a broader nursing course. Most BSN (Bachelor of Science in Nursing) programs

---

[4] Some scholars attempt to maintain a distinction between morality and ethics, but here I follow the majority of academic philosophers in using them interchangeably to refer to the study of the related concepts of good, bad, right, wrong, permissible, impermissible, and obligatory.

have a required, stand-alone ethics course, though these are often taught through philosophy departments and rarely incorporate "authentic nursing content" (Fowler, 2017, p. 292). The trouble is that many nursing education programs regard ethics as add-on information. Marsha Fowler describes this attitude as treating ethics as frosting on the cake, rather than the cake itself: "if everything else the student needs to know has been taught, and there is still room, then let's put in some ethics lectures" (2017, p. 297). Yet, this was not always the case.

From the 1870s to 1965, nursing education was primarily hospital-based, largely independent of colleges and universities. During this period, curricula included ethics training alongside technical skills and clinical knowledge, and regarded all as equally necessary for cultivating expertise in nursing. There were between 2 and 11 nursing ethics textbooks used widely at any given time (Davis & Fowler, 2018, p. 28), and Fowler (2017, p. 296) notes that these "early nursing ethics books are adamant about the need for rigorous nursing education that included scientific, professional, and moral formation. Indeed, a major role of nursing education was that of moral formation." In addition to what we might call mainstay ethical issues, such as confidentiality and conscience, textbooks often included discussions of ethical duties to oneself, such as "instruction on nutrition, sleep, recreation, exercise, . . . how to keep warm in cold homes" and "chapters on the life of the mind that included lifelong learning, reading widely and well, [and] taking courses" (Fowler, 2017, p. 298).

In 1965, the ANA called for a transition in nursing education from institutional governorship to traditional models of higher education. This split nursing education into two tracks, a technical, two-year track, overseen by junior and community colleges, and a professional, baccalaureate track, overseen by four-year colleges and universities (Donley & Flaherty, 2008, p. 2). This shift had both positive and negative implications for nurses. Confined within healthcare institutions, nursing education was subsumed under patient care, so if there were a shortage of nurses or an emergency, nurses would have to miss lectures to care for patients. Further, new medical technologies made it so that "general" nursing education was inadequate to some patient-care tasks. As part of institutions of higher education, nursing programs could be independently accredited, nurses had more control over their curriculum, and nurses could compete for jobs with better pay and working conditions (Donley & Flaherty, 2008, pp. 3–7).

Unfortunately, this shift also meant that curricula were streamlined to focus on medical skills and practices (Davis & Fowler, 2018, pp. 28–29; Sullivan & Benner, 2005, p. 79). The nursing profession came to be regarded—even by those who taught it—as a largely technical field with little need for humanistic education. Ethics courses "were pushed aside" except in baccalaureate nursing programs, which, again, are often one-off courses taught in philosophy departments rather than in nursing schools (Wlody, 1999, p. 516).

As of 2004, fewer than half of registered nurses (48.8%) had a baccalaureate education (Health Resources and Services Administration, 2004). As of 2008, 22.7% of registered nurses reported receiving no ethics training at all (Grady et al., 2008). The result, according to some nursing educators, is a workforce that is "undereducated" in ethics and, because of this, lacks the credentials to "sit at policy tables" or "participate as members of governing boards," which means "there is little opportunity for the majority of practicing nurses to engage in clinical or healthcare policy" (Donley & Flaherty, 2008; see also Davis & Fowler, 2018, pp. 28–29; Fowler, 2017, p. 297).

Streamlining nursing to remove or diminish ethics education might make sense if nurses are not expected to contribute to ethical decision-making, that is, if their roles are restricted to the technical aspects their job. Of course, this presupposes that the technical parts of their job can be cleanly separated from the moral aspects, an assumption that few who practice nursing would entertain. And as we saw above, the nursing profession expects nurses to help ensure ethical healthcare practice.

Limiting ethics in nursing education might also make sense if empirical evidence showed that studying ethics does not enhance anyone's ability to address moral challenges. Part of my aim in this chapter is to show that this is not the case. It would be little comfort to say that nursing is morally central to healthcare if nurses' moral judgments could not be improved in any meaningful way. And it would make little sense for the nursing profession to encourage ongoing professional development in ethical reasoning if ethical judgment could not be improved.

In order to answer the question of whether nurses can enhance their moral decision-making, we need some concepts for talking about what it means to be able to make good judgments about anything. And then we need to apply those concepts to explore how anyone might improve their moral judgment.

Epistemic Placement, Advantage, and Peerhood

If you know something, you stand in a "good" epistemic place with respect to what you know, where "good" means "sufficient" or "fitting."[5] For example, if you know how to remove an arterial line, you have sufficient understanding and skill to do so, and that it is fitting for you to do it rather than someone who

---

[5] I'm talking about "knowledge" in terms of what knowledge is *for*, i.e., what virtues it entails, rather than what knowledge *is*. Traditional conceptions of knowledge focus on what knowledge is, for example "justified true belief." Here, I am more concerned with how knowledge contributes to our epistemic responsibility, especially how knowledge—whether our own or someone else's, like an expert's—helps us form responsible beliefs.

lacks that understanding and skill. Of course, someone can be better or worse at something. Whereas one person may be "good enough" at performing a physical exam, someone else may be excellent at it. If two people are equally good or equally bad at something, or they know it equally well, they are equally placed, that is, they are "epistemic peers."

We have to be careful here because most philosophers talk about "epistemic peers" in a very narrow sense. They use it to describe a situation in which two people: (1) are equals with respect to their familiarity with the evidence and arguments which bear on that question; and (2) are equals with respect to general epistemic virtues such as intelligence, thoughtfulness, and freedom from bias (Kelley, 2005, p. 175).

It turns out that, in practice, this is a very high standard. When we are actually working on a problem with other people, these criteria are rarely met. We work with people from different specialties, so we have different bodies of evidence, only some of which overlaps. And, unfortunately, some people are not as thoughtful or careful with their evidence as we would like them to be. As Jonathan Matheson (2015) explains, "Regardless of how exactly we think of evidence, it is doubtful that any two individuals ever have *exactly* the same evidence pertaining to any one matter. . . . Things only get worse once we include experiences, intuitions, background beliefs, and so forth . . ." (p. 115, italics his, references removed).

This implies that, in the normal circumstances where we are working with others, whether someone has an epistemic advantage or is an epistemic peer is a rough approximation that should be approached with humility. Matheson again explains:

> In general, each opinion should be weighted in correspondence with what you are justified in believing about the epistemic position of the individual holding that opinion. You should give extra weight to an individual's opinions that you are justified in believing are in a better epistemic position than you are on the matter. (2015, p. 122)

In other words, if you are peers with someone, you may reason with them differently than if you have good reason to think they are in a better position than you. That doesn't mean that if you believe you are better positioned than someone, you may simply dismiss their concerns. Everyone is fallible. But you may ask more from them in terms of reasons or evidence. Or, in cases where time is limited, you may also ask others to help confirm or disconfirm your own judgment.

This point holds for peerhood in ethics, as well. Some people are more familiar with the evidence and arguments presented in professional and academic literature that bear on a moral question than others. Some people have more experience addressing moral concerns than others. And, of course, the more controversial an ethical case, the less likely that any of us is free from cognitive or emotional biases that influence our reasoning and conclusions. The implication is that we should regard one another's moral judgments with respect, recognizing that they may be in a better epistemic position to form a judgment on the matter. This does not mean we always have to agree with them, but it does mean that we are usually epistemically better off if we hear them out.

In those cases where you perceive that someone is in a better epistemic position than you, an important consideration is how much weight to give their advice. Should you defer to it completely, substituting it for your own judgment? Should you add it to your other evidence as one more mark for or against your own judgment? Should you ask for their reasons and then decide?

The answer depends on a further set of considerations, including how much better their position is than yours, how they acquired their position, how much time is available, how high the stakes are, and so on. Elizabeth Fricker (2006) describes two general ways that people can be unequally placed in a domain. She draws a distinction between someone's being in a different "spatio-temporal location" than another and someone's having "superior skill" over another (pp. 234–235).

In some cases, someone is better placed with respect to a proposition than another by being, literally, in the right place at the right time. If I am in my office and you are in a patient's room while they are conscious and speaking, you are in a better position than I am to know what the patient says. If the patient loses consciousness, I should defer to you on questions about what the patient said. Nurses often have this kind of advantage because of their proximity to the bedside: they talk with the patient more frequently, and they are present for many family discussions. Call this a "thin epistemic advantage." Fricker calls it "thin" because your placement could have easily been otherwise. I could just as easily have been in the room as you. You don't have any special knowledge or skill that allowed you to know what the patient said. Your placement is also thin because it is subject to more accidents in accuracy. You could have misheard the patient, or you might forget what the patient said because you believe it is not important to remember.

In other cases, someone is better placed than another if they have a greater ability to recall, discern, judge, or reason about a proposition, and these abilities come in degrees. Nurses usually have a better working knowledge of the medications they give patients than the patients or their families. And this working knowledge is acquired through years of study and practice. It involves a large set of interconnected claims that includes practices and guidelines, risks and benefits, contraindications, and so on. This means that a nurse is better positioned with respect to questions about a medication than a patient's spouse who has just looked it up on a website. This doesn't mean the spouse isn't right about any particular claim. A nurse can be wrong about a particular claim that a website gets right. But even if the website gives factually correct information, that information is isolated from hundreds of interlinked concepts that the nurse understands. The nurse's advantage is "thick" in this case because it is grounded in specialized knowledge and skill. They are *more likely* to get the right answer in the context and to recognize whether website information is correct. The nurse has a thick placement with respect to the claim at hand (cultivated through years of study), while the spouse's placement is thin (what they read on a website). It follows that nurses may also have a thick epistemic advantage over other nurses, staff, and physicians when it comes to the technical aspects of their domain of expertise—aspects they have studied and practiced that others have not. And importantly, for my purposes, it implies that nurses may also have a thick epistemic advantage over these others with respect to moral judgments.

In short, the concept of epistemic placement is important for two reasons. First, it explains *how* someone can have an epistemic advantage over someone else and *what* sort of advantage it is. Second, it explains how *expert* testimony differs from other types of testimony. Experts are thickly placed in their domains—they can explain why claims in their domain are true and explain how those claims relate to other claims and practices in their domain (Watson 2020). Thick epistemic advantage is broader and less subject to luck and coincidence than thin epistemic advantage. The possibility of having a higher degree of ethical competence—that is, a thick epistemic placement in moral matters—than someone else introduces the possibility (though certainly not the necessity)[6] that someone could become a moral expert. Further, the notions of advantage and peerhood will prove to be tools for improving moral judgment, which we will see in the penultimate section of the chapter.

The Trouble With Moral Expertise

Some are concerned about the idea that one person could be better placed than someone else to say that a clinical decision is right or wrong, better or worse, good or bad. Talk about epistemic advantage and thick epistemic placement is all well and good when we're thinking about the technical aspects of nursing. Clearly, there are better and worse nurses and nurses who are equally good. But

---

[6] There are a few domains with a range of competence but no experts, such as walking and using a smart phone. But the possibility of gaining competence opens the door for expertise. Once we define an activity narrowly enough (e.g., race walking or runway walking), then it becomes obvious that there are experts in them. Activities as seemingly mundane as memorizing and jumping rope have international competitions.

why think this is true for moral judgment? If someone were not as well placed as someone else in ethics, it would be epistemically responsible to turn to the better-placed person for advice. But we all have a general sense of what's right and wrong, so turning to a "moral expert" for advice can seem unnecessary and wrong-headed.

Historically, even philosophers—arguably, the people most interested in studying morality critically—have been uneasy with the idea that someone could speak with *authority* about what is good or bad, right or wrong, wise or imprudent. In the early 4th century BCE, Plato tells us that Socrates convinced Meno that virtue is not something one can know by pointing out that there are no reliable teachers of virtue, and if something cannot be taught, it is not knowledge.[7] Two millennia later, Enlightenment philosophers, such as John Locke and Immanuel Kant, were likewise skeptical of moral advice.[8] And this skepticism persisted into the 20th century, when philosophers like C. D. Broad (1952) claimed that "it is no part of the professional business of moral philosophers to tell people what they ought or ought not to do" (p. 244). Bernard Williams even said it is a "notorious fact" that there are no experts in ethics, and he pointed to medical ethics as an example of an especially implausible project.[9] If the people who study ethics think there are no moral experts, who could disagree?

Such sentiments persist,[10] but it is important to note that not all of the concerns are aimed at the same meaning of either "expertise" or "moral expertise." Williams's complaint presumes an authoritarian kind of expertise, where the novice can understand the expert's arguments and disagrees with them, but still feels an obligation to defer to the expert anyway, simply because the person is an expert (1995, p. 235). In standard cases, however, this is not how expertise works. More commonly, experts either have knowledge and skill that is not comprehensible to a novice (as in the case, say, of a physicist or mathematician) or, because of their experience and training, experts contribute reasons and evidence the novice wouldn't have considered on their own (as in the case of an expert counselor). Williams actually acknowledges this latter possibility, though he doesn't call it expertise (1995, pp. 235–236). However, if a medical ethicist's expertise operates in either of these ways, it is not an especially implausible project.

---

[7] Plato, *Meno* (1997). See also *Protagoras* (1997).

[8] John Locke famously doubted whether we can learn much through testimony, writing, "we may as rationally hope to see with other [people's] Eyes, as to know by other [people's] Understandings" (1689/1975, I.iv.23). The standard interpretation of Immanuel Kant is that moral authority can derive only from one's own will, not from moral testimony.

[9] Williams criticizes medical ethics in: "Who needs ethical knowledge?" (1993) and "Truth in Ethics" (1995).

[10] For more on the history of this debate, see the first seven chapters of Rasmussen (2005), which include discussions of Socrates, Aristotle, David Hume, J. S. Mill, Josiah Royce, John Dewey, and G. E. Moore.

With respect to different interpretations of moral expertise, someone might be thinking of *academic moral expertise.* An academic moral expert is someone trained to study and teach moral philosophy. Academic moral expertise is acquired by obtaining advanced degrees in moral philosophy and actively participating in academic ethics by publishing in peer-reviewed journals and presenting at conferences. Importantly, however, it is not usually within the academic moral expert's scope to speak to specific moral behaviors in highly complex environments like a patient's medical decisions. They would need extensive clinical experience and training over and above their academic training to acquire such an ability. Academic moral experts often abstract from the particular features of specific decisions to pronounce the *general* permissibility or impermissibility of, say, abortion, environmental protections, animal welfare, or euthanasia. But whether any particular instance of one of these is permissible or impermissible for a particular person in a particular situation requires a different type of training. Further, some academic moral experts aren't concerned with people's behavior at all. Those who study metaethics, for instance, are, instead, interested in what moral terms mean, how moral language functions, and how they are related to normative moral theories. Presumably, it is academic moral expertise that Broad has in mind when he writes that philosophers have no business telling people what they ought or ought not to do. But academic moral expertise is simply not the sort of competence that nurses or other health professionals should be expected to have.

Alternatively, concerns about moral expertise might be aimed at *performative moral expertise.*[11] A performative moral expert is someone who can reliably make good moral decisions for themselves. Robert Burch (1974) describes this sort of moral expert as someone who is good at telling right from wrong. They have "insight into the ways one can twist or blunt moral issues, and [they have] competence in stiffening [their] wills so that [they do] not always take the easy way out (p. 652).[12] This kind of moral expertise is relatively uncontroversial, as we can usually think of people known for living lives of moral courage, generosity, kindness, and other strengths of character.[13] No one is perfect, of course, but performative moral experts regularly direct their lives in ways that are morally admirable. As a community, we certainly hope that nurses aspire to be performative moral experts, as we do for ourselves and everyone in our lives. And it may be that a person is more credible for giving moral advice if they can also direct their lives in a morally admirable way (see Cholbi, 2007).

---

[11] There is no widespread consensus on this terminology. Cheryl Noble (1982) might call this "moral wisdom," and Bruce Weinstein (1994) calls this "expertise in living a good life."

[12] The brackets in this paragraph replace masculine pronouns with plural pronouns.

[13] For a contemporary defense of moral expertise as performative, see Hulsey & Hampson (2014).

Unfortunately, just because you can make good moral decisions for your-self doesn't mean you can speak authoritatively on someone else's moral behalf. What's possible for someone to value may be shaped by legal, social, or finan-cial constraints that you don't have. That person may understand and reason about their values through complex cultural or religious assumptions that you don't share—for example, they may prefer for a certain family member to make decisions on their behalf even if they have decisional capacity, or they may value certain religious commitments more than their life; they might prefer to endure a painful illness without pain medication due to a metaphysical belief about the moral value of pain.

The relevant question, then, is whether anyone can be competent to *help others* expertly navigate their moral path, that is, whether they have *practical moral ex-pertise*. The competence to help others think ethically likely entails some degree of both academic and performative moral competence—in other words, prac-tical moral expertise may include some background knowledge about ethics as well as the ability to make morally good decisions for yourself (see Cholbi, 2007). Nevertheless, practical moral expertise is conceptually distinct from academic or performative moral expertise. It would consist primarily in the authority to speak on moral matters on behalf of others, such as decisions about end-of-life care and whether chemotherapy is appropriate given a patient's goals of care.

A practical moral expert, if there were any, would understand important nuances and concepts in moral philosophy, the concrete complexities of a par-ticular decision, and what it feels like to face moral decisions in that domain on a regular basis. A practical moral expert in the domain of health care could draw informed distinctions between the moral and non-moral features of a case, work with clinicians and families to weigh the conflicting and complex features against one another (recognizing how much weight to confer on various moral considerations), and form moral judgments about morally preferable plans of care. This kind of expert could also convey this judgment in a manner and lan-guage useful to the clinicians, patients, and families. To make her advice useful, the moral expert would have skill in translating rich moral notions into concrete clinical recommendations.

Unlike academic and performative moral expertise, however, practical moral expertise is controversial. There are reasons to think it isn't possible to achieve, and it is worth exploring these reasons to get a sense of what is and isn't pos-sible when it comes to enhancing moral judgment. In the remainder of this section, I review three prominent arguments against the possibility of moral expertise. I show, however, that these concerns are not well founded. I leave it to others to show whether robust moral expertise can be achieved (e.g., see the essays in Watson & Guidry-Grimes, 2018), but defusing these three objections and exploring empirical research on how expertise is acquired suggest, at the very least, that nurses can enhance their moral judgment, as well as how they can do so.

For Moral Decisions, Every Person Must Judge for Themselves

The first argument against practical moral expertise aims to show that morality is fundamentally different from other domains. Unlike the technical aspects of nursing and other areas of expertise, which can be learned and enhanced, morality is an entirely personal matter that cannot be evaluated by external criteria. Thus, no one can authoritatively give someone else moral advice. Charles Hendel (1958) explains:

> To allow of any possible role for authority in the moral life of [people] is to take away its properly ethical character, no matter whether the authority be divine or regal, because morality consists in actions of an individual's own authentic choice, choice in the light of [their] own knowledge, appraisal, and conviction, without any external inducements or sanctions. (p. 7)

For a moral decision to be *authentic*, so the argument goes, it cannot be based on *advice*. You must understand and evaluate all the moral reasons relevant to a decision for yourself (see Archard, 2011; Cowley, 2005, for recent versions of this argument).

What's more, we all have a robust ability to reason ethically. So, attempts to enhance moral sensibilities or moral judgment with so-called expert moral advice just makes moral problems more difficult than they need to be. As an example, Stephen Scher and Kasia Kozlowska (2018) relate that a therapist once expressed distress to Scher about a patient who could no longer afford care (2018, pp. 49–50). The therapist felt a conflict between what she perceived as a "right" to be paid for service and the patient's "right" to treatment. Scher and Kozlowska take this to be a textbook example of how bioethics teaches clinicians to organize moral decisions into opposing positions and frame them in terms of some recognizable ethical concept, such as "rights". When Scher suggested to the therapist that there may be a third option for this patient, such as a federal assistance program, the therapist was relieved of her "no-win situation" that she had artificially constructed for herself. But if this artificial construction is the result of trying to "learn" ethics, the idea that we can improve our moral judgment is tragically mistaken.

In contrast to the idea that providers could benefit from moral expertise, Scher and Kozlowska point out that healthcare professionals have a rich background in moral decision-making that cannot be divorced from how they practice health care. Providers were raised in cultures that value honesty and integrity and that shun maliciousness and self-centeredness. They have practiced making ethical decisions in their own lives since childhood. "I soon realized," Scher explains, "that doctors, as well as other health professionals, had the capacity to use their own, existing thinking—not just about ethics, but about the personal and social milieu in which medical care is provided—to understand and analyze ethical problems in medicine" (p. 21). If Scher and Kozlowska are right, there aren't different levels of competence in ethical judgment, only a difference between people who have reflected on their commonsense moral sensibilities and people who haven't.

This argument is based on some mistaken assumptions. First, while there are, undoubtedly, plenty of ethically savvy healthcare providers, there are reasons for thinking that commonsense morality is not sufficient for acquiring or enhancing that savviness. Medical ethics, for example, arose in response to egregious practices among seasoned medical professionals, such as the horrors of the Tuskegee syphilis experiment and the Willowbrook hepatitis experiment, and expanded to respond to bedside horrors, such as lobotomies for psychiatric conditions and pelvic exams without consent.

Even when providers attempt to make conscientious, well-intended moral judgments, they often get the wrong moral answers. For example, Charles Bosk (2003) highlights that

> [t]he earliest empirical work on the process of dying in hospitals indicated that great effort was exerted to make certain that patients did not know they were dying because [doctors] felt that such information would create untoward stress, would involve patients' "flooding out" emotionally, and would, in general, make day-to-day patient management difficult. (2003, p. 151)

These anecdotes suggest that clinicians' moral intuitions seem better attuned to projecting their own moral assumptions onto their patients rather than to assessing the objective ethical demands of the situation.

In reality, ethicists' background in philosophical reasoning leads them to try to break false dilemmas like the one presented to Scher, not preserve them. If anything, the clinician stopped short of robust ethical reasoning, not recognizing that what is ethically at stake in medical decision-making is both broader and richer than "rights" claims. Further, as noted in the previous section, it is epistemically responsible to trust people who stand in a better position than we do, whether the domain is physics or ethics. Karen Jones writes that "just as borrowing scientific knowledge can enhance our capacity to discover truths about the nonmoral world, borrowing moral knowledge can enhance our capacity to understand the world of value" (1999, p. 56).

To sum up, while Scher and Kozlowska are right that healthcare professionals bring a robust commonsense morality to their work, it seems clear that this is insufficient for handling the complex moral challenges they face in practice. And since it *is* possible to handle those challenges, it is plausible that commonsense ethical competence can be enhanced.

There Is Too Much Disagreement in Ethics for Anyone to Be a Moral Expert

The second argument against practical moral expertise starts by pointing to the vast amount of disagreement over ethical issues, from abortion to euthanasia to capital punishment. For any ethical issue, one can easily find a host of scholars defending conflicting positions. But for someone to be an expert in a domain, so the argument goes, there must a shared set of methods, beliefs, and findings to be an expert about, that is, there must be extensive agreement among experts in a domain. Renford Bambrough (1967) concludes that ethicists "disagree so much and so radically that we hesitate to say that they are experts" (p. 152) (see Fiester, 2015, 2018, for contemporary versions of this argument).

Those who make this objection acknowledge that all domains of expertise allow some degree of disagreement. Experts make progress by testing hypotheses that others might demonstrate are faulty. And when the evidence is not yet adequate or admits of varying interpretations, experts may take incompatible positions. Nonetheless, it still turns out that this objection against practical moral expertise obscures the difference between *concerning* disagreement in a domain, which referes to disagreement over one or more fundamental assumptions or fundamental questions in that domain, and *expected* disagreement, which refers to disagreement over particular conclusions in a particular case.

Domains that face concerning disagreement include law, macroeconomics, and medical research (for the latter, see Prasad & Cifu, 2015). For example, disagreement among legal scholars over standards for expert testimony raises serious concerns about the use of experts in legal trials. And we do find concerning disagreement in some areas of ethics, for example, over which moral theory best underwrites moral claims and the role of metaphysics in ethical decision-making. Typically, however, as long as there is substantial agreement about basic concepts, methodologies, and how these are used to set the boundaries of the domain, disagreement is little cause for concern.

It is noteworthy that we actually find less concerning disagreement in healthcare ethics than in other domains of ethics. Ethicists in healthcare environments largely agree on the relevant issues in any given case, such as the importance of decisional capacity for autonomous decision-making, that capacitated patients have the right to make bad decisions or refuse all treatments, that the role of a surrogate is to "speak the patient's voice," and so on. Further, many cases of ethical uncertainty in health care are based on empirical or clinical uncertainty, such as whether a patient is capacitated, whether an old advance directive reflects a patient's current wishes, or whether a baby with Trisomy 18 is likely to benefit from surgery. Given that disagreement in healthcare ethics is expected disagreement and not concerning disagreement, this argument also fails to show that there is no practical moral expertise.

Even if There Were Moral Experts, There Would Be No Way to Identify Them

A final, and perhaps the strongest, objection is that, even if there were moral experts, no one who isn't a moral expert could tell that they are moral experts, and therefore, would have no reason to trust their moral judgment. The idea is that people who have a privileged perspective on an issue—in our case, experts—cannot explain that perspective to others without those others also gaining that privileged perspective. For example, an astrophysicist cannot demonstrate to a novice that they are truly an astrophysicist without explaining enough astrophysics so that the novice could see for themselves. And by that time, the novice is no longer a novice.

Michael Cholbi (2007) offers a version of this argument against moral expertise. Even if there are people who can answer ethical questions competently, it is unclear how the rest of us could recognize them and, thereby, rely on their advice. So, even if nurses could enhance their moral judgment, why should anyone listen to them?

While this argument is challenging (and it challenges many domains besides ethics), it is not intractable. For some domains, it is quite easy to tell who is competent and who isn't, even if you aren't an expert, such as sharpshooting and surgery. For others, though, even experts have trouble coming up with adequate tests for expertise. There are plenty of frauds who have passed medical certification exams and fooled legal review boards. Nevertheless, these professions have developed sophisticated mechanisms for training and identifying experts that tend to identify real experts more often than not. And as we will see in the following section, ethics has some relevant similarities to these kinds of expertise.

But even without comparing ethics with other domains, there are reasons for thinking that it is possible to recognize how those around us are epistemically placed in ethics. C. Thi Nguyen (2018) explains that, in complex moral decisions, we all have "blurry spots," that is, places where our commonsense moral sensibilities are not especially attuned. But we are not starting from pure ignorance, as we might be in astrophysics. Given that most of us do have basic competence in ethics, we can typically rely on one another to help catch general missteps in one another's moral perception or reasoning. Nguyen claims that "[m]ost of us have some trouble seeing moral flaws and errors in ourselves, or noticing applicable moral criteria. . . . Others can (and do) help me by pointing out my moral error and my obliviousness" (p. 10). This suggests that others who share our ethical competence, that is, those who are epistemic peers, can help us make better moral decisions. Elizabeth Anscombe puts this pithily: "[O]nly a foolish person thinks that [their] own conscience is the last word . . . about what to do. . . . [A]ny reasonable [person] knows that what one has conscientiously decided one may later conscientiously regret" (1981, 2008, p. 46).

How does this help solve the identification problem? The more that nurses work as epistemic peers in these blurry areas, the better they can get at recognizing their own blind spots and those of others, especially around moral issues they encounter often, such as those in nursing. Morally sensitive professionals cultivate what Nguyen calls "moral coverage networks" that "check our own worst tendencies" and help to corroborate when our moral reasoning is working properly (2018, p. 11).

Moral coverage networks also allow new nurses to easily recognize those better positioned than they are with respect to moral issues: people who are better placed to reliably, and more quickly, recognize moral error and inattention. And new nurses can test those judgments by applying them and finding out whether they resonate with their own moral sensibilities. This not only helps mitigate the identification problem, it suggests a strategy for cultivating ethical competence both in nursing education and in nursing practice, to which we now turn.

Moral Epistemic Peerhood and Working Toward Moral Expertise in Nursing

According to sociologists and psychologists who study competence and performance, there are three key requirements for improving competence in a domain: engaging with others in that domain, practice, and feedback. "Engaging with others" means being immersed in the language of a domain—learning not just what those who practice in the domain say, but *how* they say it and *how they think* about what they say (Collins, 2014; Collins & Evans, 2007). This requires listening to them talk, asking questions, and problem-solving with them. In ethics, this involves studying the central discussions around common moral decisions—such as those one finds in this volume—and talking with those who commonly have to make them. For nurses, especially those who did not receive formal, clinic-based ethics education, this may require becoming a member of their medical center's ethics committee, regularly attending ethics grand rounds, and participating in ethics sessions of nursing conferences. Gaining competence in the language of ethics can help nurses more quickly identify a moral concern, articulate that concern to others, and help the rest of the care team address it.

Practice and feedback go hand in hand; but practice boosts improvement only when feedback is a good indicator of what went wrong. And there are roughly two types of environments would-be experts face when trying to improve their competence. Some domains, like surgery or basketball, have a strong correlation between success and feedback on performance. Each mistake is immediately obvious, and years of specialized practice (called "deliberate practice"; Ericsson & Pool, 2016) can help practitioners improve. Psychologist Robin Hogarth calls learning environments where feedback is immediate and strongly correlated with success "kind" learning environments (2001, 2010).

In some domains, however, feedback is lacking or distorted so that it is not strongly correlated with success. Teaching is such an environment. If a student does poorly on an exam, we can ask whether that is because the teacher is not competent, the student didn't study, the student was distracted by serious problems at home, or the material is very difficult. Grading, it turns out, is not a strong indicator of whether a teacher is a good teacher. Hogarth (2001, 2010) calls these "wicked" learning environments.

Ethical judgment, as you might expect, operates in a wicked environment. Part of the problem with ethical decisions is that they cannot be evaluated on whether a particular outcome is achieved (e.g., shorter length of stay, fewer hospital deaths, patient satisfaction, etc.). The appropriateness of an outcome is partly what's in question, so the outcome itself will not reflect competence in ethics. A patient's dying might be the ethically best option in one case and the ethically worst in another. Thus, clinic-based ethics education is likely the most appropriate for nurses and other healthcare providers who are trying to acquire practical moral expertise. This would help explain why hospital-based nursing programs, like those predominant prior to 1965, valued ethics training so highly.

So, how do we improve competence in wicked learning environments? It's important to note that practice alone is not enough. While there is evidence that surgeons get better with more experience (Vickers et al., 2007, 2008), this is likely because feedback is immediate and strongly correlated with competence. But evidence shows that radiologists and diagnosticians, whose environments are more wicked, tend to get worse the longer they practice (Choudry et al., 2005; Elmore et al., 2009; Spengler & Pilipis, 2015). Increasing competence in wicked environments requires a different kind of training, and I close this chapter with three empirically informed strategies that can be applied directly to nursing.

First, training in wicked environments must slow down the decision-making process. In kind environments, experts have the freedom to find a rhythm or "flow" in their performance. Any deviation from what's working will be evident; immediate feedback is a check on performance. In wicked environments, feedback is lacking or distorted, so careful thinking and double-checking have to make up for the lack of immediate or reliable feedback. For this reason, epistemic peers are important for enhancing competence in wicked environments. They can provide "moral coverage," raise concerns, identify missed considerations, and help to expand our problem-solving imagination.

Second, training for wicked environments must mimic the environment for which it is needed. Didactic training can help us learn basic concepts, but even in health care, didactic education does not help professionals improve (Davis et al., 1999; Forsetlund et al., 2009). Role-play and simulation activities show marginally better results (Forsetlund et al., 2009). Resident education that occurs on rounds comes closest to a model fitting for wicked environments. Residents have the opportunity to problem-solve with peers about a real case with immediate feedback from the attending and without the distracting pressure of being the final decision-maker. Nurses who have the opportunity to participate in ethics simulation activities or to shadow ethics consultants on cases may derive similar benefits for enhancing their moral judgment (see Deem et al., 2020; Hoskins et al., 2018).

Third, and perhaps most difficult, is that would-be experts should cultivate a willingness to update and change their beliefs as they acquire new information. In his decades-long research with political forecasters (a wicked environment if any is), Philip Tetlock found that the best predictor of improved performance is a willingness to update beliefs in light of new evidence (Tetlock, 2005; Tetlock & Gardner, 2015). Whereas novices tend to double-down on preconceived notions and emphasize only the evidence and arguments that support their positions, would-be experts look for disconfirming reasons. They try to prove themselves wrong. If they find one good piece of evidence against a belief, they lower their confidence in that belief a little. If they find further evidence against the belief, they lower their confidence even more, and so on, until they either stop finding contrary evidence or find enough to warrant rejecting the belief.

In health care, it is easy to approach cases with certain biases—a spouse is "difficult," a son is "aggressive," a patient is "irrational." But an openness to being wrong can lead to asking more questions, which can reveal evidence that helps us update our beliefs. A spouse may have seemed difficult because they felt their questions weren't being answered. A son may have simply had a moment of extreme grief. A patient may be struggling with a bad reaction to a medicine or may need additional decisional support. An openness to updating our beliefs helps us avoid anchoring too quickly on features of a case that may evaporate on closer inspection, and thereby, helps us identify and address genuine ethical concerns more adequately.

Summary and Conclusions

As nurses are increasingly viewed as equal members of the clinical team, the need for competent moral judgment grows. This raises the question of whether and how nurses could enhance their moral judgment. The idea of enhancing moral competence has struck many as problematic, and there are a number of arguments against "practical moral expertise," that is, the competence to help others make good moral decisions. Happily, I have shown that these arguments are largely unfounded. And while I have left it an open question whether anyone can acquire robust practical moral expertise, there are reasons for thinking that nurses can enhance their moral judgment. The implication is that they could acquire thick epistemic placement and therefore have an epistemic advantage over other members of the healthcare team, including physicians. This would further empower nursing voices in care decisions. Thus, recent expertise research has welcome implications for ethics education in nursing, both formal curricular instruction and continuing professional development.

By understanding features of wicked learning environments, educators now have a better sense of why some domains (e.g., law, medicine, ethics) are difficult to learn through didactics and practice alone. This research also provides guidance that would allow nurse educators and ethicists to partner on strategies for enhancing nursing ethics education. An especially attractive aspect of this guidance is that it is consistent with successful pedagogical techniques already used in health care, namely, case-based, simulation-based, and rounds-based group problem-solving with epistemic peers and feedback from more seasoned professionals.

References

American Nursing Association. (2015). *Code of ethics for nurses with interpretive statements*, American Nurses Association.

Anscombe, E. (1981). Authority in morals. In M. Geach & L. Gormally (Eds.), *Faith in a hard ground* (pp. 92–100). Imprint Academic.

Archard, D. (2011). Why moral philosophers are not and should not be considered moral experts. *Bioethics*, 25(3), 119–127.

Bambrough, R. (1967). Plato's political analogies. In R. Bambrough (Ed.), *Plato, Popper, and politics: Some contributions to a modern controversy* (pp. 152–158). Cambridge University Press.

Benjamin, M., & Curtis, J. (2010). *Ethics in nursing: Cases, principles, and reasoning.* Oxford University Press.

Bosk, C. (2003). The licensing and certification of ethics consultants: What part of "No!" was so hard to understand? In M. P. Aulisio, R. M. Arnold, & S. J. Younger, (Eds.), *Ethics consultation: From theory to practice* (pp. 147–162). Johns Hopkins University Press.

Broad, C. D. (1952). *Ethics and the history of philosophy.* Routledge.

Burch, R. W. (1974). Are there moral experts? *The Monist, 58*(4), 646–658.

Cholbi, M. (2007). Moral expertise and the credentials problem. *Ethical Theory and Moral Practice, 10*(4), 323–334.

Choudry, N. K., Fletcher, R. H., & Soumerai, S. B. (2005). Sytematic review: The relationship between clinical experience and quality of healthcare. *Annals of Internal Medicine, 142* (4), 260–273.

Collins, H. (2014). *Are we all scientific experts now?* Polity Press.

Collins, H., & Evans, R. (2007). *Rethinking expertise.* University of Chicago Press.

Cowley, C. (2005). A new rejection of moral expertise. *Medicine, Health Care and Philosophy, 8*(3), 273–79.

Davis, D., O'Brien, M. A. T., Freemantle, N., Wolf, F. M., Mazmanian, P., & Taylor-Vaisey, A. (1999). Impact of formal continuing medical education: Do conferences, workshops, rounds, and other traditional continuing education activities change physician behavior or health care outcomes? *JAMA, 282*(9), 867–874.

Deem, M. J., Vogelstein, E., & Glasgow, M. E. S. (2020). Integrating ethics across the curricula: Innovations in undergraduate and graduate nursing education. In E. Emerson & M. Celeste (Eds.), *Innovative strategies in teaching nursing: Exemplars of optimal learning outcomes* (pp. 59–65). Springer.

Donley, R., & Flaherty, M. J. (2008). Revisiting the American Nurses Association's first position on education for nurses. *Online Journal of Issues in Nursing, 13*(2).

Dubler, N. N., & Liebman, C. B. (2011). *Bioethics mediation: A guide to shaping shared solutions.* Vanderbilt University Press.

Elmore, J. G., Jackson, S. L., Abraham, L., Miglioretti, D. L., Carney, P. A., Geller, B. M., Yankaskas, B. C., Kerlikowske, K., Onega, T., Rosenberg, R. D., & Sickles, E. A. (2009). Variability in interpretive performance at screening mammography and radiologists' characteristics associated with accuracy. *Radiology, 253*(3), 641–651.

Ericsson, A. K., & Pool, R. (2016). *Peak: Secrets from the new science of expertise.* Mariner.

Fiester, A. (2015). Teaching nonauthoritarian clinical ethics: Using an inventory of bioethical positions. *Hastings Center Report, 45*(2), 20–26.

Fiester, A. (2018). Clinical ethics expertise & the antidote to provider values-imposition. In J. C. Watson & L. Guidry-Grimes (Eds.), *Moral expertise: New essays from theoretical and clinical perspectives* (pp. 245–258). Springer.

Forsetlund, L., Bjørndal, A., Rashidian, A., Jamtvedt, G., O'Brien M. A., Wolf, F., Davis, D., Odgaard-Jensen, J., & Oxman Andrew, D. (2009). Continuing education meetings workshops: Effects on professional practice and health care outcomes. *Cochrane Database of Systematic Reviews, 2009*(2), CD003030.

Fowler, M. D. (2017). Why the history of nursing ethics matters. *Nursing Ethics, 24*(3), 292–304.

Fricker, E. (2006). Testimony and epistemic autonomy. In J. Lackey & E. Sosa (Eds.), *The epistemology of testimony* (pp. 225–250). Oxford University Press.

Grady, C., Danis, M., Soeken, K. L., O'Donnell, P., Taylor, C., Farrar, A., & Ulrich, C. M. (2008). Does ethics education influence the moral action of practicing nurses and social workers? *The American Journal of Bioethics, 8*(4), 4–11.

Hamric, A. B., & Blackhall, L. J. (2007). Nurse-physician perspectives on the care of the dying patients in intensive care units: Collaboration, moral distress, and ethical climate. *Critical Care Medicine, 35*(2), 422–429.

Health Resources and Services Administration. (2004). The registered nurse population: National survey of registered nurses, March 2004. U.S. Department of Health and

Human Services, Health Resources and Services Administration, National Center for Health Workforce Analysis, Nursing Workforce Research.

Hendel, C. (1958). *The absurdity of Christianity, and other essays*. Liberal Arts Press.

Hogarth, R. M. (2001). *Educating intuition*. University of Chicago Press.

Hogarth, R. M. (2010). Intuition: A challenge for psychological research on decision making. *Psychological Inquiry, 21*(4), 338–353.

Hoskins, K., Grady, C., & Ulrich, C. M. (2018). Ethics education in nursing: Instruction for future generations of nurses. *The Online Journal of Issues in Nursing, 23*(1).

Hulsey, T. L., & Hampson, P. J. (2014). Moral expertise. *New Ideas in Psychology, 34,* 1–11. https://doi.org/10.1016/j.newideapsych.2014.02.001

Jameton, A. (1984). *Nursing practice: The ethical issues*. Prentice-Hall.

Jones, K. (1999) Second-hand moral knowledge. *The Journal of Philosophy, 96*(2), 55–78.

Kelly, T. (2005). The epistemic significance of disagreement. In T. Gendler & J. Hawthorne (Eds.), *Oxford Studies in Epistemology* (Vol. 1, pp. 167–196). Oxford University Press.

Locke, J. (1689/1975). *An essay concerning human understanding*. Clarendon Press.

Matheson, J. (2015). *The epistemic significance of disagreement*. Palgrave Macmillan.

Nguyen, C. T. (2018). Cognitive islands and runaway echo chambers: Problems for epistemic dependence on experts. *Synthese, 197*(7), 2803–2821.

Noble, C. (1982). Ethics and experts. *The Hastings Center Report, 12*(3), 7–15. doi:10.2307/3561822

Perregrini, M. (2019). Combating compassion fatigue. *Nursing, 49*(2), 50–54.

Prasad, V. K., & Cifu, A. S. (2015). *Ending medical reversal: Improving outcomes, saving lives*. Johns Hopkins University Press.

Rasmussen, L. (2005). *Ethics expertise: History, contemporary perspectives, applications*. Springer.

Robb, I. (1900). *Nursing ethics: For hospital and private use*. Koeckert.

Scher, S., & Kozlowska, K. (2018). *Rethinking health care ethics*. Palgrave MacMillan/Springer Nature.

Spengler, P. M., & Pilipis, L. A. (2015). A comprehensive meta-analysis of the robustness of the experience-accuracy effect in clinical judgment. *Journal of Counseling Psychology, 62*(3), 360–378.

Sullivan, W., & Benner, P. (2005). Challenges to professionalism: Work integrity and the call to renew and strengthen the social contract of the professions. *American Journal of Critical Care, 14*(1), 78–80.

Tetlock, P. E. (2005). *Expert political judgment: How good is it? How can we know?* Princeton University Press.

Tetlock, P. E., & Gardner, D. (2015). *Superforecasting: The art and science of prediction*. Crown.

Theofanidis, D., & Sapountzi-Krepia, D. (2015). Nursing and caring: An historical overview from ancient Greek tradition to modern times. *International Journal of Caring Sciences, 8*(3), 791–800.

Turgut, M. (2011). Ancient medical schools in Knidos and Kos. *Child's Nervous System, 27*(2), 197–200.

Ulrich, B. T., Lavandero, R., Hart, K. A., Woods, D., Leggett, J., & Taylor, D. (2006). Critical care nurses' work environments: A baseline status report. *Critical Care Nurse, 26*(5), 46–57.

Vickers, A. J., Bianco, F. J., Gonen, M., Cronin, A. M., Eastham, J. A., Schrag, D., Klein, E. A., Reuther, A. M., Kattan, M. W., Pontes, J. E., & Scardino, P. T. (2008). Effects of pathologic stage on the learning curve for radical prostatectomy: Evidence that recurrence in organ-confined cancer is largely related to inadequate surgical technique. *European Urology, 53*(5), 960–966.

Vickers, A. J., Bianco, F. J., Serio, A. M., Eastham, J. A., Schrag, D., Klein, E. A., Reuther, A. M., Kattan, M. W., Pontes, J. E., & Scardino, P. T. (2007). The surgical learning curve for prostate cancer control after radical prostatectomy. *Journal of the National Cancer Institute, 99*(15), 1171–1177.

74   JAMIE CARLIN WATSON

Volbrecht, R. M. (2002). *Nursing ethics: Communities in dialogue.* Prentice Hall Health.

Wlody, G. S. (1999). Critical care nurses: Moral agents in the ICU. In J. P. Orlowski (Ed.), *Ethics in critical care medicine* (pp. 513–545). University Publishing Group.

Watson, J. C. (2020). *Expertise: A philosophical introduction.* Bloomsbury.

Watson, J. C., & Guidry-Grimes, L. (Eds.). (2018). *Moral expertise: New essays from theoretical and clinical perspectives.* Springer.

Weinstein, B. D. (1994). The possibility of ethical expertise. *Theoretical Medicine, 15,* 61–75. https://doi.org/10.1007/BF00999220

Williams, B. (1995). Truth in ethics. *Ratio, 8*(3), 227–242.

Williams, B. (1993). Who needs ethical knowledge? *Royal Institute of Philosophy Supplement, 35,* 213–222.

5

Patient Best Interest

Why Nurses Cannot Be Expected to Know What Is Best for Their Patients

Robert M. Veatch

Classical ethics generated by the health professions centers on the maxim that the health professional should always strive to do what is best for the patient. The moral mandate was to pursue the patient's best interest. Contemporary, 21st-century ethics for the health professions rejects that maxim. This chapter analyzes the concept of *patient best interest* and attempts to explain why most have found it necessary to abandon the traditional professional norm.

Professional ethics typically traces the norm of patient best interest back to the Hippocratic Oath. That classic oath for physicians has the physician pledge to "apply measures for the benefit of the sick according to my ability and judgment, I will keep them from harm . . ." (Edelstein, 1967, p. 6). The similar late 19th-century oath for the nursing profession, the oath named in honor of Florence Nightingale, has the nurse pledge that "I will abstain from whatever is deleterious and mischievous . . . and devote myself to the welfare of those committed to my care" (The Florence Nightingale Pledge, 1911, p. 596). Both have the health professional commit him- or herself to striving to benefit the patient and protect the patient from harm.

Four Problems With the Traditional Patient-Benefiting Ethic

That core principle can be called Hippocratic. It dominated health professional ethics as generated from within the professions for 24 centuries until the mid-20th century, when we began to discover why it is so problematic. Four problems have emerged that now lead every commentator—both from within the health professions and outside of them—to reject the core Hippocratic ideal. First, at least in its physician-generated Hippocratic form, it has the physician commit to benefiting the patient *according to his ability and judgment*. In addition to the now-conspicuous masculine pronoun, the Hippocratic Oath has the physician determine patient benefit based on the individual's professional ability to discern patient benefit by relying on his personal judgment. This ignores the fact that not only may others within the profession disagree about what will benefit the patient; it more importantly ignores the fact that the patient may disagree that the physician's chosen course is beneficial. For instance, we discovered in the late 20th century that sometimes when the physician believed that preserving the life of a terminally ill, octogenarian, metastatic cancer patient was best for the patient, the patient might not agree. The original Hippocratic Oath was aggressively paternalistic, and most interpretations of the Florence Nightingale Pledge were similarly slanted.

Second, the original professional codes for both physicians and nurses were single-mindedly individualistic. They ignored the question of any duties to benefit other people in society. Although most professional ethics insists on maintaining a primary focus on the patient, more recent codifications have found it necessary to acknowledge some duty to consider benefits to others in society. The American Medical Association (AMA) by 1957 had incorporated the principle that "responsibilities of the physician extend not only to the individual, but also to society" (American Medical Association, 1978, p. 1751). Similarly, by 1976 the American Nurses' Association *Code for Nurses* commits the nurse to "promoting community and national efforts to meet the health needs of the public" (American Nurses' Association, 1976). Nurses, like physicians, could no longer ignore the interests of other members of society. To hold otherwise would make public health nursing immoral. It would also condemn other aspects of healthcare that do not focus primarily on a single, isolated patient, such as healthcare research, organ transplant, the rights of those outside the healthcare system, and the ethics of health-resource allocation.

Third, the original professional codes for both physicians and nurses failed to recognize that ethics in lay-professional relations was much more than simply promoting benefits and avoiding harms for patients. Beginning in the 1970s, the rights of patients began to take center stage. The right to consent to treatment and to refuse consent emerged, as did many other rights. These rights were increasingly recognized as grounded in ethical principles other than beneficence and nonmaleficence (i.e., benefiting the patient and protecting the patient from harm). The principles of autonomy, veracity, fidelity, and justice were acknowledged, and many also affirmed an independent principle of avoiding killing or the sacredness of life (Veatch, 1981). Critically, these rights and associated principles were morally relevant even if they did not result in benefit to the patient. For example, the patient was seen as possessing a right of confidentiality even if disclosure of patient information in no way harmed the patient. The patient was acknowledged to have a right to refuse medical treatment even if that treatment really would produce benefit for the patient according to the health professional's judgment or even the patient's.

These three problems with classical patient-benefit ethics—its pater-nalism, its individualism, and its ignoring of rights and duties others than benefit production—have been decisive in the evolution of non-Hippocratic professional ethics for nurses as well as for the other health professions. There is a fourth problem with traditional patient-benefit ethics that requires attention and will be the focus of this chapter: the inherent subjectivity of the notion of patient benefit that makes it impossible to assume that nurses and other health professionals can even know what will benefit their patients. Only gradually have we realized the radical pervasiveness of this problem.

Late 20th-Century Healthcare Ethics and the Ethically Exotic Case

In the last decades of the 20th century, these problems began to emerge. They did so in a deceptive way that focused on what can be called the "ethically ex-otic case." These appeared to be relatively rare cases that required taking time out from the health professional's pursuit of the patient's best medical interest. These cases involved issues like abortion, sterilization and contraception, test tube babies, gene modification, euthanasia, and heart transplants.

In one of my first real-life bioethics experiences, I got a call from a young lawyer who had a client who was 21 years old. She had consumed alcohol and a minor tranquilizer and didn't know they potentiated. The combination caused respiratory depression and left her permanently unconscious. After a long pe-riod of reflection and consultation with the family priest, her parents decided it was appropriate to withdraw life-support. Her physician, a man named Robert Morse, believed that it was in her best medical interest to continue ventilating her. He felt he had a duty to preserve life. The moral dilemma for the nurses caring for her was that they were trapped between the decision of the parents and the judgment of Dr. Morse.

The young woman's name was Karen Quinlan (*In re Quinlan*, 1976). We de-veloped the ethical arguments for the right of such patients to forgo life support. In doing so, we claimed not only that Dr. Morse had an unusual view of what was in Karen's best medical interest. We also claimed that even members of the healthcare professions at the time did not concur that it was in a permanently unconscious patient's best medical interest to have life preserved by mechanical ventilation. In doing so, we challenged the traditional view that the physician's own judgment was decisive in such matters. More critically, we claimed that even if the entire medical profession (and the other health professionals as well) believed that ventilation of such patients was in their medical interest, that was not decisive. The first decisive question was whether the patient (or those empowered to speak for the patient) believed it was in her medical interest. The second question was whether the patient has other interests that might override the medical, even if somehow ventilation was in the patient's interest. The ultimate question was whether patients or those empowered to speak for them have a right to forgo treatment regardless of whether they consider it in their interest.

In such a case, the nurse's dilemma was how to encourage this out-of-date physician to do the right thing for his patient rather than continuing to pursue what he thought was in her medical interest. Unfortunately, it took a court action to resolve the matter. Eventually, the courts determined that there was evidence that she would not have wanted this treatment continued and that her parents had a right to speak on her behalf (*In re Quinlan*, 1976).

Bioethicists of the past generation cut their teeth on cases like this one. They made clear that there was more to healthcare ethics than merely pursuing the best medical interest of the patient. In fact, they made clear that there was more to healthcare ethics than pursuing the patient's best interest, whether medical or non-medical. They made clear that the physician's ability and judgment about the patient's best interest were not all there was to the ethics of the patient/professional relation.

These occasional ethically exotic cases forced both health professionals and laypeople to come to terms with the fact that there was more to ethically correct decision-making than having the health professional paternalistically pursue what he or she thought was in the patient's best interest, but they had an unfortunate, unintended side effect. They left people with the sense that this was only an occasional problem. Once in a while, health professionals would have to call time-out from doing the day-to-day work of clinical healthcare pursuing the best medical interest of their patients to address some profound moral problem about which patients might have religious or other convictions that supersede their medical interests. On even more rare occasions, they may even have convictions that supersede their other, non-medical interests. They may, for instance, want to refuse life-support—even life-support they desire and consider in their interest—in order to preserve resources for their children or to spare family caregivers.

The problem with the ethically exotic cases of the late 20th century was that they could leave us feeling that going beyond patient best interest was a relatively rare event. In such rare moments, the nurse might have to confront a physician, like Dr. Morse, who had an unusual view about the patient's best interest or refused to recognize other non-medical interests and moral convictions beyond interests that should be shaping the patient's judgment about what constituted appropriate care. For the everyday practice of nursing, however, nursing practice could be differentiated from the sphere of physician decision-making, and physicians could be expected to determine what was medically best for their patients, while nurses determined what was in the patient's nursing interest.

In the latter decades of the 20th century, we were still in what could be called the era of "modern medical ethics." In the modern period (as contrasted with the ancient era of science and medicine), the physician was still responsible for not only diagnosis, but also medical treatment decisions. We gradually abandoned the old Hippocratic idea that it was the individual doctor's judgment that was decisive. We objectified medical decision-making relying on good science, tested and confirmed by peer review. Similarly, in nursing we developed concepts of good nursing practice that were subject to professional consensus and peer review. Thus, we shifted to objective standards for good medical and nursing practices. By the mid-20th century, the goal was to benefit the patient according to the best available, most objective standard of what is beneficial. We shifted to peer review and treatment protocols. The texts used terms like "medically indicated treatment" and "treatment of choice." The doctor was to do what was best for the patient according to objective medical science. The nurse was to follow the nursing protocol that was best for the patient according to objective nursing standards. Only on rare occasions did we deviate from these seemingly objective standards to accept patient judgments grounded in religious or philosophical views about what was morally right.

Let me illustrate with a case from the 1970s. I was consulting at a hospital in New York City. I was in a conference room with several nurses when I heard screams coming from down the hall. Finally, it bothered me to the point that I asked the nurses what was going on. One of them explained to me that they had a terminally ill geriatric patient who didn't have long to live. She had osteogenesis imperfecta (brittle bone disease). The nursing protocol called for turning the patient every two hours in order to prevent decubitus ulcers. Her bones were so fragile that every time they turned her, the bone injury made her scream in pain.

Now, some 40 years later, it is hard to image that nurses would feel so duty-bound to a protocol that they would torture a patient. It is particularly hard to imagine in a case of a terminally ill patient who will, in all likelihood, not live long enough to develop ulcers, and even if she did, it seems legitimate to ask whether their prevention was really in her interest as she would perceive it.

It appears we were still making a serious mistake in our model of decision-making. We were making a "fact/value" error. We were assuming that matters of nursing, as well as medicine, are factual and can be known by objective science. We now know that this "objective fact" model is true for some aspects of medicine and nursing. It probably true, for example, that this woman was terminally ill. Even that begs the ambiguity of what "terminal" means. Regardless, it is totally untrue for the value judgments necessarily involved in nursing and medical decisions, like whether preventing bed sores is worth it, for instance.

These value judgments in a clinical decision cannot be based on medical or nursing science. In the late 20th century we began discovering the irrationally of basing decisions on healthcare professionals' knowledge of the relevant science. We first discovered this with some of the ethically exotic cases. In the 1960s, women could get an abortion only on a doctor's orders. A woman had to have a medical reason for an abortion—a genetic diagnosis in the fetus or some concern about a woman's physical health (and eventually a woman's mental health). Two physicians had to endorse the abortion. At the same time, if this was a matter of professional judgment, we did not know what to do with a woman confronting a physician's recommendation for termination of a pregnancy if the woman decides she does not want to abort.

We soon recognized that this required value judgments, for example that the genetic disease did or did not justify killing the fetus, or that a certain level of physical or mental health risk justified the abortion. Most critically we began to recognize that, if a health professional made this judgment, it had to be based on the professional's personal religious or philosophical values, not on science.

21st Century Healthcare Ethics and Patient Best Interest

We also recognized the value judgments in euthanasia, organ transplant, and the other exotic cases. Only slowly did we recognize that this could not be limited to the ethically exotic cases, and here is the radical part that will change healthcare ethics in the 21st century. We are beginning to recognize that literally every healthcare decision, both medical and nursing, requires a value judgment. This means that every healthcare decision requires an element that cannot be based on medical or nursing science.

This moves us to a postmodern or contemporary era of medical decision-making, and this is where postmodern bioethics work will reside. If literally every clinical decision requires a set of value judgments to be superimposed on the medical and nursing facts, we can't treat ethics as a special, occasional moment in medicine and nursing. Value judgments will be required constantly for every case we face. Let me illustrate with two examples and then offer some reflection on the basic language of postmodern clinical decision-making.

A patient was hospitalized with a history of mitral valve prolapse, congestive heart failure, and respiratory distress that appeared to be secondary to pneumonia. The attending physician told her that she was too weak to get out of bed, or even to go to the bathroom. That evening when a different attending was on the floor, the patient was told that it was important for her to get up and exercise when possible, including going to the bathroom. Both recommendations had some basis in fact. They were, however, clearly incompatible.

The nurse was caught in the middle. At first, it seemed like one of the physicians was wrong, that one of the physicians didn't perceive correctly what was best for the patient. Under this assumption, the nurse would have the task of politely asking the two physicians to determine which approach was best.

Twenty-first-century healthcare ethics perceives this story very differently. In a postmodern perspective, both getting up and staying in bed have risks. Both also have benefits. At least in borderline situations, the patient's values will be critical in deciding how to balance the risks and benefits. In these situations, the clinicians, whether physicians or nurses, cannot know which is in the patient's best interest.

It turns out that this patient absolutely hated having to stay in bed. Her back ached. She felt trapped. She had terrible trouble using a bedpan. She wanted to get up now and then, the way she had been doing at home a few hours earlier. The nurse's ethical dilemma is now entirely different. It is not a matter of figuring out which doctor is right. It is now a matter of using her nursing skills to convey to the doctors how miserable the patient felt being trapped in bed, and how much better she felt following the night attending's view rather than the daytime attending's. Of course, she needs to know of the risks of pursuing the night attending's recommendations, the risks of falling, fainting, and so forth. The advocates for both getting up and staying in bed need to articulate their concerns and why each thinks it might be in the patient's interest to follow the recommended course. But the idea that one recommendation or the other is definitively correct and can be proven to be correct based on medical and nursing science is simply false.

It is conceivable that a particular patient may have a set of value preferences that so jeopardizes the interests of other parties that the patient's choice cannot be tolerated. The nurse may feel too compromised if the patient is permitted to get out of bed and wander the halls. He or she might feel responsible for an anticipated injury. The nurse may feel that the interests of other patients might be compromised, particularly if the patient's infection could be transmitted. Similarly, each of the physicians may feel that they are failing in their duty to protect patient interests, perhaps even feeling that they cannot remain in a professional/patient relationship given the choice that the patient might make. Those are all problems to be anticipated when we confront the implications of a postmodern healthcare ethic in which there is no rational, objective, scientific basis for determining the interests of the patient. What cannot occur in postmodern healthcare, however, is the claim that the patient must follow the "orders" of the physician or the nurse because the professional has a basis for knowing the patient's interest and has a right to impose that conception of the patient's interest on the patient.

Consider another example. About 20 years ago, right at the transition point from the modern medicine of the 20th century to the postmodern medicine of the 21st, three faculty members at a major university shared a work-study student who did routine office tasks for them, such as logging in mail, photocopying, and so forth. One afternoon the work-study student appeared somewhat ill. She had a sore throat, cough, and achy muscles. She thought it was a cold. By the next day she had spiked a high fever and was admitted to the hospital. By that evening she had died. Her diagnosis was bacterial meningitis, a highly contagious disease.

The three faculty members seemed to share a similar level of exposure. She had been in the offices of all three the previous day and had handled their mail. There was no further exposure besides standing on the other side of their desks. All were disturbed by the tragedy. They were also advised to talk to their personal physicians to determine if any further action was required.

They each saw their physicians. It turns out that the physicians had separate practices and didn't know each other. All three faculty appear to have been told reasonable factual information and given a recommendation. The first was told that the likelihood of transmission of the bacterium was low and that the standard antibiotic drug that could be given had significant side effects: nausea, vomiting, liver toxicity, cerebral hemorrhage, psychoses, and visual disturbances. Moreover, at the societal level there was concern about quick development-resistant strains so that the drug might become ineffective for cases of more substantial exposure.

The second faculty member was told that bacterial meningitis is a serious, potentially fatal disease and that a standard regimen of the drug rifampin, 600 mg twice daily, would be protective. That physician recommended taking the drug.

The third faculty member was told similar information, including the potential therapeutic benefit of rifampin as well as its side effects. That physician recommended an intermediate course of a lower dose of rifampin, 300 mg.

None of these physicians was obviously wrong. None appeared to state any incorrect medical facts. Yet, they gave significantly differing recommendations. In postmodern medicine, none of those recommendations is implausible. None was definitively correct or incorrect. The correct postmodern conclusion is that the physician cannot know what is in the patient's best interest here. That will depend on the patient's risk preferences, how worried each is about meningitis, and how comfortable with the risk of side effects of rifampin. While none of these physicians was definitively incorrect, none was correct either.

Clearly, not all of these physicians can be definitively right. I suggest that none of them was. In the world of postmodern healthcare, they should have explained the range of options and explained that the correct choice for the patient will depend on idiosyncratic value orientations of the individual patients. Physicians can't know which is in the best interest of the patient or which is right for the patient.

Thus, the thesis of this analysis is that clinical decision-making changes radically once we realize that literally every healthcare choice requires value judgments. Decisions require the integration of good medical and nursing science (about which physicians and nurses are the obvious experts) with totally non-medical value judgments (about which they cannot be expected to be an expert). Hence, order giving is irrational in ignoring the fact that non-medical values need to be incorporated into every clinical choice.

The nurse's task is not to determine which nursing practices are best for the patient; it is to consider the plausible alternative nursing practices and figure out which best fits the patient's values. Is it staying flat on your back, or carefully getting out of bed to go to the bathroom? The physician's task is not to determine which dose of rifampin is best for the patient, or whether no dose is preferable. It is figuring out which risk profile best fits their patient. The even more challenging nurse's task is to grasp the value choices in the physician's recommendations and gently advocate for the choices that best fit the patient's values.

The Problem of Pursuing the Patient's Best Medical or Nursing Interest

This has radical implications for the idea that the health professional should be committed to pursuing the patient's best medical interest. The real problem is that there is no basis for assuming that the health professional can know the patient's best interest, even the patient's best medical interest. To compound the problem, no rational person wants solely to maximize his or her health or medical well-being. There is decreasing marginal utility as one approaches maximally healthy choices, and approaching maximum healthy lifestyle comes at greater and greater expense in terms of other goods. Rational people want to be "very" healthy—not "perfectly" healthy. The most important question is one a health professional cannot answer: How far should a patient back off from maximal health?

Each of us holds a complex set of value preferences and trades off medical well-being against other goods. If we jog a mile a day, we face the question whether it would be better for our health to jog two miles a day. If we jog two miles a day, we face the question of whether it would be a little better for our health to jog three miles a day. If we eat a healthy diet, we face the question whether it would be better for our health to eat a slightly healthier one. Thus, not only is it inherently subjective to determine what constitutes medical well-being, it is also irrational to strive for maximal health.

There is still a third problem. Nurses and other health professionals probably "over-value" health. If one thinks about it, our values shape our career choices. Those who most value intellectual life choose academic and similar mentally oriented careers. Those who place greater value on physical activity choose more physically demanding careers. It stands to reason that those who most value health in comparison to other interests will tend to choose a health profession for a career. Thus, if a health professional's recommendations reflect their comparative evaluation of alternatives based on how important health is compared to other goods, we should expect the health professional's recommendations to be "off."

There is a fourth problem: Even within the health sphere, there are competing values. The health professional who modestly says to the patient, "I can't make the trade-offs for you; I can only tell you what will serve your health or physical well-being," makes another kind of mistake. "Health" or "physical well-being" is not a univocal concept. A legitimate goal of medicine, perhaps the "gold standard" as it was once believed, is preservation of life. But the goal of preserving life may come at the expense of other goods, including avoidance of pain and suffering. Different medical courses will serve different medical values.

Consider four medical values: preservation of life, cure of disease, relief of suffering, and promotion of health. Different medical choices will serve these four goals in differing proportions. All are medical goods and yet, at least in some cases, they are contradictory. Pursuing one will come at the expense of one of the others. For instance, preserving life may come at the expense of relieving suffering. There is no definitively correct mix of medical goods any more than there is a definitively correct mix of medical and non-medical goods. The health professional cannot be expected to know the patient's values preferences and cannot know what mix of outcomes will maximize the patient's medical interest, let alone the patient's total well-being.

The real contribution of bioethics in the 21st century is at this fundamental level of recognizing that health professionals cannot know what is in the patient's interest, as well as affirming that the patient's interest may not be definitive in the face of the rights of patients and the rights and interests of others. This will require a change in the basic way we think about healthcare decision-making. It will impact literally every doctor/patient interaction and nurse/patient interaction. It will change the way physicians and nurses talk.

This change must start with the fundamental concept of "doctor's orders." "Order" is a rather strange and harsh word for a lay-professional interaction. It is the mode of speaking of military officers and prison wardens. Most professionals do not give "orders." College professors don't give "orders" to their students. Professors may say, "the paper is due on Tuesday." That is different from saying, "I order you to submit the paper on Tuesday." We need a better and more respectful language than referring to "doctor's orders." We can talk about "doctor's advice" or "proposals."

For what I will call "postmodern bioethics," bioethics of the 21st century, there is a more basic and more radical point. Changing the tone of professional communication from "orders" to "advice" begs the question of how the physician can know what advice to give. If we are correct, the physician or nurse cannot be expected to know what is in the patient's best interest. Even if they somehow could know what is in the patient's interest, we live in a free country: no patient has to follow a healthcare professional's advice. But more importantly and more fundamentally, doctors and nurses are normally not in a position to know what advice to give. Even the concept of "doctor's advice" or "doctor's proposals" contains a logical flaw. They are "irrational" in the sense that there is good reason that doctors cannot know what is in a patient's interest, cannot know what to recommend or suggest.

The nurse gets caught in the middle of this, between the physician who believes he or she can know, based on his or her medical knowledge, what is good for a patient and therefore what to "order" or "advise" and a patient who, based on personal values, has a very different perspective on what is best.

It turns out that there are similar problems with many of the other standard terms used in clinical decision-making. Once the radical impossibility of a health professional being expected to know the best interest of the patient is recognized, it becomes impossible to speak about a "medically indicated treatment." It turns out that medicine does not indicate which treatments are appropriate. Only by taking the basic facts of medicine, such as diagnosis, prognosis, pharmacology, and other matters of medical science, and superimposing on them someone's value framework can we know what is appropriate, and the newly discovered problem is that there is no reason to believe that the clinician is justified in using his or her values in making those judgments. Good medical and nursing science can tell us a diagnosis. It can tell us the predicted effects of various interventions and the probabilities of those effects. It can also tell us the predicted side effects and their probabilities. It cannot tell us whether those effects are worth it given the range of side effects, the economic and other costs, and the alternatives that are available. There is simply no such thing as a medically indicated treatment.

Exactly the same point needs to be made for nursing. There are standard nursing practices, such as the protocol for turning patients. Good nursing science can tell us the predicted effects of following such protocols and their probabilities. It can also tell us the predicted side effects and alternatives. What it cannot do is tell us whether the effects are worth it given the range of side effects, the economic and other costs, and the alternatives that are available. There is simply no such thing as an "indicated" nursing procedure. A similar analysis can be provided for other traditional language in medicine and nursing. There can be no such thing as a "treatment of choice," or a "standard nursing practice."

One final example is worth reflection. In the era of modern healthcare we often spoke of patients being "discharged" from the hospital. That is another anachronism. In an era in which health professionals could be expected to know what is in a patient's best interest and were operating under a moral mandate to promote that best interest according to their ability and judgment, perhaps it was understandable that we spoke as if patients, once they were on the grounds of the hospital, were in the custody of the professional caregiver. If patients were conscripted into healthcare the way soldiers were conscripted into the army, it might make sense to speak of discharging them. If patients were committed to the hospital the way prisoners were committed to a prison, it might make sense to speak of discharging them. But once we realize that the goal of hospitalization is patient-centered, it no longer makes sense to believe that the only goal of hospitalization is patient best interest as perceived by the health professional, and it no longer makes sense to speak of "discharging" them as if they were in the custody of the professional.

Conclusion

There is an aesthetic unattractiveness with terms like "doctors' orders," "medically indicated treatment," "treatment of choice," and "discharge" of a patient. The hospital is not a prison, and neither the doctor nor the nurse has custody of a patient. The real issue is far more basic: conceptually the doctor and the nurse cannot know what to "order." The problem is just as great if we change to more polite language and speak of doctor's "recommendations" or "suggestions." The doctor and nurse cannot know what to recommend. The logic of literally every clinical decision is that we start with descriptions of the facts. Some facts are medical. Others are not. Some are nursing facts, but others come from outside the health professions. They are economic, legal, religious, and aesthetic. We presume that the physician is the expert on the facts that are medical. We presume that the nurse is the expert on the facts that are in the nursing sphere. But the problem is that, in the era of postmodern healthcare, we cannot get from a description of the relevant facts to a conclusion about an appropriate healthcare choice without superimposing a set of value judgments. Those value judgments will be unique for each patient. We cannot assume that the physician or the nurse is an expert on the values. In the world of postmodern bioethics, the nurse is going to get caught in the middle of this. Some old-school physicians practicing 20th-century modern medicine will continue to believe that they have the authority to order the best treatment for the patient: the ventilator for Karen Quinlan, the rifampin for the professors exposed to meningitis, the bed rest or exercise for the patient with cardiac insufficiency. The nurse is the health professional most likely to see physicians ordering treatments that may not fit a patient's values. The nurse is the health professional best positioned to mediate between the physician giving orders and the patient whose values may not fit with the orders that are given. It is the nurse who is in the best position to bring healthcare into the postmodern period, where it is practiced based on the premise that the professional cannot know what is in the patient's best interest.

References

American Medical Association. (1978). Principles of Medical Ethics (1957) with reports and statements. In W. T. Reich (Ed.), *Encyclopedia of bioethics* (Vol. 4, pp. 1750–1751). Free Press.

American Nurses' Association. (1976). *Code for nurses with interpretive statements*. American Nurses' Association.

Edelstein, L. (1967). The Hippocratic Oath: Text, translation and interpretation. In O. Temkin & C. L. Temkin (Eds.), *Ancient medicine: Selected papers of Ludwig Edelstein* (pp. 3–64). Johns Hopkins University Press.

The Florence Nightingale Pledge. (1911). In: Editorial comment. *The American Journal of Nursing, 11*(May), 596.

In re Quinlan, 70 N.J. 10, 355 A. 2d 647 (1976), cert. denied sub nom., *Garger v. New Jersey*, 429 U.S. 922 (1976), overruled in part, *In re Conroy*, 98 NJ 321, 486 A.2d 1209.

Veatch, R. M. (1981). *A theory of medical ethics*. Basic Books.

6

Revisiting Moral Agency

Jennifer L. Bartlett and Carol Taylor

Today there is no guarantee that healthcare will work for anyone when it is needed. A precondition of safe, quality healthcare is the moral agency of professional caregivers. Every nurse, from the newest graduate to the most experienced, must be intentional about developing the moral agency that will enable them to competently meet each day's ethical challenges. Nurses' moral agency, which is rooted in the development of trusting relationships, needs to be cultivated like any other human excellence. Development of moral agency requires consideration of the underlying motivation and analysis of the associated action that should be grounded in moral principles that are focused on what is good, right, and just. Actions attributed to moral agency must accurately depict the image that the profession of nursing intends to project and who the public trusts nurses to be. While many define nursing agency as the abilities or capacities nurses possess in order to authentically *live* the profession's moral identity, this chapter emphasizes the importance of cultivating these abilities or capacities in order for nurses to secure the public's trust. Ultimately, both the nurse's abilities and trustworthiness are instrumental in creating the types of partnerships with individuals, institutions, and societies which promote health and well-being. Nurses with moral agency individually prove themselves trustworthy, but equally important, collectively prove the profession trustworthy—no small accomplishment in today's world. It should not be a surprise that national Gallup polls in the past 20 years rank nurses as the country's most trusted professionals—with exception of the year following 9/11 when firefighters merited the top award. This chapter bases its assumptions and recommendations on care ethics (Gilligan, 1982; Noddings, 1986) that are widely adopted by nurses to explain why trust matters in every professional encounter. The elements of nursing agency have been identified inductively by studying everyday ethical challenges in nursing practice and exploring those habituated dispositions, Aristotle's human excellencies or virtues, necessary to meet these challenges with integrity. Three cases will be used to illustrate this conception of moral agency and its development. We respect the role that reflective inquiry plays in

developing and enhancing the moral agency of the nurse, and we suggest reflective practice questions to facilitate the development of moral agency. The case-
based approach provides context for the professional formation of nurses as
moral agents. Liaschenko and Peter (2016) emphasize the importance of moral
community in developing nurses' moral identity and moral agency. The three
cases that we have selected illustrate situations in which moral agency becomes
relevant in ways that are outside the more typical nurse-patient relationship.
Our aim is to invite readers to reflect on the critical role that moral agency plays
in diverse situations where the outcomes at stake are at least partially determined
by the agency of the nurse(s) involved. With this in mind, the chapter concludes
with a call to action to those most able to promote and support the development
of the moral agency of nurses, nurse educators, system/institutional leaders, and
nurse researchers/scientists.

Moral Agency: A Definition

Once professional nurses understand what is reasonable for the public to expect of them (see the following section on the moral identity of nursing), the
next step is to determine if one has the capacity to meet these expectations (i.e.,
"Am I trustworthy?"). What makes a nurse trustworthy is not holding a creden-
tial that is publicly recognized or bestowed by the requisite credentialing body.
Rather, trustworthiness is proved in every clinical encounter when the nurse
demonstrates that they are able to be trusted, in the moment, with the challenge
at hand. It may be as simple (relatively speaking) as a change in the plan of care,
transitioning from curative to purely palliative goals. Or it could be as complex as
rethinking obligations to critically ill patients in a pandemic when a shortage of
personal protective equipment (PPE) forces choosing between the patient's need
for cardiopulmonary resuscitation and the health and continuing well-being of
frontline caregivers. It is never a given. Nurses who view the ethics of care as the
foundation for nursing's ethical obligations recognize that the nurse-patient relationship is central to care-based ethics and thoughtful, person-centered care.
Care directs attention to the specific situations of individual patients, viewed
within the context of their life narratives, and directs that how nurses choose to
be and act in each encounter is a matter of ethical significance. This is an ethics of
responsiveness. Characteristics of the care perspective include:

- Centrality of the caring relationship
- Promotion of the dignity and respect of patients as unique humans
- Attention to the particulars of individual humans

- Cultivation of responsiveness to others and professional responsibility
- A redefinition of fundamental moral skills to include virtues like respect, kindness, attentiveness, empathy, compassion, and reliability (Taylor, 1993).

Moral agency is therefore the ability to be what is professed: a moral human, a moral citizen, a moral professional nurse, such that one is trusted—even with another's very life and well-being. Moral agency may be defined as the capacity to be ethical and to do the ethically right thing for the right reasons. It requires personal and professional motivation to practice well and make good choices. Moral agency in any specific situation requires more than knowing what is right to do. It also entails (Taylor et al., 2023):

- *Moral character*: Cultivated dispositions that allow one to act as one believes one ought to act, such as respect, kindness, attentiveness, empathy, compassion, accountability, and reliability;
- *Moral motivation and valuing*: Valuing in a conscious and critical way what squares with good moral character and ethical integrity; for nurses this is a primary commitment to patient well-being and a degree of altruism;
- *Moral sensibility*: The ability to recognize the moral moment when an ethical challenge presents;
- *Moral responsiveness*: The ability and willingness to respond to the ethical challenge such that trust is engendered;
- *Ethical reasoning and discernment*: The knowledge of, and ability to use, sound theoretical and practical approaches to thinking through ethical challenges and to ultimately decide how best to respond to this particular challenge after identifying and weighing alternative courses of action; using these approaches to both inform and justify moral behavior;
- *Moral accountability*: The ability and willingness to accept responsibility for one's ethical behavior and to learn from the experiences of exercising moral agency;
- *Transformative moral leadership*: Commitment and proven ability to create a culture that facilitates the exercise of moral agency—a culture in which individuals are supported in doing the right thing simply because it is the right thing to do.

For the professional nurse, moral agency is the capacity to be trusted to meet the reasonable expectations of the public we serve, as articulated in the American Nurses' Association's Social Policy statement (2010), Code of Ethics for Nurses (ANA, 2015), Nursing: Scope and Standards of Practice, 4th edition (ANA, 2021) such that others are able to entrust their very life and well-being to the nurse.

Situating Moral Agency

With a clear definition of moral agency it is helpful to clarify related terms and briefly address how to develop and assess moral agency.

Moral Identity, Moral Agency, Moral Integrity, Moral Distress, Moral Resilience

Given the moral nature of nursing, which entrusts the well-being of society's most vulnerable to nurses in every clinical encounter, the need for moral agency seems self-evident. The opposite of our ability to strengthen, comfort, and heal, however, is our capacity to do harm, even lethal harm. In order to understand the significance of moral agency, it is helpful to establish the links among moral agency and moral identity, integrity, distress, and resilience. One of the primary challenges of the nursing profession is articulating and communicating a robust notion of the moral identity of the professional nurse. This assumes even greater importance as nursing attracts individuals who seek job security in today's economy, as opposed to drawing individuals to the profession based solely on the notion that nursing is a sacred vocation or calling. Kennedy (2018) questions how we could form nurses' professional identity, realizing that it is not enough to *do* nursing; rather, we must *be* nurses. How can we transform nursing students into nurses who have a professional sense of self that is influenced by the characteristics, norms, and values of the nursing discipline and that results in an individual who thinks, acts, and feels like a nurse? Primarily through its educators, the profession ensures that the nurses it licenses have the character, motivation, and values—in a word, the moral agency—that deserve the public's trust. When a nurse's everyday moral behavior and decision-making align with nursing's moral identity, the nurse has moral integrity. Pask (2003) studied moral agency in nursing by focusing on nurses' accounts of how they see intrinsic value in their work and believe that they make a difference to patients in terms that leave their patients feeling better. The nurses' moral agency is intrinsically linked to, and dependent upon, their capacity to see good in the work they do.

When individual or institutional factors create barriers to a nurse's acting ethically, moral distress results. Nurses who believe they know the ethically right course of action who find themselves unable to act on these beliefs and values can suffer great distress with serious consequences. The large literature on moral distress is now creating the demand for the profession and health care leadership to be more intentional about developing resources to foster each nurse's moral integrity and resilience (Rittenmeyer & Huffman, 2012). Rushton (2016) defines moral resilience as "[t]he capacity of an individual to sustain or restore their integrity in response to moral complexity, confusion, distress, or setbacks" (p. 112). Character, resilience, and moral fortitude support the development of moral agency, which requires the ability to recognize an issue and the ability to act and impact change. Recently, the Rest Four-Component Model (Narváez & Rest, 1995; Rest, 1982, 1984, 1994; Rest et al., 1999) had made a resurgence in practice and research models primarily because it provides a clear, integrative framework for describing moral reasoning development that undergirds *role formation* in nurses. The development of functional ability in each of the four components (ethical sensitivity, moral judgment, moral motivation and identity formation, and moral character) provides the foundation and impetus for moral behavior. Agency requires the development of who we *are* as nurses that goes well beyond scope of practice, assigned roles, and a laundry list of tasks. But agency also requires internal and demonstrated motivation, professional support rooted in nursing's norms and values, and an environment where action is possible. Agency requires tenacity, courage, resilience, and perseverance. The Clinical Ethics Residency for Nurses (CERN) developed by Robinson and others (2014) sought to strengthen nurses' moral agency as an antidote to moral distress. One of the key insights of the faculty members was the recognition that clinical ethics is not enough to develop moral agency. The CERN utilized a variety of methods based in adult learning theory, such as active application of ethics knowledge to patient scenarios in classroom discussion, simulation, and the clinical practicum, in addition to lecture-style classes. Feedback from participants (67 over three years of the program) indicated that CERN achieved transformative learning.

Developing and Assessing Moral Agency

Let's explore moral agency through the lens of a few pointed and challenging cases. In the three scenarios that follow, nurses are confronted with ethical challenges whose outcomes are dependent on the moral agency of the nurse. In the first scenario, a nurse researcher, under some pressure to recruit subjects for a clinical trial, suspects that a potential subject arrived for the interview under the influence of an illegal substance. Not only are they unable to consent to the clinical trial, but they tell the nurse they need to leave to pick up their three-year-old grandson. In the second scenario, an emergency department (ED) nurse is asked to initial that he completed 15-minute checks on a patient with a psychiatric history who is being boarded in the ED in a seclusion room until a bed on the psychiatric unit can be secured. The nurse did not complete the checks because he was with a patient who was being resuscitated. In the third scenario, a nurse broaches a conversation with her state representative about her patients' concerns over the potential impact that new religious conscience objections may have on healthcare access for the LGBTQIA+ community. In this chapter, these cases will be analyzed as individual, institutional, and sociopolitical moral agency is explored. Rather than use these cases to conduct a general ethical analysis of an ethically challenging situation, the cases are used to demonstrate the critical importance of moral agency. For each case, take a moment to reflect on the following questions before moving to the discussion:

1. How would you describe the ethical challenge?
2. What elements of moral agency are most applicable in this case? What is needed to earn the trust of all participants?
3. What will successful moral agency "look like" in this scenario, and what are the probable consequences of deficient or absent moral agency?
4. What guidance (if any) does the ANA Code of Ethics provide in this specific situation?
5. What resources exist to facilitate the development of moral agency and drive subsequent action?
6. What responsibilities do the professions of nursing, nurse educators, and healthcare leadership have to develop the moral agency of nurses? What is the individual nurse's responsibility to develop moral agency?
7. How do the individual moral identity of the nurse and the collective identity of the profession impact on the moral reasoning and action?
8. How do we develop a moral culture in healthcare that is rooted in agency and that is responsive to the power differentials in local, national, and global trends?

Case One (Individual)

The Case

Laura McLoughlin is a research nurse, currently recruiting individuals for a pain study. Inclusion criteria include being currently enrolled in a methadone program and being free of any illegal drugs. Recruitment is going slowly, and Laura is excited about the possibility of meeting a new potential subject. This particular morning, she is scheduled to meet a 62-year-old female, Jane White. When Jane presents to the research unit, Laura suspects that they are "high" because of their considerable drowsiness and difficulty attending to the conversation. Laura begins to explain the research study, hoping to enroll Jane, but is concerned about Jane's capacity to make valid decisions. Laura informs Jane that they will need to do a drug screen, at which point Jane tells Laura that they shot up with

heroin that morning. Laura explains that Jane is welcome to come back the following month, but that Jane is unable to be considered for participation at this
time. If the drug screen is negative next month, Jane can consent to participate
at that time. Jane then informs Laura that they should leave soon because they
have to pick up their grandson from his day school. Laura is uncomfortable letting Jane leave while they are under the influence of heroin and is also concerned
about Jane's ability to care for their grandson.

Discussion

Clinicians doing research with human subjects have an inherent conflict. The
goal of the clinician is the health, well-being, or good dying of the patient; the goal
of the researcher is to generate knowledge that will be used to benefit others in
the future. If Laura is a non-nurse research employee hired to recruit individuals
for a clinical study, a good day might translate into successful recruitments for
the study. As a *nurse* researcher, Laura must balance her job requirements as a
research recruiter with the moral identity and responsibilities of the professional
nurse. The relational nature of the nurse-patient dyad involves connection, trust,
and implicit obligations. This relationship exists even when the nurse is engaged
in parallel work that is not necessarily patient-focused. The nurse's professional
obligations exist in tandem with the task-driven obligations, extending to the
consideration of patient well-being and safety. Nurses frequently integrate professional standards with task-based requirements and are trusted to advocate for
the patient as needed. Moral agency requires nurses to not only recognize a potentially dangerous or unhealthy situation; they are professionally obligated to
act. Providing nurses the structure and framework within which they can act
promotes their ability to be moral agents in the moment, even when that action
requires extra work and follow-through.

In the case presented, as Laura broadens her role to consider the person
along with the task of recruitment, she integrates: (1) adhering to the research
protocol and other research standards (such as verifying capacity) to ensure
ethical research; (2) considering the potential benefit of participation for Jane
and recommending Jane come back at a later time; and (3) taking a moment
to consider the current situation and the potential safety ramifications for Jane
and their grandson. As professional nurses, saving the world is not our personal or professional objective, but we are obligated, at the very least, to keep
people in our care safe. This case is interesting because Laura does not have
the classic nurse-patient relationship with Jane and certainly not with Jane's
grandson, which is stretching her thinking about her responsibilities and the
prerequisite moral agency. Nurses tend to be more comfortable considering

advocacy or moral agency in the context of caring for patients assigned to them. Based on the structure of the healthcare environment, nurses, and other health-care professionals, are privy to and entrusted with patient information that is protected and not available to the general public. Appropriately balancing confidentiality and privacy, the prescriptive nature of the research protocol, and consideration of the psychological and physical safety of the potential participant requires training and is not necessarily unique to a nurse in this consent role. However, the relational nature of nursing often provides insight into person-specific nuances that may motivate or even compel the nurse to take additional intervening action. The nurse is professionally obligated in some situations to gather additional information, enumerate potential resources, notify or report, and/or collaborate with the interprofessional team. This motivation and duty to act reflect moral agency. The challenge for the nurse revolves around determining the overlap between the role of researcher and overarching professional obligations. Exploring the tension between role-based, person-centered, and professional-based obligations drives the development of agency. This example extends the expectations for the nurse in the nurse-patient relationship to all persons with whom the nurse comes into contact in the context of their professional roles.

Chances are good that this situation is not unique or a one-time event for this nurse. The repetitive nature of ethical issues that challenge moral agency often result in the nurse experiencing moral distress, which further affects the agency of the nurse. Retaliation against nurses is unacceptable, especially when used as a bludgeon to silence an individual professional. Trusting the process and relying on policies, assuming the policies are well-designed, provides the individual with a recourse and rationale for some decisions. In other words, if the policy mandates notification and triggering of a system-level response, the nurse must activate the response to comply with policy. This takes the burden off the individual, but this only works if the structure is in place, and if the individual consistently follows said policy and does not make exceptions that can be perceived as bias or discriminatory practice. In the case presented, research protocols guide decisions regarding recruitment, but addressing follow-up or the current safety issue is not likely outlined in the protocol and may or may not be addressed at the facility level. If institutional or personal variables create obstacles for Laura translating her ethical beliefs and convictions into action, she is likely to experience moral distress and will have to balance remaining in this position with preserving her moral integrity. Ideally, Laura's moral agency will be sufficiently developed to equip Laura to navigate this conflict. What is immediately apparent is that Laura feels a sense of accountability for the safety of Jane and their grandson. Absent a formal relationship, she will need some creative leadership to strategize about how best to keep Jane safe while high. Clearly Laura has the motivation to respond and values responding, and she may need the support of colleagues and leadership to determine how to do this most effectively.

Individual moral agency is essential, especially when structures or procedures do not exist. This came to the forefront during the early days of the COVID-19 pandemic. Due to a paucity of resources and a lack of a national plan, resource-allocation decisions and the enforcement of policies related to myriad things, including visitation and mandating that patients also wear masks, fell to the individual clinical healthcare provider. The lack or delay in development of uniform, enforceable policies, coupled with inadequate resources and public distrust of evolving science, resulted in nurses and other healthcare professionals addressing issues in individual patient interactions, acting as the face of health-care to the public, and scrambling to create individual institution-based crisis plans. In these instances, nurses chose to be moral agents and do the best they could to care for their patients, while protecting the public, even if that protec-tion meant nurses separating from their personal families and making dramatic changes to their daily routines.

Application of the Code of Ethics for Nurses

Provisions one, two, three, and four of the Code (focusing on compas-sion and respect for patients, the primacy of the patient, the nurse's advocacy responsibilities, and the nurse's authority, accountability, and responsibility for nursing practice; American Nurses Association [ANA], 2015) are all applicable in this scenario. The role of the nurse varies depending on the setting, but the nurse as a professional has an individual responsibility to patients and the public. The trust required for the development of the patient-nurse dyad can be applied to the relationship nurses have individually and collectively with the public.

Case Two (Institution/System)

The Case

Carlos Gomez is an ED nurse practitioner in a busy community hospital. Because of inadequate inpatient beds for psychiatric admissions, patients with mental health challenges are frequently boarded in the ED in a seclusion room while they await a bed. Hospital policy requires that boarded patients be assessed every 15 minutes, with formal documentation required. Because the ED is fre-quently understaffed and the acuity is high, it is not unusual for a nurse to be un-able to make and document these required 15-minute checks. In these instances, management asks the nurse to sign their initials as if they were doing the checks to avoid problems during the state and Joint Commission visits. Carlos is hesitant to lie to protect the hospital, but he wants to be a team player.

Discussion

This scenario could be rewritten for so many settings where professional nurses practice. Given that staffing and resource allocation remain common challenges for nurses, it can be difficult to muster and sustain the moral outrage and agency required to enact change, especially when the issues are so pervasive across all healthcare settings.

Institutions control aspects of the environment including development, evaluation, and enforcement of everything from policies, procedures, guidelines, and protocols, to interpersonal and intra/interprofessional conflict-resolution tactics, and the establishment of norms. Institutions exhibit moral agency when they claim responsibility for the outcomes stemming from these control mechanisms and consider these outcomes with respect to their institution's values and goals (Charles, 2017). The impact of these regulatory mechanisms must also be considered in relation to the healthcare professionals who fall under their purview. Charles (2017) considers this specifically through the lens of patient autonomy and highlights how policies and processes can increase or decrease professional autonomy and authority (within scope of practice), resulting in the establishment of an environment that can either recognize or stifle the agency of the individual. Pressure points include staffing ratios and their well-documented link to moral distress and burnout, the hierarchies that persist in healthcare that place nurses subservient to other professionals and belie the clinical expertise of nurses, and power imbalances that are exacerbated when policy interferes with nursing judgment (Charles, 2017). This thinking transcends issues related to patient autonomy and can be applied to myriad other situations where the institution's moral agency impacts the professional's moral agency, and then trickles down to patient agency and, ultimately, patient outcomes. Moral agency does not exist in a vacuum. We need to do a better job differentiating issues that require personal responsibility from institutional issues that require system-level reform. Wocial (2020) eloquently writes about the inadequacy of the individual nurse's resilience as a strategy for coping with moral distress. See also Epstein, Haizlip, Liashenko, Zhao, and Bennett's (2020) call for moral community to address traumatic stress in provider burnout.

We cannot wish or will away the basic premise that an individual's moral agency can either be fostered or squashed by the confines of an institution. The ill-conceived notion that an individual can easily enact moral action in spite of an oppressive institution exemplifies a very American value and sets the stage for individual and systematic failure. Can one person make a difference? Sure. Social media touts these exceptional individuals and their stories every day—right alongside examples of institution-driven whistleblower retaliatory practices. Changing the culture from within is challenging, to say the least, but the value of bottom-up *and* top-down promotion of agency results in an expectation of accountability from the individual professionals, their leaders, and the institution itself. Consider Carlos's situation. He wants to be a team player, but being a team player does not mean accepting less than what you or your patients deserve. Doing your job should not involve lying to convince yourself that the ends justify the means. A true team player elevates their team by maintaining personal and professional accountability for following the rules, but also by questioning those rules as needed, and engaging in the hard work of forcing change, which exemplifies moral agency.

In this scenario we begin to see the importance of administration in a practice site setting a tone/environment which communicates that integrity matters—or that it does not. Every nurse would have to decide whether sacrificing moral integrity to be a team player is a reasonable trade-off. Leadership at every level in an institution or health system is responsible for creating an ethical environment that supports everyone's ability to be ethical, to do the right thing simply because that is the right way to be.

This is where initiatives like shared governance are exceedingly important, but they are only as effective as their constituents demand. Working within the confines of a system lends itself to forward progression, but if the system is broken, role modeling, completing a report, or being vocal only with peers (who can appreciate, but not independently impact change) are not going to have the desired effect. Nurses and other healthcare professionals do not have to wait for someone else to shake up the process. Think of agency as *having a say*. It is an oversimplification, but it gets at the root of institution-based disenfranchisement. Experienced nurses and bioethicists know that those who do the work get to make the decisions. Promote an environment and build structures and processes where professional practitioners get involved, do the work, and make the decisions.

Application of the Code of Ethics for Nurses

Provisions four, five, and six of the Code (focusing on the nurse's authority, accountability, and responsibility for nursing practice; duties to self, including the responsibility to preserve wholeness of character and integrity; and responsibility to improve the ethical environment and conditions of employment conducive to safe, quality healthcare; ANA, 2015) are all applicable for this scenario. The Code applies to leaders in nursing, whether they be formal administrator or informal leaders. The establishment of a moral environment that supports individual and collective moral agency is a team sport.

Case Three (Sociopolitical/Professional)

The Case

Katherine Hill is a practicing nurse in the United States where a rule was announced in May 2019 outlining specific religious conscience protections for healthcare professionals. Although rules and laws change depending on the administration and their views regarding separation of legislation and service entities, staying abreast of proposals, rules, and laws is important to Katherine, who works with vulnerable populations. Right now, Katherine is focused on two specific rules that are germane to her work. One rule titled *Protecting Statutory Conscience Rights in Health Care; Delegations of Authority* (45 CFR Part 88-RIN 0945-AA10) replaces a 2011 rule and is housed within a division of the Health and Human Services (HHS) Office for Civil Rights (OCR) referred to as the Conscience and Religious Freedom Division that was established in 2018 (U.S. Department of Health & Human Services, 2018). This final rule specifically covers moral and religious protections related to: abortion and (involuntary) sterilization (performance, training, referral, and accreditation standards); "assisted suicide, euthanasia, and mercy killing" (U.S. Department of Health and Human Services, Office for Civil Rights, 2019, p. 23170); exemptions to the individual mandate (healthcare plans, Medicare Advantage, and Medicaid managed care organizations); the performance of advanced directives; Global Health Programs and other federal funding administered by the secretary of HHS; compulsory healthcare related to hearing screening, occupational illness testing, vaccination, and mental health treatment; and religious non-medical healthcare providers and their patients from requirements under Medicare and Medicaid (U.S. Department of Health and Human Services, Office for Civil Rights, 2019). An objection to this rule was heard in the courts in November 2019. Despite public pushback (115,966 public comments; Centers for Medicare and Medicaid Services, 2019), another HHS rule on *Nondiscrimination in Health and Health Education Programs or Activities: Delegation of Authority* was finalized on June 12, 2020 (U.S. Department of Health and Human Services, & Centers for Medicare & Medicaid Services, 2020). This rule revises the Affordable Care Act, Section 1557. These rollbacks effectively eliminate protections for persons based on gender identity, eliminate insurance protections for transgender persons, adopt blanket abortion and religious freedom exemptions for health-care providers, weaken protections surrounding interpreter/translation serv-ices, and affect other protections for people with disabilities and prohibition of discrimination on the basis of gender identify or sexual orientation at the fed-eral level. Although hospitals, healthcare systems, insurance companies, and providers can add these categories of nondiscrimination if they desire, they are not mandated at the federal level (Mattinson et al., 2020). Katherine finds it sig-nificant that this rule went into effect in the middle of the COVID-19 pandemic because in her personal and professional opinion, potentially limiting healthcare during a pandemic is inhumane. She also has patients in her practice who would be directly affected by these changes. Katherine broaches a conversation with her state representative about her patients' concerns over the potential impact on healthcare access for the LGBTQIA+ community.

Discussion

Although laws may change, new bills may be passed, and the Supreme Court may deliver rulings, the point is that we need to pay attention to the world around us and not become complacent or inured to things within our environment that affect the people and communities that nurses serve. Enacting the nurses' code of ethics may involve voting, lobbying, advocating, activism (in all forms), and educating on a larger scale. Nurses promote health, human rights, social jus-tice, health diplomacy, and the reduction of disparities (ANA, 2015). Enacting change requires engagement and involvement in the development and imple-mentation of health policy.

Contextual elements provide nuance and variability to any ethical situa-tion. The challenge with the *Protecting Statutory Conscience Rights in Health Care; Delegations of Authority* rule is that although it is concerned primarily with abortion and end-of-life issues, the verbiage seems to allow discriminatory practice. Therefore, there are two major considerations: (1) moral and religious objection to abortion and anything that hastens death, and (2) the ability of the individual and organization to refuse to care for *any* patient on the basis of religious or moral objection. Pro-choice and pro-life stances are generally considered dichotomous and mutually exclusive. As healthcare professionals, we may need to separate what we would do in a situation from what is pos-sible for a patient to do in the same situation. Whether we place arbitrary or ra-tional parameters around our decision-making (e.g., abortion is permitted/not permitted in rape or incest), or we ascribe to dichotomy narrative, the devel-opment of professional moral agency requires a deep exploration. This entails a willingness to use one's moral agency to engage in deep reflection on one's role and personal conscience related to an issue, and then take that conclusion and advocate for patients as these laws are developed. Deep moral reflection and refined moral agency are essential to help the nurse reach a careful and thoughtful conclusion about their own position in light of the need for public trust and nondiscrimination. This has become much more complicated in light of the 2022 Supreme Court's decision in *Dobbs v. Jackson Women's Health Organization* regarding federal protections surrounding abortion rights. These rights, which have been in place since 1973, no longer have even the veil of federal protection. Although the wide-reaching ramifications are yet to be fully realized, what we already know is that the provider's role in providing medical care and protecting the privacy of the individual is now legally in question in some states.

Although we will not consider abortion within the larger context of women's reproductive healthcare in this section, let's take a moment to explore other potential applications of this rule. What if a nurse who is a member of the Catholic Church agrees with recent proclamations from the Church and morally objects to the idea of *transgender*? Can this nurse refuse care to the patient who presents to the ED for complications related to gender-affirming surgery? Does the individual who is transgender not have the right to access medically necessary care based on some else's religious belief? Can the patient be denied care by the facility itself? Can the patient legally be denied healthcare coverage? According to this rule, the simple answer to each of these questions is "yes."

As nurses, we must stay abreast of political developments and educate ourselves and our peers—go to the actual rule, instead of relying on a politician's, journalist's, or other individual's interpretation of a rule that directly affects our profession and the patients we serve. Staying abreast of elements in politics, government, and healthcare administration that directly affect the work of healthcare professionals is part of our job—we must stay vigilant and informed to develop moral sensibility. Legislation does not happen to us; we are invited to be an integral part of that process. We need to accept the invitation to lobby, to join advocacy groups, and to work through our professional organizations to demand change. Nurses have always had the ability to choose where we work or to refuse to participate in a specific procedure. This rule has simply cast our professional choices in a different light, forcing public comment and conversation. But nothing gives the nurse the right to discriminate by refusing care of a patient based on their gender, sex, sexual orientation, race, ethnicity, or a myriad of other factors. Nurses have a unique responsibility to the public—the public trusts nurses. This responsibility extends to moral agency in the sociopolitical environment. This call applies to clinicians, leaders, educators, and researchers alike. Having moral character enhances the profession as a whole, but we need to create a transformative moral leadership path to ensure that nurses retain their voice in our society and maintain our commitment to the health and well-being of the people we serve.

Application of the Code of Ethics for Nurses

Provisions seven, eight, and nine specifically address health policy, health diplomacy, and social justice, which provide the impetus for moral agency (ANA, 2015). Provision 8 in particular reads, "The nurse collaborates with other health professionals and the public to protect human rights, promote health diplomacy, and reduce health disparities" (ANA, 2015, p. 31). We cannot enact change on these fronts without agency, knowledge, and motivation to take action. The words *right* and *good* are often used when considering ethical situations, but the collective definition of what is right or good may not reflect an individual nurse's perspective. That nurse has an opportunity—no, a mandate—to formulate an opinion and to take actions that support reaching a desired outcome. This requires more than a tweet or a post. Agency drives us to do the work required. Provision 8.1 states, "health is a universal right" (ANA, 2015, p. 31). It includes provisions related to reproductive health and is an excellent example of how a professional organization (ANA) has clearly articulated the position of its members. Provision 9.4 encompasses social justice and the need for nurses to engage in policy formation and enforcement.

Call to Action

Moral agency is a universal human experience. Within the context of everyday life, people make judgments about what is right and wrong, act based on that judgment, and then bear responsibility and accountability for their decisions and actions. We may not routinely notice the judgment, related action, and accountability in every moment, but there are instances where humans become acutely aware of these internal processes. Adversity is the great illuminator—when there is unity and no perceived conflict, we are blissfully unaware of our decision-making processes and the associated ramifications. But when there is disagreement between what is right and wrong—systemic racism that results in significant health disparities, staffing issues that result in medical errors, the disconnect between science and policy regarding the social contract of masking during a pandemic—the tenets of moral agency are illuminated, articulated, and important. Nurses and other healthcare professionals have been articulating the relationship between moral judgment and clinical decision-making for years. We talk internally about moral conflicts and resolutions from the bedside to the boardroom; we engage in advocacy for our patients and communities. But let's think a bit bigger about moral agency. There is sufficient evidence in 2020 to support the claim that systemic racism leads to health disparities (related to access and treatment) that result in negative outcomes for disenfranchised, marginalized, and socially stigmatized groups. As nurses and healthcare providers, this influences our daily practice, and if it does not, it should. As a profession, nurses have a collective identity that is rooted in serving individuals and communities. This identity is ever-evolving, but manifests in our Code, professional organizations, nursing education standards, and public discourse. Engagement at the individual, system, and sociopolitical levels requires intentionality and stamina—nurses are entrusted to do this work.

It is impossible to discuss moral agency without mentioning what we are doing right, and where we are still making mistakes. We need to stop using *empowerment* as a synonym for *moral agency* in programs geared toward nurses. Empowerment implies that one needs to be given power—agency is not bestowed by another, it comes from within. It is the drive to address a wrong, the willingness to step up, the need to advocate in a situation, and the enhanced ability to bring about change. Nurses already have individual and collective power. Robinson et al. (2014) are correct in their assertion that knowledge is not enough to develop moral agency. Transformative learning requires that education also intentionally address attitudes and develop skills through discussion, reflection in clinical practice, simulation, case study, and other modalities requiring the nuanced application of knowledge (Lee et al., 2020; Robinson et al., 2014). Moral agency is foundational to professional identity formation. Nurses, especially new nurses, require support as they transition to clinical practice because the development of moral agency requires success. Continued futile attempts that never lead to change cause frustration, discouragement, exhaustion, and other demoralizing outcomes. We talk about nurses having burnout, becoming jaded, or giving up the good fight in response to the relentless pressures of microaggressions, everyday ethical issues, and the experience of moral distress. Rushton (2018) discusses moral distress, moral outrage, and moral injury as forms of moral suffering, and identifies integrity as the core of resilience. The parallels between resilience and agency cannot be denied—agency comes from who we are as professionals and as people. Agency is the antidote to moral distress. Creating environments where moral successes are encouraged and recognized maintains the professional's integrity and allows for the space required for the development of moral agency.

Clinical Nurses

Ideally, every nurse can use the resources in this chapter to assess their moral agency and ability to be trusted. Once the development of moral agency is prioritized, individual nurses can begin by analyzing the adequacy of their moral identity. How easily can I articulate what is reasonable for the public to expect of me? When did I last review the ANA Code of Ethics for Nurses? Have I read the American Nurses Association's *Nursing: Scope and Standards of Practice* (2021)? Is my moral agency such that practicing congruently with what the profession describes as our moral agency is my norm? What are our options when we are practicing in healthcare environments that prioritize profit over care and require heroic virtue and courage of nurses to advocate for the health and well-being of patients and the public? Physician colleagues writing about professionalism [substitute: moral agency] offer an insight that seems particularly germane here and in keeping with the earlier comments of Wocial (2020), Liashenko and Peter (2016), and Milliken (2018) about moral community and context. Professionalism [moral agency] needs to evolve from being conceptualized as an "innate character trait or virtue . . . [to] sophisticated competencies that can and must be taught and refined over a lifetime of practice (Lesser et al., 2010, p. 2733). Furthermore, "professional behaviors are profoundly influenced by the organizational and environmental context of contemporary medical practice, and these external forces need to be harnessed to support—not inhibit— professionalism in practice" (Lesser et al., 2010, p. 2733). This perspective on professionalism provides an opportunity to improve the delivery of healthcare through education and system-level reform (Lesser et al., 2010).

Moral agency development is a process, much like the process of developing professional practice or developing compassion or empathy. One does not simply *have* moral agency; one develops the habituated dispositions congruent with moral agency, and one *engages* as a moral agent in an encounter-specific context engendering trust.

Nurse Educators

Nurse educators are uniquely positioned to impact the future of nursing. There is a general understanding that educators influence and shape the development of future nurses, but we must not minimize the impact of their individual and collective voices on educational norms, accreditation standards, licensure decisions, and the expected knowledge, skills, and attitudes of clinical nurses. Educators can influence the direction of education by participating in, for example, task forces dedicated to the revision of accreditation, education, or licensure standards. This can be through formal engagement in professional organizations or professional volunteer opportunities, or through less formal avenues. For example, a work group recently provided input to the two major accreditation bodies in nursing, imploring the explicit articulation of ethical principles in education standards using a structured process based on the Rest Four-Component Model (Rest, 1994; Robichaux et al., 2022). A gap was identified by the group of nurse educators, and they recognized their moral agency and chose to speak up regarding the importance of articulating ethical competence as a core component of education. Educators have an obligation to their students to stay abreast of developments in ethics to better enable meaningful and intentional integration of ethics in nursing curricula.

Nurse educators also need to consider global volunteerism with respect to students. Although there are plenty of opportunities for experienced nurses to engage in mission trips or other opportunities, mission trips have become synonymous with service-learning and global outreach, according to many institutions nationwide. The 2019 position statement from the American Nurses Association supports short-term activities that focus on partnering with the community to be served, demonstrating that principles of social responsibility and cultural humility are mutually beneficial and can result in the development of sustainable outcomes (ANA, 2019).

Institution/System Leaders

Nurse leaders are often in a precarious situation. Formal and informal leaders face the challenge of integrating traditional definitions of *good* care with evolving societal pressures and norms, the need to consider the logistics of implementation, and the consideration of both the individual nurse-patient relationship (micro) and healthcare as a whole (macro). Maintaining the delicate balance between professional accountability and institutional structure requires fortitude. But what about their role in cultivating and even demanding moral agency in the nurses who report to them? Are advocacy, agency, and activism specifically articulated on the annual performance review? These formal leaders are positioned to encourage nurses who face situations that require moral agency. From supporting them in difficult interactions to facilitating advocacy and promoting action, those in leadership roles have an obligation to the profession. Let's update those competency checklists and start including measures of integrity, accountability, and agency.

When stressed, as leaders have been during the COVID-19 pandemic, a re-examination of the ethical duties resulted in their identification as: (1) duty to plan, especially in light of rapidly evolving science and guidelines;

(2) duty to safeguard, which applies to both healthcare employees at all levels and populations deemed vulnerable; and (3) duty to guide and provide clear identification of contingency plans related to evolving levels of care and, more importantly, crisis standards of care that took into account the availability of resources, offset with the needs of any given population (Berlinger et al., 2020). Leaders had to make their voices heard and embrace their roles as moral agents in balancing patient-centered focus with equality and equity factors that inform the decision-making process that occurred at every institution across the Unites States.

Nurse Researchers and Nurse Scientists

The term *evidence-based practice* is a mainstay in healthcare today, but this was not always the case. Nurses are driving the generation and analysis of sound data to support clinical and educational decisions. We are challenging traditional processes and lobbying for change at institutional and system levels. For example, how can we reasonably view shootings as a public health crisis without data? How can we create meaningful plans to prevent mass shootings and to mitigate potential/actual negative ramifications on individuals and our communities without data? Commentaries and reports on school shootings and mass shootings are remarkably data-light. Scientific investigation has been stifled by a lack of funding for firearm research, a lack of standard definitions and comparison of like data, and fatigue or apathy of the public (Galea et al., 2018). Nurse researchers have a unique opportunity to provide insight into ongoing health disparities and to integrate evolving public views on policing and incarceration, gerrymandering that skews representation, and voting rights—these concepts are interconnected and must be considered together as symptoms of a ubiquitous issue in the United States that citizens are ready to address. Opportunities for nurse researchers exist outside the bounds of an acute care setting—we need to share our knowledge and perspective as leaders in healthcare and in our communities.

Summary

Whether nurses view their profession as a calling or as a job, we have an obligation to serve those entrusted to our care and to design systems that promote health and health equity. The absence of moral agency—the motivation, the requisite action, and associated reflection—limits the nurse's ability to impact necessary change that ultimately affects the health and well-being of those they serve. Developing a professional identity rooted in the core values of nursing as a profession requires development of the ethical self, who is ready, willing, and able to take a stand. Georgia Representative John Lewis, who died in 2020, profoundly stated in 2019, "When you see something that is not right, not just, not fair, you have a moral obligation to say something. To do something.... We have a mission and a mandate to be on the right side of history." Representative Lewis (2018) was known for being a civil rights freedom fighter alongside other civil rights leaders, and encouraged people to "[n]ever, ever be afraid to make some noise and get in good trouble, necessary trouble." He challenged citizens to be moral agents and worked to change the systems he rallied against from the inside by becoming a congressman. His work exemplifies the interconnectedness of individual, system, and sociological agency.

Mark Lazenby (2017b) writes that nursing "is a profoundly radical profession that calls society to equality and justice, to trustworthiness, and to openness. The profession is, also, radically political: It imagines a world in which the conditions necessary for health are enjoyed by all people" (p. 1). To realize Lazenby's (2017a, 2017b) vision, every nurse, from the newest graduate to the most experienced, must be intentional about developing the moral agency that will enable them to competently meet each day's ethical challenges head on. As the preceding cases illustrate, these challenges assume many forms, from simple to complex, mundane to profound.

References

American Association of Colleges of Nursing. (2020). Essentials task force. Retrieved November 29, 2020, from https://www.aacnnursing.org/About-AACN/AACN-Governance/Committees-and-Task-Forces/Essentials.

American Nurses Association. (2010). *Nursing's social policy statement: The essence of the profession* (3rd ed.). American Nurses Association.

American Nurses Association. (2015). *Code of ethics for nurses with interpretative statements*. http://www.nursingworld.org/DocumentVault/Ethics_1/Code-of-Ethics-for-Nurses.html.

American Nurses Association. (2019). *Ethical considerations for local and global volunteerism*. Retrieved July 15, 2020, from https://www.nursingworld.org/~4a346d/globalassets/practi ceandpolicy/nursing- excellence/ana-position-statements/social-causes-and-health-care/ ethical-considerations- for-local-and-global-volunteerism_final_nursingworld.pdf.

American Nurses Association. (2021). *Nursing: Scope and standards of practice* (4th ed.). American Nurses Association.

Berlinger, N., Wynia, M., Powell, T., Hester, M., Milliken, A., Fabi, R., Cohn, F., Guidry-Grimes, L. K., Watson, J. C., Bruce, L., Chuang, E. J., Oei, G., Abbott, J., & Jenks, N. P. (2020, March 16). Guidelines for institutional ethics services responding to the coronavirus pandemic: Managing uncertainty, safeguarding communities, guiding practice. The Hastings Center. https://www.thehastingscenter.org/ethicalframeworkcovid19/.

Centers for Medicare and Medicaid Services (2019, June 14). Nondiscrimination in health and health education programs or activities [Agency/Docket

No.: HHS-OCR-2019-0007; RIN: 0945-AA11 Document Number: 2019-11512]. https://www.federalregister.gov/documents/2019/06/14/2019-11512/nondiscriminat ion- in-health-and-health-education-programs-or-activities.

Charles, S. (2017). The moral agency of institutions: Effectively using expert nurses to support patient autonomy. *Journal of Medical Ethics, 43*(8), 506–509.

Dobbs v. Jackson Women's Health Organization, 597 U.S. 19–1392 (2022). https://www.supre mecourt.gov/opinions/21pdf/19-1392_6j37.pdf.

Epstein, E. G., Haizlip, J., Liaschenko, J., Zhao, D., Bennett, R. (2020). Moral distress, mattering, and secondary traumatic stress in provider burnout: A call for moral community. *AACN Advanced Critical Care, 31*(2), 146–157.

Galea, S., Branas, C. C., Flescher, A., Formica, M. K., Hennig, N., Liller, K. D., Madanat, H. N., Park, A., Rosenthal, J. E., & Ying, J. (2018). Priorities in recovering from a lost generation of firearms research. *American Journal of Public Health, 108*(7), 858–860.

Gilligan, C. (1982). *In A different voice: Psychological theory and women's development.* Harvard University Press.

Kennedy, M.S. (2018). To be a nurse. *American Journal of Nursing, 118*(11), 7. doi:10.1097/ 01.NAJ.0000547640.70037.f6.

Lazenby, M. (2017a). *Caring matters most: The ethical significance of nursing.* Oxford University Press.

Lazenby, M. (2017b). Why caring matters most. *Yale Nursing Matters, 17*(1), 16. https://nurs ing.yale.edu/sites/default/files/25783_nursing_web.pdf

Lee, S. M., Robinson, E. M., Grace, P. J., Zollfrank, A., & Jurchak, M. (2020). Developing a moral compass: Themes from the Clinical Ethics Residency for Nurses' final essays. *Nursing Ethics, 27*(1), 28–39.

Lesser, C. S., Lucey, C. R., Egener, B., Braddock, C. H., Linas, S. L., & Levinson, W. (2010). A be-havioral and systems view of professionalism. *JAMA, 304*(24), 2732–2737.

Lewis, J. [@repjohnlewis]. (2018, June 27). *Do not get lost in a sea of despair. Be hopeful, be opti-mistic. Our struggle is not the struggle ... #goodtrouble* [Tweet]. Twitter. https://twitter.com/ repjohnlewis/status/1011991303599607808.

Lewis, J. (2019, September 24). *Moral obligation* [Speech video recording on the floor of the U.S. House of Representatives]. Vox. https://www.vox.com/2020/7/18/21329556/john-lewis-speeches.

Liaschenko, J., & Peter, E. (2016). Fostering nurses' moral agency and moral identity: The im-portance of moral community. *Hastings Center Report, 46,* S18–S21.

Mattinson, J. M., Wethall, J., Fosheim, G. E., & Solomon, T. A. (2020, June 18). HHS finalizes anti-discrimination revisions to ACA Section 1557. *The National Law Review, X*(170). https://www.natlawreview.com/article/hhs-finalizes-anti-discrimination-revisions-to-aca-section-1557

Milliken, A. (2018). Refining moral agency: Insights from moral psychology and moral phi-losophy. *Nursing Philosophy, 19*(1), 10.1111/nup.12185. https://doi.org/10.1111/nup.12185

Narváez, D., & Rest, J. R. (1995). The four components of acting morally. In W. Kurtines & J. Gerwitz (Eds.), *Moral behavior and moral development: An introduction* (pp. 385–400). McGraw-Hill.

Noddings, N. (1986). *Caring: A feminine approach to ethics and moral education.* University of California Press.

Pask, E. J. (2003). Moral agency in nursing: Seeing value in the work and believing that I make a difference. *Nursing Ethics, 10*(2), 165–174.

Rest, J. R. (1982, February). A psychologist looks at the teaching of ethics. *Hastings Center Report, 12*(1), 29–36.

Rest, J. R. (1984). The major components of morality. In W. M. Kurtines & J. L. Gerwitz (Eds.), *Morality, moral behavior and moral development* (pp. 24–38). Wiley.

Rest, J. R. (1994). Background: Theory and research. In J. R. Rest & D. Narváez (Eds.), *Moral development in the professions: Psychology and applied ethics* (pp. 1–26). Lawrence Erlbaum Associates.

Rest, J. R., Narváez, D., Bebeau, M. J., & Thoma, S. J. (1999). *Postconventional moral thinking: A Neo-Kohlbergian approach.* Lawrence Erlbaum Associates.

Rittenmeyer, L. & Huffman, D. M. (2012). How professional nurses working in hospital environments experience moral distress: An updated systematic review. *Critical Care Nursing Clinics, 24*(1), 91–100.

Robichaux, C., Grace, P., Bartlett, J., Stokes, F., Lewis, M. S., & Turner, M. (2022). Ethics education for nurses: Foundations for an integrated curriculum. *Journal of Nursing Education, 61*(3), 123–130. https://doi.org/10.3928/01484834-20220109-02

Robinson, E. M., Lee, S. M., Zollfrank, A., Jurchak, M., Frost, D., Grace, P. J. (2014). Enhancing moral agency: Clinical ethics residency for nurses. *Hastings Center Report, 44*(5), 12–20.

Rushton, C. H. (2016). Moral resilience: A capacity for navigating moral distress in critical care. *AACN Advanced Critical Care, 27*(1), 111–119.

Rushton, C. H. (2018). *Moral resilience: Transforming moral suffering in healthcare.* Oxford University Press.

Taylor, C. (1993). Nursing ethics: The role of caring. *AWHONN's Clinical Issues in Perinatal and Women's Health Nursing, 4*(4), 552–560.

Taylor, C. (2023). Values, ethics, and advocacy. In C. Taylor, P. Lynn, & J. Bartlett, *Fundamentals of nursing: The art and science of person-centered care* (10th ed., pp. 116–142). Wolters Kluwer.

U.S. Department of Health and Human Services (2018, January 18). *HHS announces new conscience and religious freedom division.* https://www.hhs.gov/about/news/2018/01/18/hhs-ocr-announces-new-conscience-and- religious-freedom-division.html.

U.S. Department of Health and Human Services. (2019, May 21). *Protecting statutory conscience rights in health care: Delegations of authority* (45 CFR Part 88-RIN 0945-AA10). https://www.federalregister.gov/documents/2019/05/21/2019-09667/protecting-statut ory- conscience-rights-in-health-care-delegations-of-authority.

U.S. Department of Health and Human Services & Centers for Medicare & Medicaid Services. (2020, June 19). *Nondiscrimination in health and health education programs or activities: Delegation of authority* (Document Number: 2020-11758). https:// www.federalregister.gov/documents/2020/06/19/2020-11758/nondiscriminat ion- in-health-and-health-education-programs-or-activities-delegation-of-authority.

Wocial, L. D. (2020). Resilience as an incomplete strategy for coping with moral distress in critical care nurses. *Critical Care Nurse, 40*(6), 62–66.

7

Designing a Culture of Ethical Practice in Healthcare

A New Paradigm

Heather Fitzgerald and Cynda Hylton Rushton

Healthcare is reeling from escalating complexity, competing interests, and patients challenged by increasingly diverse and severe health conditions. Clinicians, including nurses, feel the external pressure of regulations, documentation to recover financial resources, efficiency and throughput mandates, alongside inner conflicts about their ability to practice in ways that reflect their professional values. Emerging data reflect that this often leads to moral distress and burnout (National Academies of Sciences, Engineering, and Medicine et al., 2019). Leaders struggle with decisions about material and human resource allocation, and wrestle with how best to uphold their fiduciary responsibilities and obligations to provide safe, compassionate care. Patients and families desire access to relational, quality healthcare, yet many are dissatisfied or disillusioned with the healthcare they receive. Surrounding these issues are societal trends that reflect a deepening divide among citizens, lack of consensus about the priorities of healthcare, and widening disparities—social factors exacerbated by the global COVID-19 pandemic. These ethical challenges have intensified, and pandemic-associated shifts in practices, processes, and decisions have threatened the moral core of healthcare and society.

Across the United States, where we practice and teach, the ripples of these dynamics are felt from the bedside to the boardroom. Many leaders are struggling to find and maintain a coherent individual moral compass as the morass of ethical issues accumulates and persists. Clinicians at the frontlines and the people they serve are reporting alarming levels of disengagement and despair in an ever-chaotic culture that reflects broader societal disempowering norms and systems. Our damaged healthcare cultures are reflected in our narrative as continuous distraction, reactively putting out fires, focusing on what's not working, engaging in turf battles, and thinking that solutions lie in more training programs. Far too often our focus is on solutions to the symptom rather than the underlying problem. We ponder why, when there are so many "good" people with "good" intentions, we cannot make a significant dent in solving recalcitrant problems. The answer is clear and simple—but not simplistic. We must attend to the deeper dimensions of these problems, rather than focus on surface-level interventions, if we want to meaningfully address complex challenges. Partial, unsustainable approaches fail to integrate our core professional commitment: to act with integrity in healthcare. This requires both individual moral resilience and an organizational culture that supports ethical practice. Moral resilience, "the ability to preserve or restore integrity in response to moral adversity" (Rushton, 2018, p. 127), is an enabling resource that is amplified in a culture where ethical practice is routine (Rushton et al., 2022). It is cultivated through discernment and embodiment of fundamental values, ethical competence, buoyancy, self-regulation, mindfulness, and self-stewardship (Holtz et al., 2018). These have been outlined in depth in *Moral Resilience: Transforming Moral Suffering in Healthcare* (Rushton, 2024) and provide the basis for this chapter.

We must learn to hold multiple perspectives, to source solutions from our own wisdom and inner capacities, to do what we are already doing—but differently. A new paradigm is needed that leverages core ethical values, shifts patterns that undermine integrity, produces meaningful and sustainable results, and offers a vision of hope for the future. What if we were able to create a healthcare system where ethical practice is routine? A system where decision-making processes at all levels are transparent and aligned with core values. Where organizational values are lived rather than talked about. Where healthcare professionals' alignment of personal and professional values invigorates moral agency and integrity. Where it is safe to speak up without risk of reprisal or repercussions. Where everyone is accountable for their choices and behaviors and there is a robust infrastructure to identify, address, and resolve ethical concerns. Where there are ongoing education, systems, and tools to leverage creative solutions to the patterns that create moral distress and burnout. Where reinforcing structures promote ethical reflection, moral inquiry, perspective-taking, and solution-oriented action committed to safety, dignity, and respect for ourselves and those we serve. Where individual and organizational values are aligned to produce compassionate, equitable healthcare.

An ethical practice environment, populated with people who are aligned through values, commitments, and wisdom, enables ethical discernment and action and fosters individual and collective moral resilience (Delgado et al., 2021). Creating a culture that promotes and sustains ethical practice requires a multipronged approach. Many factors must be considered and weighed. Evaluating the role of leadership and a balance between personal and professional obligations are essential. Assessing and evaluating the tension between clinical and organizational ethics, including corporate structure, policies and procedures, and risk management, are also critical to developing values-based, real-world solutions.

This chapter applies a practical model of full-spectrum change—the conscious full-spectrum (CFS) model (Sharma, 2017)—to create cultures of ethical practice in healthcare by leveraging our moral resilience and intentionally designing solutions that reflect our core values. After defining moral resilience and describing the CFS model, we highlight several key shifts that are necessary to begin the process of individual and organizational transformation. These include shifts in individual and collective mindsets, new ways of designing that address the patterns that are no longer working, and using design principles to produce strategic results. Promising practices to enable these shifts and exemplars from healthcare settings engaged in this work are included.

Moral Resilience

Moral resilience, "the capacity of an individual to restore or preserve integrity in response to moral adversity" (Rushton, 2018, p. 127), reflects an evolving awareness of oneself individually and collectively within our moral communities. The foundation of moral resilience is personal and professional integrity, combined with robust relational integrity that acknowledges the interconnectedness of everyone within the moral community where we reside. It leverages the capacities for self-regulation and moral efficacy to regain moral stability and balance in the aftermath of perceived threats or violations of our integrity (Holtz et al., 2018). Importantly, it includes investment in self-stewardship, a recognition of our inherent dignity as human beings and the necessity to invest in fostering our own health and well-being in order to fulfill our professional responsibilities while compassionately acknowledging our needs, resources and limitations (Holtz et al., 2018; Rushton, 2024).

Moral resilience is foundational to a culture of ethical practice. It fuels wholeness and integrity-preserving action aimed at restoring one's moral agency after it has been degraded so that one is able to choose words, behaviors, and actions that reflect our core values (Rushton, 2018). It is not complacency, nor does it suggest that the responsibility for integrity-preserving actions resides only with the individual (Sala Defilippis et al., 2019). As conceptualized by Rushton (2018), it acknowledges that our moral communities are made up of individuals who are capable of and oriented toward wholeness and the dynamic interplay with others, including patients and their families, interprofessional colleagues, and leaders, that create the ethical climate within which we practice. It presumes that human beings strive for wholeness and that everyone has innate resiliency that can be amplified and supported (Rushton, 2023).

Moral resilience is an ongoing practice; it is not a fixed state, nor does it imply that once one has been morally resilient in one situation that it will necessarily transfer into all others. Like other forms of resilience, our capacities may be expanded or contracted depending on our personal resources and capabilities, the circumstances of the situation, and the environment where moral adversity is arising. Instead of seeing ourselves as morally deficient, the orientation of moral resilience invites us to consider how we can leverage our moral conscientiousness in ways that reflect who we are and the values we stand for within the constraints of the situation. The potential to transform our moral suffering "by releasing its grip and discovering an alternative path" (Rushton, 2018, pp. 69–70) offers clinicians a means for discovering a path toward constructive change.

The Conscious Full-Spectrum Model

The CFS model provides the conceptual basis for designing individual, team, and organizational interventions aimed at cultivating moral resilience in its members and a culture that enables ethical practice (Sharma, 2017). It is a design methodology that solves problems, supports integrity, shifts patterns that undermine moral resilience and ethical practice, and sources the innate inner potential of the healthcare team and organization to produce impactful, sustainable results that benefit all.

The CFS framework is useful in addressing the sources of moral adversity within complex healthcare systems. It helps us to "align who we are, how we function and what we do into a synergistic whole" (Rushton, 2018, p. 221). This design template aligns our values, purpose, and actions to tap healthcare professionals' inner capacities and full potential to craft breakthrough initiatives and create new patterns of engagement. It has the potential to transform our healthcare systems by understanding that the situations that cause moral suffering are embedded in the moral ecosystem that was designed (intentionally or unintentionally) to produce the results that occur. Rather than focusing on a symptom of the problem and designing partial solutions that do not account for the complexity and interconnection among various forces within the system, the CFS framework invites us to step back to see the situation holistically with fresh eyes.

Shifting the culture by using the CFS model to enable and sustain healthcare professionals' integrity despite moral adversity has been described elsewhere (Rushton, 2018). We highlight aspects of the model here. Figure 7.1 is the framework which aligns overlapping spheres labeled *be*, *understand*, and *do* which nurture individual moral resilience and actualize a culture of ethical practice. This model provides guidance to align purpose, values, and actions

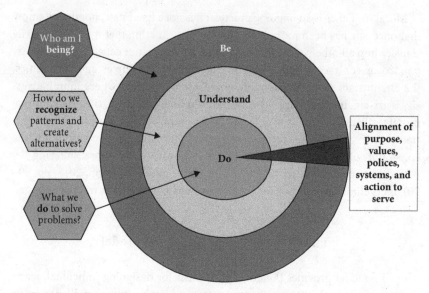

Figure 7.1 Moral Resilience and Ethical Practice Template©.

Based on the conscious full-spectrum framework (Sharma, 2017). Used with permission from Oxford University Press.

into a coherent whole. The triangle, or pie-shaped figure, illuminates a different approach for design and action from that which is customary in healthcare. Rather than addressing an issue or challenge with an action plan, the CFS model prompts us to begin *first* with our inner capacities, reflected at the wide base of the triangle figure.

The outer sphere, labeled *be*, engages individuals to identify and live out the values and commitments that comprise their moral core or compass, and reflects the essence of who they essentially are—their character and basic goodness. Embodying, rather than speaking about, our values and what we stand for in life and work provides an essential grounding for solution design and drives our choices and behaviors. It is also the realm where discernment and insight reside. This outer sphere permeates the other two spheres and infuses our understanding and action with the wisdom and essential values that are foundational to our work. In this sphere, the capacities necessary for moral resilience are nurtured, providing the source for our creativity and power to solve problems and shift culture.

The middle sphere, labeled *understand*, harnesses one's moral compass, insights, and discernment that arise from the outer sphere of *be*, to recognize and name the patterns of decisions and behaviors that have contributed to the underlying conditions shaping our current reality in healthcare. From this

Table 7.1 Potential Shifts to Create a Culture of Ethical Practice

From		To
Resignation	→	Engagement
Inattentive	→	Mindful
Victimized	→	Capable
Separation	→	Collaborative
Silence	→	Voice
Exclusion	→	Inclusion
Unworthy, disrespect	→	Self-esteem, dignity
Disparity	→	Fairness

Used with permission from Oxford University Press.

vantage point, alternatives can be identified to design specific shifts to create the conditions for ethical practice. This can stimulate pattern thinking to identify systems levers and strategic drivers to transform unworkable processes and norms to solve problems. Identifying current dynamics that can be shifted is necessary to develop specific tactics or interventions for culture change. Table 7.1 lists examples of potential shifts to support a culture of ethical practice.

The inner circle, labeled *do*, focuses on action. This inner sphere is where the specific tactics, initiatives, or interventions are implemented. In most models we tend to start here, in action, rather than in the outer sphere of who we are being in each moment. By aligning all aspects of this model, our tactics arise from the values, insight, and wisdom of the outer circle, combined with the detection of patterns in the middle circle, to focus on specific ways to achieve the results we are seeking. Instead of a series of disconnected initiatives that are likely to be unsustainable, there is an opportunity to harness the power of this alignment to create transdisciplinary strategies for action that deliver productive solutions.

Personal Transformational Learning

There's a tendency when considering how to create a culture of ethical practice in healthcare to assume that the process begins with dismantling the system. The 2019 report of the National Academies of Medicine (NAM), *Taking Action Against Clinician Burnout: A Systems Approach to Professional Well-Being*, calls for sweeping reforms of healthcare and health services learning organizations to address the very real systemic contributions to the erosion of clinician well-being and ultimately patient care. While systemic change is urgently needed, this alone will not sufficiently contribute to the shifts necessary to create cultures of ethical practice. Organizational investment in transformational learning which invites clinicians to further develop their own capacity to cultivate moral, emotional, and social intelligence is also essential to create and sustain systemic change.

What fuels and sustains large-scale culture change is beginning with ourselves (Sharma, 2017). All systems are made up of the people who inhabit them. The responsibility for organizational change resides with both the system and its leaders and the people who deliver care and services, yet we first need to cultivate the conditions for authentic and wise solution design in everyone in the system. Investing in processes that focus on the ethical practices and behaviors of the people who make up the system is vital to shift the current culture in health-care. Energy is generated when there is resonance in values, commitments, decisions, and actions that can be aligned and leveraged for large-scale reforms. This inside-out process is vital, as it connects us to our fundamental values, so we design solutions from a place of discernment rather than reaction or outdated rote methods that are incompatible in today's complex environment (Rushton, 2018). Transformational learning is foundational to leveraging the full potential of those within the system, as it provides an expanded repertoire of practices, tools, techniques, and skills which enable clinicians to enhance and value their contributions to patient care, to their team, and to the organization.

When clinicians believe that moral adversity and unhealthy work environments are immutable, feelings of victimization, powerlessness, and res-ignation are reinforced (Rushton, 2018). As a result, examples of compassionate action and integrity-preserving decisions, though present, can go unnoticed. Over time, this type of "moral blindness" (Bauman & Donskis, 2013) reinforces a negativity bias, eroding recognition of the courage, skillful effort, and wisdom routinely manifest in clinical practice, and diminishes our confidence, moral agency, and self-efficacy. When our moral sensitivity, conscience, and engage-ment in our work flounder, we are more vulnerable to a "we-versus-they" atti-tude, blaming each other and the system for the conditions in which we practice (Rushton, 2018). The urgency to fix these problems often leads healthcare organ-izations to invest in programs that develop technical skills, for example, one-off programs focusing on communication or customer service that require manda-tory participation. A common outcome is a cost-benefit mismatch, as the im-pact of these trainings is unsustainable despite significant financial investment. Of particular concern is that these approaches can make things worse. Instead of increased engagement and behavior change, cynicism and resistance can inten-sify, and disengagement often follows, creating a perpetual cycle that maintains the status quo.

Alternatively, transformational learning, "the process of deep, constructive, and meaningful learning that goes beyond simple knowledge acquisition and supports critical ways in which learners consciously make meaning of their lives" (Simsek, 2012), unleashes the human potential to care for others. This is a powerful strategy which fuels clinicians to commit to action and effect change at the point of care and beyond. Transformational learning leverages direct and active learning experiences to become critically aware of one's assumptions and biases to assess their relevance and to shift from mindless or unreflective acceptance of information to conscious choices that are aligned with our moral core. Engaging in experiential learning allows us to discover, rather than be told what we should learn; it has the potential to change our worldviews and how we inhabit the world. It occurs through dialogue, reflective practices, and critical reflection within a psychologically safe, supportive, and trusting environment. Transformational learning is synergistic with the qualities and competencies needed to foster moral resilience in individuals, teams, and organizations, as the foundation of moral resilience is stability of mind, body, and emotions, along with skills in self-regulation and the ability to remain flexible and whole in the midst of moral adversity. From this stable foundation, integrity flourishes.

Cultivating Moral Efficacy

Our ability to meet the ethical challenges that arise in our work requires us to see ourselves as capable of responding to them with competence and integrity. Moral efficacy "is the belief in one's ability to bring about desired and beneficial results through one's efforts and the exercise of one's moral agency individually and collectively" (Rushton, 2018, p. 133). This involves having the awareness, skills, and tools to be able to recognize ethical issues, to reason and deliberate about them, and to act in accordance with our values and commitments. The foundation of our moral efficacy is a well-developed sense of our self-conception, moral identities, social-ecological context, and the boundaries of authority and freedom to enact our values through our choices and decisions (Pavlish et al., 2014). Being able to articulate and leverage our values when they are threatened or violated allows us to remain in alignment with them as moral agents even when the stakes are high or uncertain.

Cultivation of self-awareness is also central to moral efficacy. Self-awareness attunes us to how rapidly thoughts and feelings shape our inner state, which can risk reactivity due to real or perceived threats, versus connecting to the values and commitments that inform our work. Moral efficacy invites us to account for the emotional and distressing aspects of the situation and use them as information to inform our inquiry, discernment, and action. Often emotions can point us to what is at stake in a particular situation, and the meaning that various courses of action have for us. Part of this process includes honing our awareness to the signals of conscience and using them to more fully appreciate the contours and consequences of the situations we find ourselves in. This emotional attunement and ethical sensitivity offer us additional resources to draw upon as we consider the range of ethically permissible options and the strategies that can be engaged when ethical tensions and conflicts arise. Expanding our capacity to hold multiple perspectives without feeling our own are eclipsed can stabilize us amidst these tensions and conflicts. From this space of awareness, we begin to notice our patterns of responsiveness or disengagement so that we can amplify our ability to choose our responses rather than remain in an autopilot or unreflective mode.

Developing moral efficacy is not a static process; it evolves as our experience and awareness evolve. This requires an ongoing investment in processes that continue to expand our repertoire of individual and collective capacities. It's tempting to reduce the development of moral efficacy to the simple application of a few ethical principles or to a profession's Codes of Ethics. While both are valuable, what is also needed is a nuanced and rigorous method for recognizing and examining the ethical tensions that arise in our clinical practice. Using approaches such as James Rest's framework for addressing ethical questions goes beyond cognitive reasoning to integrate commitment and action (Rest, 1986). Likewise, going beyond the nine provisions of the 2015 American Nurses Association *Code of Ethics for Nurses with Interpretive Statements* to understand the application of the interpretive statements to complex situations develops moral sensitivity and ethical awareness, and grounds moral agency in clinical practice (Robichaux, 2012).

Creating an Enabling Work Environment

Cultivation of the moral efficacy necessary to create cultures of ethical practice is not determined solely by individuals. We influence, are dependent upon, and are vulnerable to the moral ecosystems within which we practice. In a culture of ethical practice, this dynamic interchange between and among individuals, teams, leaders, and the organization reinforces shared values and yields normative, integrity-promoting behavior in a bolstering work environment (Rushton, 2018).

To create a culture that fosters ethical practice, we must engage in understanding this interplay between individuals and the systems in which we work. Recognizing the structures and processes within healthcare organizations that enable or disable moral efficacy is vitally important to begin aligning individual, collective, and organizational values and processes. This requires assessing policies, strategy, and change through the ethical lens of organizational values. The assessment can draw on discerning questions; for example, how does this policy/strategy/change support or undermine our commitment to create and sustain a culture of ethical practice? How are our values informing this decision? Are our values in tension, and if so, are we communicating transparently about how we plan to address that tension? Who will be affected by this policy/strategy/ change, and are their values in alignment with organizational values in this case? Have we fully considered the intended and unintended consequences of this policy/strategy/change, and have we worked to mitigate any negative effects which could undermine a culture of ethical practice? Developing questions for discernment and applying them at the unit, team, and systems levels supports cultural continuity and roots values integration at the micro- to macro-levels.

Working with interprofessional colleagues, engaging with professional organizations, and serving as a unit-based ethics champion begin to leverage individual moral agency to contribute to the collective moral agency of our work settings and profession. Leveraging our individual moral efficacy within our teams acknowledges our interconnectedness and the importance of fostering processes to support everyone's relational integrity (Rushton, 2018). In doing so, we ultimately impact the health and well-being of the people we are called to serve.

Assuring Reflective Moral Spaces

Creating cultures of ethical practice requires recognizing and shifting patterns through regular inquiry into ethically challenging, morally distressing aspects of care (Liaschenko & Peter, 2016). Prioritizing time and space for intra- and interprofessional discussion and reflection on ethical challenges is shown to diminish moral distress and cultivate moral efficacy (Trotochaud et al., 2018). Nursing studies reflect that positive perceptions of ethical climate—settings in which ethical inquiry is normative—have an inverse relationship to moral distress and promote retention. The greater the perception of ethical climate, the less likely nurses were to experience moral distress to the degree it would prompt leaving a position (Karakachian & Colbert, 2019; Pauly et al., 2009).

Emerging programs such as unit-based ethics conversations, ethics liaisons or champions, clinical ethics residencies, and comprehensive ethical practice series create moral spaces in which participants deepen ethical sensitivity, foster moral imagination, and create moral community (Austin, 2007; Carter et al., 2018; Hamric & Wocial, 2016; Robinson et al., 2014; Traudt et al., 2016; Trotochaud et al., 2018; Wocial, 2018; Wocial et al., 2010; 2023). These inspired approaches hone moral reasoning, deepen moral efficacy, and activate moral agency (Burston & Tuckett, 2013; Sauerland et al., 2014). Wisdom, respect, compassion, and individual and relational integrity bloom in these spaces, creating the conditions for moral resilience in healthcare settings.

Supporting Principled Change-Makers and Risk-Takers

It is essential to support clinicians who, often quietly but steadfastly, consistently work from their core values and take principled action (Rushton, 2018). Whether formal or informal leaders and whether virtuous by nature or development, these ethics advocates engage challenges through a lens of possibility. To operationalize solutions, they appeal to others' moral efficacy to influence collective efforts in service to enable a culture of ethical practice. These principled change-makers and risk-takers engage beyond individual clinicians or frontline teams to also connect with unit and organizational leadership in sustainable strategies to mitigate workplace conditions which undermine ethical practice. This bottom-up and top-down collaboration meaningfully activates shared governance and anchors the understanding that integrity-preserving action is the normative response to problematic patterns (Rushton, 2018).

These clinicians model values of alignment and embodiment of ethical commitments and must be supported through establishing organizational processes for escalation of challenges or concerns. System-level policies that endorse clinicians' responsibility and right to speak up and raise concerns at the patient, unit, and organizational levels without fear of retribution are essential. To embed what is valued in the organization, recognition practices should include honoring and highlighting exemplars of those whose behaviors animate core organizational values. Organizational communication strategies and platforms should regularly feature these recognitions and expand coverage of similar accounts to enculturate ethical practice from the unit level to the systems level. Organizational policies to address persistent behaviors which are out of alignment with core values should incorporate fair and firm processes that clarify expectations and assure that realignment behaviors are sustained in order to prevent undermining the conditions necessary for a culture of ethical practice to flourish.

Application of the CFS Framework for Nurses

Two initiatives designed and informed by the CFS model feature the key stanchions we've described—*personal transformational learning, cultivating moral efficacy, creating an enabling work environment, assuring reflective moral spaces*, and *supporting principled change-makers and risk-takers* (details in Tables 7.2a and 7.2b). These efforts demonstrate the practical impact of the CFS *be, understand,* and *do* framework.

The Mindful Ethical Practice & Resilience Academy (MEPRA) for nurses was designed at Johns Hopkins University using the CFS approach. Its core structure includes (1) a 24-hour experiential, discovery learning foundational curriculum,

Table 7.2a Applying the CFS *Be*, *Understand*, and *Do* Framework

The Mindful Ethical Practice & Resilience Academy (MEPRA)

	Be	Understand	Do
Program launch: MEPRA	Values which guide the program: respect for the diversity of participants/project team; compassion toward ourselves and others; integrity in our process and structure.	Iterative process—literature review, key informant interviews and collective experience of the project team revealed issues and patterns that we sought to shift, including victimization, disrespect, disengagement, voicelessness. Design approach: creating a focus on leveraging individual transformation to propel system change.	Process, content, and practices were designed to enable desired shifts to produce sustainable results from the beginning; developed a measurement strategy to capture impact of interventions using a multipronged approach.
Personal transformational learning	Curriculum cultivates mindful awareness with daily guided mindfulness and reflective practices to foster positive emotions; aligns essential and professional values and commitments to be authentic advocates for themselves and their patients; builds awareness of what enables/impedes moral efficacy and authentic advocacy; develops skills and tools for constructive, effective communication.	Key skills, tools, and practices were designed to facilitate competence and confidence in recognizing, responding, taking action to address ethical issues, transform ethical challenges and moral distress into moral resilience through experiential and reflective practices, role-play, simulation, and multimedia platforms.	Exploring the sources of moral suffering, expanding awareness of the consequences and contributing factors in the system and leveraging moral resilience to restore or preserve integrity aligns values, pattern shifts, and facilitates action aimed at system change.

(continued)

Table 7.2a Continued

	Be	Understand	Do
Cultivating moral efficacy	Springing from alignment of personal and professional values, nurses build on this strong foundation to (re)connect to their purpose in being a nurse and the ethical foundations of care. Participants' insights deepen their own ethical practice and inform and positively influence others.	To shift from silence to voice, participants learn skills and tools to communicate their concerns confidently and clearly. They learned skills in applying Rest's framework for analyzing ethical concerns using clinical cases.	Appling decision-making frameworks and other tools (e.g., E-Pause) to situations in clinical practice. High-fidelity simulation using trained actors to portray challenging scenarios where nurses must speak up about ethical concerns supports participants' recognition of ethical issues and how to source their inner capacity to engage in dialogue and solution. Through this application of skills and tools for constructive and effective communication, participants trust they can speak up with confidence and competence.
Creating an enabling work environment	When MEPRA participants graduate, they have opportunities for Renewal Retreats to replenish and rejuvenate their connection with their essential values and commitments, deepening their sense of self and their capacity for moral resilience. These "refresh and reset" opportunities fuel their efforts in the settings they serve to engage in solutions to the ethical issues within their sphere of influence.	Scanning for patterns in the work setting and sources of moral adversity illuminated opportunities for priority shifts in these conditions and identification of individual, team, and system levers which can meaningfully transform the work environment.	The MEPRA foundational program culminates in engaging participants to apply the CFS model to an aspect of their unit culture that is amenable to shifting and is within their sphere of influence, leveraging their capacity for culture change. MEPRA Champions, unit-based and highly visible team members, leverage their knowledge and skills to engage others, proactively recognize and address ethical issues that arise at the unit level that contribute to moral distress and burnout, creating the work environment conditions necessary to thrive.

Assuring reflective moral spaces	Moral spaces for participants to reflect on the alignment of their purpose and essential values and embody them in their choices, actions, and behaviors to create the conditions for ethical practice.	Regular experiential sessions and participation in the Community of Practice as a forum to apply skills, tools, and practices. Participants reflect on the patterns of ethical challenges and moral distress and build ethical competence and competencies to transform them.	Having experienced what is possible by creating reflective moral spaces, participants are equipped to replicate those qualities in their clinical settings and with those whom they serve. They are prepared to share the skills and tools with others to shift key patterns that undermine integrity and ethical practice.
Supporting principled change-makers and risk-takers	Authentic advocacy and moral courage of nurses are honored and fueled by connecting who we essentially are, our professional values and commitments, and leveraging them for personal transformation and system change.	Opportunities to reflect on qualities and patterns of authentic advocacy (e.g., the importance of awareness of exerting one's own agenda); serving with "egoless" engagement to serve others while sourcing action from wisdom and purpose-reinforced risk-taking and principled action. Patterns to shift the ethical climate at the unit level were identified.	Nurses as courageous moral agents were supported to manifest action on behalf of others in ways that embody integrity-preserving choices. Proactive identification of ethically challenging situations that require unit-level engagement and participation in the MEPRA Community of Practice established connections across the hospital, extending the reach of these ethics influencers. These nurses modeled for themselves and others that we are always at choice points for ethical action.

Table 7.2b Applying the CFS *Be, Understand,* and *Do* Framework

An Ethics Nurse Liaisons Program

	Be	*Understand*	*Do*
Program launch	Professional values, framed in the ANA *Code of Ethics for Nurses*, ground the program.	Recognized patterns of moral distress in ICUs, ED, transplant, hematology/oncology settings, which dampened pediatric nurses' moral agency. Identified gaps in knowledge of clinical ethics, ethical decision-making models, ethics resources in the organization, which shaped the initial educational curriculum.	Approached clinical leadership about nurses who exemplify professional values and character to invite participation in the program, with an initial focus to further cultivate ethical competence and shift out of moral distress and into moral agency.
Personal transformational learning	Initial orientation and ongoing ethics education include a focus on awareness of mindset and cultivating ethical sensitivity, acknowledging that we all have biases and lenses through which we view the world. Cultivating an expanded capacity to hold a plurality of viewpoints without feeling destabilized, and to support others who may be challenged by fixed lenses, is foundational to this role.	Recognizing the importance of a shift out of the powerlessness so often experienced with moral distress into moral agency, practices which facilitate this shift are taught during periodic workshops and retreats. Monthly education sessions are designed to integrate ongoing skill-building to shift from drama and reactivity to sustainable, resourceful agency.	Participants practice the Three Vital Questions framework thempoewrmentdynamic.com) in their settings, drawing on the skills and tools to compassionately shift themselves and others into engagement and dialogue on ethical issues, rather than feeling "stuck" in reactivity or disruption. Participant successes are shared at monthly meetings or unit-based ethics rounds to inspire others and seed ideas for practice.

Cultivating moral efficacy	Quarterly attendance at the hospital ethics committee meeting for education and skill-building provides opportunities for ethics liaisons to connect to individual and collective purpose for this work in the organization.	These quarterly "deep dives" into discussion of complex ethical issues across the system provide perspective-expansion about patterns and how experienced ethicists consider solutions. This sparks new understanding about how unit-based issues may relate to larger systems issues, clarifying what is within the liaisons' sphere of influence, what is not, and what new strategies might be possible.	Insights and experience gained from ethics committee attendance provide the ethics liaisons with opportunities to bring new solutions to their respective settings. For example, the ethics liaison in the cancer center advocated to bring a Jehovah's Witness Hospital Liaison who had presented to the ethics committee on parental decision-making and blood transfusion refusal to share the same, illuminating information at an interdisciplinary unit staff meeting. The ethics liaison recognized that there were widespread and conflict-oriented misperceptions about this issue which could be shifted through accurate information and dialogue.
Creating an enabling work environment	The ethics liaisons meet twice annually for educational, half-day retreats for the sustaining opportunity to share and hear new skills, build new wisdom, and affirm their inner capacities to positively influence the settings in which they serve.	Ethics liaisons share observations during the retreats about ethical challenges encountered, noting contributing, modifiable factors which can be shifted to create the conditions in which ethical practice is possible. The perspectives of their ethics liaisons colleagues frequently build on successful strategies and illuminate new possibilities for solution.	Frequently, ethics liaisons are inspired to "import" approaches that have been impactful in others' settings. An ethics liaison in the pulmonary unit invited the ethics faculty to facilitate monthly interdisciplinary moral distress rounds centering on a particularly ethically challenging and chronic patient situation. New strategies at the patient, unit, and systems levels were identified each month, which shifted the team from a despairing lens on the situation to a more solution-oriented approach, energizing what had been an emotionally exhausted team into agency and greater capacity for the inherent complexity of the case. Other ethics liaisons adopted this approach to moral distress rounds, both standing and ad hoc in their settings, which resulted in a growing norm of leadership support for team members' time in these resilience- and moral

(continued)

Table 7.2b Continued

	Be	Understand	Do
Assuring reflective moral spaces	A programmatic commitment to create safe spaces in which to cultivate ethical competence, grounded in core values, evolved over time from standing monthly educational meetings to rounding with ethics liaisons in their respective settings. The opportunity to connect with each ethics liaison about particular, local issues and patterns makes ethical reflection visible in the moral space of his/her/their work setting.	The clinical nurse ethicist connects regularly with ethics liaisons through ethics rounds in their settings. The increased visibility and awareness this brings to both the role of the ethics liaisons and available organizational ethics resources activate discussion with local teams. Unit-specific opportunities for transformation from a problem orientation or distress to engagement and agency are considered.	Recognizing that moral spaces happen wherever and whenever focused attention is directed to potential solutions to ethical challenges, the ethics liaisons confidently engage interdisciplinary colleagues in ethical reflection on complex cases. They model that even micro-moments of engaged, mutually respectful discussions can positively inform the ethical climate of their clinical settings.
Supporting principled change-makers and risk-takers	Regularly exploring each participant's "why" and identifying personal and professional connection to nursing values and the ANA *Code of Ethics for Nurses* with Interpretive Statements are foundational to ongoing development in this role. This affirms participants' resourcefulness and capacity to cultivate cultures of ethical practice and see the impact of values alignment and principled action.	Meeting agendas include time to reflect on patterns in participants' respective units that can shift to support a more robust ethical climate. Discussions center on framing these shifts in possibility versus powerlessness. Ethics liaisons support each other through brainstorming ideas for sustainable change in their respective settings.	Participants engage unit leaders in discussion about patterns identified, inhibiting patterns and associated opportunities to develop sustainable plans to impact the ethical climate. In some cases, ethics liaisons lead ethics education and discussion on particular topics with their teams to build individual and collective ethical competence. In other cases, targeted approaches to address specific issues, for example assuring a process that includes nurses in ethics consultations for their patients and assures freedom from retribution, have been employed.

(2) community of practice, and (3) a unit-based Champion program (Rushton et al., 2021). The starting point for the program was alignment of purpose, essential values, and processes—who we are being—that would inform the development of the program. These values included respect for the diversity of participants and project team, compassion toward ourselves and others, and integrity in our processes and structure.

Next, through literature review, key informant interviews, and the collective experience of the project team, the Hopkins team came to understand, through identification of the issues within the healthcare system and associated patterns, what patterns they sought to shift. This process of pattern recognition was iterative and ongoing throughout the development and delivery of the program. Patterns of victimization, disrespect, and disengagement of the nursing staff within the organization; nurses feeling incapable to speak up about their ethical concerns, or their stated concerns not being taken seriously; and constant distraction of their attention away from their core purpose as nurses were elements that guided program development. Intentionally designing processes, content, and practices to enable the shifts they sought to achieve focused attention on sustainable results from the beginning. Concurrently, the design team developed a measurement strategy to capture the impact of this intervention, using a multipronged approach. The pre/post intervention results demonstrate statistically significant improvements in ethical confidence and competence, mindfulness, resilience, and work engagement, and decreases in depression, anger, and intent to leave (Rushton et al., 2021).

A similar strategy in a Colorado pediatric setting, an ethics nurse liaisons program, was launched in order to shift out of the perceived powerlessness related to moral distress experienced in high-risk settings and into ethical competence and moral agency (Trotochaud et al., 2018). In the Colorado approach, the ethics nurse liaisons serve as recognizable, known, and trusted colleagues in their respective settings, extending the reach and resources of the hospital ethics committee to support ethical practice at the bedside. Activating the practical guidance in the American Nurses Association *Code of Ethics for Nurses with Interpretive Statements* (2015), this program is designed to deepen nurses' knowledge, understanding, and application of ethics and our core ethical commitments to shift from a problem orientation to an empowered solution orientation. Cultivating the capacity for ethical discernment, stability amidst conflict or uncertainty, clarity about ethically permissible options and commitment to ethical action promotes and preserves individual and relational integrity despite moral complexity (Trotochaud, et al., 2018). This approach to intentional development of ethical competence contributes to mitigating moral distress, responding to moral adversity in new ways, cultivating ethical practice, and improving the ethical climates in which the ethics nurse liaisons serve (Trotochaud et al., 2018).

These programs center on intentionally aligning our essential values and commitments with our choices, behaviors, and actions, which are key to our personal and professional integrity. This alignment transcends our roles and identities to connect with who we most essentially are as persons, illuminating what we stand for in our life and work and supporting us as we engage with the various sources of moral adversity in healthcare (Rushton, 2018). The process of discovering and claiming our core ethical values (e.g., dignity, compassion, justice) goes beyond cognitive knowing to embodying or living our values in each moment and encounter. In living our values, we gain experience accessing and trusting our inherent capacity for resilience and creativity. We learn to tap our inner wisdom through methods such as mindfulness, self-regulation, honest and accurate self-appraisal, and inquiry into how our fundamental values and commitments shape integrity-preserving moral agency. This enables us to have an intentional awareness of the contours of our conscience so that we are able to distinguish when we are acting in alignment with what we profess as our values and when we are not. This ongoing and proactive process invites self-compassion for our vulnerabilities, fears, and default responses; helps us recognize occasions when our actions arise from courage even when fear is present; and draws upon our inner strength to take action when non-negotiable values are threatened or compromised.

Creating a New Narrative

These two programs aim to create and nurture a culture of ethical practice which requires shifting the way we think and speak about our work and the language we use to engage others in our work. The pervasive narrative about our moral suffering in healthcare is largely dominated by themes of victimization, powerlessness, and despair (Moss et al., 2016; Rushton, 2016). Rarely do we notice or amplify the moments of integrity-preserving action that occur alongside the distress. It stands to reason that if we continue to reinforce and repeat the current narrative without a clear vision for what else is possible, it will become a self-fulfilling prophecy. The MEPRA and ethics nurse liaisons programs encourage participants to consider how they might see situations with fresh eyes and begin to choose a new narrative that offers hope and possibility rather than despair and discouragement. While moral distress is pervasive in many settings, not all clinicians experience the same frequency or magnitude of impact from it. Instead of exclusively focusing on the distress clinicians are experiencing, these programs support participants in developing the skills and practices to remain engaged without becoming disabled or overwhelmed by their distress. This

Table 7.3 Guidance for Creating a New Narrative

- Begin by expanding heart space and inner potential.
- Adopt personal reflection and insight as the pathway to concise, clear expression.
- Be bold; behold possibility.
- Invite engagement without competition.
- Name the shift you want to see and be it.
- Inspire yourself and others.
- Connect your initiatives with a shift to a larger purpose.
- Let go of limiting beliefs and assumptions.
- Help others see their own possibilities for co-creation.
- Make the invisible visible without polarizing.
- Celebrate and embrace what's working.
- Transcend seeming dichotomies by embodying ethical values and actions.
- Break the "hero" archetype of today and build the archetypes required for a paradigm shift.
- Choose words with intention and care. Language must authentically reflect the new paradigm.
- Connect local courageous actions to the differences they make in the world.
- Foster full potential for action now, not later.
- Open and foster space for synergy to emerge.
- Focus on and magnify your connection to what you stand for in life.
- Enable risk in connecting to your moral compass.
- Disrupt patterns that no longer serve a useful purpose.

Used with permission from Oxford University Press.

offers the possibility of letting go of the disempowering narratives of the past and embracing a more life-giving vision for the future.

There are myriad ways to begin the process of shifting the current narrative about moral suffering in healthcare. Table 7.3 includes ways individuals can begin the process through diverse entry points. Using the CFS process, we may begin with exploring how our core values connect to universal values, and draw on those to identify the shifts that are necessary to change our mindsets and vocabulary toward a vision of integrity in healthcare that leverages moral resilience and ethical practice. Like other shifts illuminated by the CFS model, we must also identify the shifts that are needed to make our vision a reality.

An additional enabler of a much-needed paradigm shift is to intentionally notice and document the ways that clinicians are acting with integrity and leveraging their experiences with moral adversity to fuel constructive and meaningful change. We can ask new questions; for example, what new patterns of how we speak and think about the ethical challenges that arise in clinical practice might we notice? What new patterns of responsiveness might we adopt? Can we begin to link these new narratives to the changes we want to see in ourselves and our systems? How do we translate this new awareness into organizational policies, practices, and program design?

A potent narrative shift is to transform the typical request for ethics consultation from "why are we doing this?" to "how do we live our professional values in this ethically complex situation?" This might lead to a clarification about what ethical values are in conflict and why they matter. What assumptions are we making and what needs to be clarified? Can we acknowledge the individual and collective commitment to do the "right thing" by various team members, and the efforts that individuals and teams have taken to attempt to fulfill their commitments, regardless of the outcome? Can we detect patterns in the system that have contributed to the ethical challenges and take focused and intentional steps to address them? Instead of reinforcing that there is nothing that can be done to change the situation, there is an opportunity to see beyond the distress to integrity-preserving actions that *can* be taken. Therein lies the heart of this new paradigm which creates cultures of ethical practice in healthcare: confidence in our capacity to shift from feeling victimized to feeling empowered, from cynicism to hope, and from scarcity to trusting we have what we need to sustain ourselves in our work and provide high-quality care.

Acknowledgment

Portions of this chapter are adapted from Rushton, C. H. (2018).

References

American Nurses Association. (2015). *Code of ethics for nurses with interpretive statements* (2nd ed.). American Nurses Association.

Austin, W. (2007). The ethics of everyday practice: Healthcare environments as moral communities. *Advances in Nursing Science, 30*(1), 81–88.

Bauman, Z., & Donskis, L. (2013). *Moral blindness: The loss of sensitivity in liquid modernity.* Polity Press.

Burston, A. S., & Tuckett, A. G. (2013). Moral distress in nursing: Contributing factors, outcomes and interventions. *Nursing Ethics, 20*(3), 312–324.

Carter, B., Brockman, M., Garrett, J., Knackstedt, A., & Lantos, J. (2018). Why are there so few ethics consults in children's hospitals? *HEC Forum, 30*(2), 91–102.

Delgado, J., Siow, S., de Groot, J., McLane, B., & Hedlin, M. (2021). Towards collective moral resilience: The potential of communities of practice during the COVID-19 pandemic and beyond. *Journal of Medical Ethics, 47*(6), 374–382. medethics-2020-106764.

Hamric, A. B., & Wocial, L. D. (2016). Institutional ethics resources: Creating moral spaces. *Hastings Center Report, 46*(Suppl 1), S22–S27.

Holtz, H., Heinze, K., Rushton, C. (2018). Interprofessionals' definitions of moral resilience. *Journal of Clinical Nursing, 27*(3–4), e488–e494.

Karakachian, A., & Colbert, A. (2019). Nurses' moral distress, burnout and intentions to leave. *Journal of Forensic Nursing, 15*(3), 133–142.

Liaschenko, J., & Peter, E. (2016). Fostering nurses' moral agency and moral identity: The importance of moral community. *Hasting Center Report, 46*(5), S18–S21.

Moss, M., Good VS., Gozal, D., Kleinpell, R., & Sessler, CN. (2016). An official critical care societies collaborative statement: Burnout syndrome in critical care healthcare professionals: A call for action. *Critical Care Medicine, 44*(7), 1414–1421.

National Academies of Sciences, Engineering, and Medicine; National Academy of Medicine; & Committee on Systems Approaches to Improve Patient Care by Supporting Clinician Well-Being. (2019). *Taking Action Against Clinician Burnout: A Systems Approach to Professional Well-Being*. National Academies Press.

Pauly, B., Varcoe, C., Storch, J., & Newton, L. (2009). Registered nurses' perceptions of moral distress and ethical climate. *Nursing Ethics, 16*(5), 561–573.

Pavlish, C., Brown-Saltzman, K. A., Jakel, P., & Fine, A. (2014). The nature of ethical conflicts and the meaning of moral community on oncology practice. *Oncology Nursing Forum, 41*(2), 130–140.

Rest, J. R. (1986). *Moral development: Advances in research and theory*. Praeger.

Robichaux, C. (2012). Developing ethical skills: From sensitivity to action. *Critical Care Nurse, 32*(2), 65–72.

Robinson, E., Lee, S., Zollfrank, A., Jurchak, M., Frost, D., & Grace, P. (2014). Enhancing moral agency: Clinical ethics residency for nurses. *Hastings Center Report, 44*(5), 12–20.

Rushton, C. H. (2016). Moral resilience: A capacity for navigating moral distress in critical care. *AACN Advanced Critical Care, 27*(1), 111–119.

Rushton, C. H. (2018). *Moral resilience: Transforming moral suffering in healthcare*. Oxford University Press.

Rushton, C. (2023). Transforming moral suffering by cultivating moral resilience and ethical practice. *American Journal of Critical Care, 32*(4), 238–248.

Rushton, C. (2024). Self stewardship: An ethical imperative for nurses. *AACN Advanced Critical Care, 35*(2), 193–198.

Rushton, C., Nelson, K. Antonsdottir, I., Hanson, G., & Boyce, D. (2022). Perceived organizational effectiveness, moral injury, and moral resilience among nurses during the COVID-19 pandemic: Secondary analysis. *Nursing Management, 53*(7), 12–22.

Rushton, C., Swoboda, S., Reller, N., Skrupski, K., Prizzi, M., Young, P., & Hanson, G. (2021). Mindful Ethical Practice and Resilience Academy: Equipping nurses to address ethical challenges. *American Journal of Critical Care, 30*(1), e1–e11.

Sala Defilippis, T. M. L., Curtis, K., & Gallagher, A. (2019). Conceptualizing moral resilience for nursing practice. *Nursing Inquiry, 26*(3), e12291.

Sauerland, J., Marotta, K., Peinemann, M. A., Berndt, A., & Robichaux, C. (2014). Assessing and addressing moral distress and ethical climate, Part 1. *Dimensions in Critical Care Nursing, 33*(4), 234–245.

Sharma, M. (2017). *Radical transformational leadership: Strategic action for change agents*. North Atlantic Books.

Simsek, A. (2012). Transformational learning. In N. M. Seel (Ed.), *Encyclopedia of the sciences of learning* (pp. 3341–3344). Springer.

Traudt, T., Liaschenko, J., & Peden-McAlpine, C. (2016). Moral agency, moral imagination, and moral community: Antidotes to moral distress. *The Journal of Clinical Ethics, 27*(3), 201–213.

Trotochaud, K., Fitzgerald, H., & Knackstedt, A. D. (2018). Ethics champion programs. *American Journal of Nursing, 118*(7), 46–54.

Wocial, L. (2018). In search of a moral community. *The Online Journal of Issues in Nursing, 23*(1).

Wocial, L. D., Hancock, M., Bledsoe, P. D., Chamness, A. R., & Helft, P. R. (2010). An evaluation of unit-based ethics conversations. *JONA'S Healthcare Law, Ethics and Regulation, 12*(2), 48–54.

Wocial, L. D., Miller, G., Montz, K., LaPradd, M., & Slaven, J. E. (2023). Evaluation of interventions to address moral distress: A multi-method approach. *HEC Forum*. https://doi.org/10.1007/s10730-023-09508-z

8

An Ethics Lens for Nursing Leadership

Katherine Brown-Saltzman

The nature of healthcare places its leaders in the crucible of ethics, whether in creating an environment for ethics to thrive or in responding to ethical conflicts as they are escalated up the chain of command. The *Oxford Dictionary* defines crucible as "[a] ceramic or metal container in which metals or other substances may be melted or subjected to very high temperatures. A situation of severe trial, or in which different elements interact, leading to the creation of something new" (*Oxford English and Spanish Dictionary*, n.d., n.p.). That container, whether the intensive care unit, the operating room, the emergency room, or a clinic, is the place where multiple factors swirl under high pressure that often prevents ethical concerns from being addressed. As patients and their families, healthcare teams, and administrators are "melted" together, those factors and conditions—whether differing values, highly efficient environs, hierarchical power structures, biases and disparities, resource and financial constraints, differing goals, unrealistic expectations, or views of obligations—create a slurry that may be difficult to see through (Bartlett & Finder, 2018; Kelly & Porr, 2018; Leuter et al., 2013; Pavlish et al., 2011b, 2015c, 2015d, 2019, 2020; Scherer et al., 2019). This is layered with the history of our professions and how each individual handles conflict. The valued efficiency of our settings means they are not created for reflective, process-oriented, or even relational interactions. Each day within any given institution, ethical concerns could be imagined as icebergs, dangerous but barely visible obstacles that can be ignored. Yet when conflict escalates, those submerged, silenced, or discounted concerns/interests or unease can be detrimental to everyone, especially those who are most vulnerable. Yet, bioethics asks just that of us; to invite the incredibly hard and complicated question, "What ought we to do?" and then to slow down enough so that the many voices join in thoughtful and contemplative discussions, which can then lead to insightful responses. Nursing leaders typically have the greatest number of clinicians reporting to them, and if they are listening, their perception and understanding will be enhanced and are critical to this process. Whether ethics is flourishing within an institution depends upon so many factors, but leadership is key. It is not having all the answers. Rather, it is how one responds to the questions that sends messages through the entire system and into the community. A difficult example of this has been the 2020 COVID-19 pandemic. How does a nursing leader respond to the crucible of a highly infectious deadly virus, knowing that there would not be adequate personal protective equipment for the staff? The resource issues can be worked on, but how that nurse leader takes those first steps will establish the conditions of this severe trial. Once again, this must happen under crisis and in a highly efficient way, and yet without those reflective moments, panic and mistrust will reign. Then how does a leader respond to the multitude of other needs that escalate rapidly, whether it is planning for short staffing, developing timely policies, attending to new ethical issues that may be arising, or whether it be escalating moral distress, making decisions that rule out family visiting at the critical juncture of a patient's dying, or addressing concerns of contagion for nurses returning home to their own families? And what of the knowledge that there would be nurses, with their proximity and time with patients, that predictably would have the highest incidence of infection of healthcare professionals (Kambhampati et al., 2020), and worse yet, that some would die? How does one acknowledge the truth and yet inspire and support others, to commit to caring with full knowledge of the risks? Are the staff who die honored, or is the news silenced? What is being done to address their emotional toll during the crisis? What is the response for those who are broken by the weight?

The American Organization for Nursing Leadership (AONL) did an online Nursing Leadership COVID-19 Challenges survey over 10 days in July 2020, with 1,811 respondents finding that trust was a primary challenge. Staff emotional health and well-being were identified as one of the hospitals' four biggest challenges. Nurse leaders rated their effectiveness of addressing this challenge at only 3.33 on a 1–5 scale (5 being very well), their rating falling below their effectiveness in accessing PPE and supplies (AONL, 2020). Additionally, are nurses asked to show up, yet easily laid off to protect the economics of the institution? Are pregnant nurses protected? All these questions with ethical underpinnings come fast and furiously. How does one keep the ethical lens in focus, even at a time of crisis? Perhaps this is why integrating ethics throughout the everyday practice of nursing leadership is so important. A habituated ethical way of seeing and assessing will then be the lens that will help to assimilate the many dimensions of ethics. If we revisit the analogy of the environment being the crucible, the etymology of the word returns us to the symbol of nursing and the goal of its leadership. "Crucible" comes from Late Middle English, originating from medieval Latin, *crucibulum*, the night lamp (*Oxford English and Spanish Dictionary*, n.d.). In healthcare it is critical that nursing leaders hold a light, not only to uncover the darkness and dangers, but as a beacon of transparency and inspiration for the most trusted of professions (Reinhart, 2020).

Some nursing organizations have recognized the importance of ethical direction and competency for nurse leaders. Yet not all codes of ethics for nurses specifically address nursing leaders. The American Nurses Association (ANA) revision of the *Code of Ethics for Nurses* (2015) is an exception, as it incorporated more ethical responsibilities for nurse leaders. Schick-Makaroff and Storch (2019), in their review of nursing codes, recommended integrating leadership guidance, as it "not only informs nurses about what they can expect of nurse leaders but also allows formal nurse leaders to use the code with their own senior leaders, conveying what their professional body expects of them in their formal leadership roles" (p. 71). The nine provisions of the *Code of Ethics* are an architectural structure for the profession and provide a lens for the ethical comportment of the practice, for clinical nurses, leaders, educators, and researchers. One example where nurse leaders are specifically addressed is in Interpretive Statement 4.3, Responsibility for Nursing Judgments, Decisions, and Actions: "Nurse executives are responsible for ensuring that nurses have access to and inclusion on organizational committees and in decision-making processes that affect the ethics, quality, and safety of patient care" (ANA 2015, p. 16). In the same year, the American Organization of Nurse Executives (AONE, 2015) competencies refer to two specific ethical proficiencies:

1. Integrate bioethical and legal dimensions into clinical and management decision-making (p. 6).
2. Uphold ethical principles and corporate compliance standards. Hold self and staff accountable to comply with ethical standards of practice. Discuss, resolve, and learn from ethical dilemmas (p. 9).

While professional codes and competencies can inform nurse leaders, an exploration of an ethics lens as an effective tool requires an understanding of the intersection of leadership qualities, trust, the challenges of voicing ethical concerns, the nature of conflict, and the necessity of supporting moral agency and creating an ethical climate.

Leadership Qualities and Establishing Trust

When trust is present, it is almost always formed out of relationship, the experience of respect, and the history of fidelity within the institution. If a nurse leader can create an environment of trust, then crucial communication will flow more easily in both directions—between the leader and their followers. This trust is a reciprocal relationship that requires the leader to be vulnerable enough to reveal their own limitations, inviting authentic relationships without further burdening either party. This creates the conditions for a healthy work environment, where each nurse is supported in their moral agency, and with that comes improved quality of care (Grossman & Valiga, 2020; Hamric & Wocial, 2016). Along with trust, ethical leaders have been found to be fair, people-oriented, and willing to provide ethical guidance (Kalshoven et al., 2011, 2013). An Ethical Leadership at Work Questionnaire, developed by Kalshoven et al., utilizes the concepts of fairness, integrity, ethical guidance, people orientation, power sharing, role clarification, and concern for sustainability to evaluate leadership qualities (Kalshoven et al., 2011). In addition to these, others have ascribed further attributes, such as courage, competency, stewardship, empathy, honesty, and the ability to both affirm and challenge values (Barkhordari-Sharifabad et al., 2018; Conner, 2020; Grossman & Valiga, 2020). With the rapid changes that are occurring in healthcare, financial constraints, higher and important expectations for quality and safety, and patient and family satisfaction, these leaders must also be highly skilled change agents that have credibility within the organization. If they are to model change, they must be willing to risk failure themselves. Within the realm of ethics, ethics consultants are sometimes perceived as having "failed" in resolving the ethical issue; this can also happen with leaders as well. The complexity of undertaking ethical conflict or disagreement requires an understanding, by both the leader and others, that the nature of ethics is rarely black and white. It is in fact messy, without the crisp fixed edges that allow one to feel one has mastered the problem. If one has hoped for a tidy outcome when addressing an ethical dilemma, the leader and the team may have a sense of failure. More often there is a reconciling for the better decision, one that has landed on the side of beneficence and has avoided as much harm as possible. A leader must appreciate these nuances and help others to understand them as well.

System Issues, Ethical Conflict, and Ethical Environments

Ethical concerns are the fiber of everyday encounters in healthcare. Recognizing methods that leaders can pursue to create ethical environments, for themselves as well as those they serve, takes a greater awareness of both the existence and nature of ethical conflicts, the root causes of those conflicts, and institutional responses to conflict. For example, one large international study of nurses and physicians found that 71.6% reported encountering an ethical issue in their intensive care unit (ICU) environments during the previous week (Azoulay et al., 2009). The routine clinical ethics issues in the ICU settings are well documented in literature: end-of-life issues, disagreements about the plan or goals of treatment, non-beneficial treatment, capacity, patient suffering, moral distress, surrogate decision-making, and decision-making for the unrepresented

(Meyer-Zehnder et al., 2021; Swetz et al., 2007; Wasson et al., 2016). These issues are also found on the general care floors in hospitals, outpatient clinics, and extended care facilities. They include patient-centered issues such as health inequities, biases, unaddressed language barriers, competency and decision-making, autonomy violations, informed consent, discharge disposition, resource issues, managing addiction issues, difficult encounters with patients or their families, mental health issues, and misunderstandings of cultural aspects of care. In one study, nurses relayed other ethical challenges, "the precariousness of competing obligations, navigating the intricacies of hope and honesty, managing the urgency caused by waiting, straining to find time, and weighing risks of speaking up in hierarchal structures" (Pavlish et al., 2012, p. 592).

There are professional or multidisciplinary concerns, such as incompetence, role conflicts and/or lack of appreciation of others' moral obligations, power issues, bullying and abusive behavior, less than healthy workplace environments, safety issues, burnout, and compassion fatigue, that can all lead to ethical conflict (Connor, 2020; Garon, 2012; Pavlish et al., 2019; Vincent et al., 2020). These, as well as many other issues, can fuel conflict if not preempted with careful attention. Disagreement should be anticipated, given the nature of the differences in values and approaches to these issues and the complexity in which they arise. Interventions, however, can mitigate escalation of conflict, which otherwise may back people into defensive corners that can create lasting breaks in relationships, whether between clinicians and the patient/family or within the healthcare teams. A critical incident study with nurses identified risk factors and early indicators for evolving ethical conflicts with patients, their families, clinicians, and healthcare systems (Pavlish et al., 2011a). Nurses in this study and others sighted lack of limit setting, unclear policies, and limited resources (McKenna & Jeske, 2021). Physicians also are tuned into risk factors. A survey of physicians identified multiple-system risk factors for ethical conflicts, such as resource concerns (inadequate or unequal), insufficient institutional support, limited time and space, unhealthy work environment, and the frequent rotation of teams (Pavlish et al., 2015a).

System issues are often discovered when repetitive ethical conflict is explored and provides an opportunity to respond not only to each individual case as they unfold, but also to the larger environment. In nursing, moral distress is often the cue that there is a system-level issue (Hamric & Epstein, 2017).

These issues may stem from policies when: there is an absence of them, or the existing policies lack clarity, have not had input from all of the stakeholders, are not publicized, or are poorly utilized, especially if this is due to intimidation. Other system issues, such as frequent rotation of attending physicians, staffing problems, focusing on the patient satisfaction scores without the setting of limits, or communication problems (e.g., a unit that ignores the need for routine family conferencing), or a culture of silencing and hierarchal power structures, can allow conflict to fester (McAndrew & Hardin, 2020; Pavlish et al., 2015b).

When there are inadequate ethics resources or underutilization of good ethics resources, or a lack of opportunities to build ethical skills, whether in assessment, analysis, or dialogue, the scarcity of systems will allow ethical conflict to escalate. Nursing leadership given advance practice and education, as well as the nature of their role, can have a broader perspective, as well as the knowledge, networks, and organizational power to address these system issues that have allowed for the burgeoning of conflict. The U.S. Department of Veterans Affairs (VA) National Center for Ethics in Health Care has attributed the primary source of ethical conflicts as stemming from system and process issues. They have made significant advances in addressing these sources of ethical concerns. An example of this is the institution of a system-wide innovative approach for long-term opioid therapy for pain; introducing a consent process that informs about the risks and benefits, as well as alternative therapies and patient responsibilities (VA, 2020). Establishing this system-wide procedure provides patients and clinicians with clearer expectations in care that is often laden with ethical concerns.

In the corporate world, ethical climate is defined as the "shared perceptions of what ethically correct behavior is and how ethical issues should be handled" (Victor & Cullen, 1987, p. 51). In healthcare, Olson used Schneider's (1987) definition, "individual perceptions of the organization that influences attitudes and behavior and serves as a reference for employee behavior" (cited in Olson, 1998, p. 346). Olson's milestone research developed and validated the Hospital Ethical Climate Survey (HECS), in part utilizing Brown's assessment of the ethical climate, evaluating both the process of ethical resolution and the practice of ethical reflection, which required certain conditions to transpire: power, trust, inclusion, role flexibility, and inquiry (Brown, 1990; Olson, 1998). The understanding of the environment in this way provides the ability to assess when that climate is amiss. But more importantly, it allows for the building of preventive strategies that can improve the ethical climate and have far-reaching effects such as decreasing moral distress, enhancing ethics education, improving quality of care, enriching interdisciplinary relationships, decreasing medical error, resolving ethical concerns in a timely way, decreasing turnover, and developing skilled conflict management (Hakimi et al., 2020; Hamric, 2000; Van den Bulcke et al., 2020; Victor & Cullen, 1987). Kish-Gephart et al. (2010) prepared a meta-analytic review of the evidence of unethical decisions at work. While not focused on healthcare, it does provide insight into an organization's influence on ethical behavior or intention. The study affirmed that a stronger ethical culture was associated with fewer unethical choices. Instrumental climates are recognized as focusing on self-interest, either organizational or individual, that create an environment where those conflicts of interest may advance personal interests, as opposed to benevolent ethical climates and principled climates. As in other studies, ethical climates were found to promote ethical behavior (Tangirala et al., 2013). Hakimi et al. (2020) described a process of moral neutralization that occurs when ethical climates were poor. In a recent study with 285 nurses, Simha and Pandey (2020) noted that while both the principled and benevolent ethical climates were found to decrease turnover intention indirectly through trust, it was only the principled climate that impacted that intention directly. By the very nature of healthcare, one might presume benevolent and principled climates, yet the adapted business model and increasing competition can shift the climate. Importantly, leaders can question how these competing needs are assessed and managed. Are there intentional decisions and actions to create an ethical environment?

Voice

Perhaps one of the areas that can provide the greatest impact on deescalating ethical conflict and improving an ethical climate is addressing the practice of voicelessness in nursing (Pavlish et al., 2012). Unfortunately, voicelessness by its very nature can be invisible and yet can have profound and far-reaching effects (Gaudine & Beaton, 2002; Hamric, 2000; McCarthy & Gastmans, 2015; Moss et al., 2016; Pavlish et al., 2011a; Pavlish et al., 2013b; Pavlish et al., 2014; Pavlish et al. 2015b; Rushton et al., 2016). In receiving the Sydney Peace Prize, Arundhati Roy stated, "There's really no such thing as the 'voiceless.' There are only the deliberately silenced, or the preferably unheard" (Roy 2004, n.p.). Catlin et al. (2008), in surveying neonatal intensive care unit (NICU) and pediatric intensive care unit (PICU) staff regarding conscientious objection, found that 52% wanted to object but did not, while of the 45% who had objected, only 17% voiced their opinion to their physician colleagues. Other responses included refusing the order, at times covertly, or asking another nurse to cover the patient. Only a small percentage requested consultation with the ethics committee or documented the concern. Pavlish et al. (2012) found this as well; while some nurses' actions included directly addressing the ethical issue, others "looked the other way, remained silent, murmured to each other or created other avenues" (p. 592). Similarly, Newton et al. (2012) noted "four themes regarding nurses' voice: choosing to be silent, not being heard, difficulty articulating unthink-able aspects of practice and lacking skills to use one's voice" (p. 92). At times when nurses have felt powerless to raise ethical issues, fearing repercussions such as dismissal, damage to their reputations, or creating an antagonistic relationship with a physician, they have demonstrated acts of resistance by "challenging existing power imbalances through speaking up, confrontation, reporting to a higher authority and whistleblowing" (Peter et al., 2004, p. 412).

Within an organization, it is not only those at the bedside who may feel silenced; it can also occur among managers and executive nurses at the highest levels in the system. Healthcare institutions can be highly politicized cultures, where power hierarchies and avoidance of conflict can be motivated by maintaining the status quo (Cathcart, 2008; Gaudine & Beaton, 2002; Hamric, 2000; Pavlish et al., 2016; Peter et al., 2004). Newton et al. (2012) recognized "that attending to power relations is an important aspect of building ethical climate" (p. 99) and protecting patient safety. Anderson (2018) has addressed this failure of voice as a moral problem stemming from the conflict of interest (COI) that the employee straddles, essentially between personal interests/self-preservation and the moral task of speaking up. "It is leadership's responsibility to ensure that this COI is properly managed. When silence is widespread, this indicates a lack of moral leadership and organizational failure" (p. 67). Yet, this failure can be inherent, given that many nurse leaders are positioned within strong hierarchical environments. They are often compressed in the middle as they represent patients and staff, essentially upholding the caring work of the institution, and all the implications of financial, stewardship, and management responsibilities that can collide with the caring needs. They are a minority on the ladder of power. Cathcart (2008), in reflecting on Benner's work, reveals this compression on a chief nursing officer (CNO) who takes the risk of advocating:

> he or she serves at the pleasure of the chief executive officer whereas his or her physician colleagues are more firmly anchored to their positions by virtue of academic appointments or contributions to the organization's economic base. But understanding what is at stake when caring practices are abandoned can bring clarity to a situation when a difficult stand must be taken. (p. 91)

Tangirala et al. (2013) recognized in their research that employees have an inherent orientation toward either duty or achievement. Employees with a duty orientation integrate speaking up as a moral obligation in their roles. Those who are positioned toward achievement are concerned with the potential self-harm of speaking up. For those with an achievement orientation, a modifier for voice efficacy (to take risks with speaking up) was a sense of psychological safety. For those with a duty focus, Tangirala et al. (2013) believe that managers can enhance voice efficacy through the building of communication skills, while recognizing that the achievement orientation group benefited from an environment that affirmed speaking up and inventive attitudes (Tangirala et al., 2013).

While there have been improvements in the education of nurses in ethics and support of nurses in participating in the multidisciplinary ethics discussions, in general there is still a tremendous gap in nursing's presence at the table. Studies have found that nurses have felt powerless in the face of ethical conflict (Gaudine & Beaton 2002; McAndrew & Hardin, 2020; Pavlish et al., 2011b; Peter et al., 2004). They often believed their voices were quieted, and many felt they did not have the skill or vocabulary for moral deliberation. A qualitative, descriptive study in five intensive care units at a large academic medical center relayed that "nurses are marginalized during ethical conflict in the intensive care unit"; they also found that 64.8% had contemplated leaving their position (McAndrew & Hardin, 2020). Descriptions of physician retaliation for calling an ethics consult and ethics committees where nursing representation was limited added to this sense of powerlessness (McAndrew & Hardin, 2020).

In an advanced practice leadership class, a nurse relayed a story of her first year in nursing, working in an emergency room (ER). A preschooler had drowned, and every effort was made to resuscitate him, while his parents waited outside the room. When it was clear the child could not be revived, the medical team called the code and the young nurse walked in from the hallway where the parents were awaiting news and found the medical students practicing intubation on the dead child while the attending coached them. She courageously spoke up, respectfully pointing out their morally egregious behavior. With her adamancy they stopped and went to inform the parents that the child had died. Yet this nurse was not commended in any way; instead, she was called in to explain and defend her actions. She has never forgotten it. The consequences of the shame and confusion have lived within her for years. These are cultures of avoidance, where voices are held at bay to hold up the hierarchal structures. And those who are silenced and those who witness the chastisement quickly learn to mute themselves, or at least understand the risks and consequences of taking action. Technically, moral distress ensues when one feels constrained, yet this nurse achieved not only speaking out, but also successfully impacting the morally inapprehensible behavior. Still, she was tainted by this experience in a powerful way. The nursing leaders intervening with what felt like an interrogation to the new nurse may have been attempting to keep the peace, or possibly to placate a physician who believed that a nurse who had stepped out of line needed to be disciplined, yet those undercurrents ultimately live through time and place, sending an institutional message. This experience impacted an individual nurse so powerfully that she relays it with the emotion and pain of that moment so many years ago. In these situations, nurses learn not to trust those in charge. Repeatedly, studies have found that nurses do not feel supported by leadership (McAndrew & Hardin, 2020). In one study, nurses described feeling supported when speaking up and then subsequently abandoned by both peers and nursing leaders when they needed backing (Ludwick & Silva, 2003).

An article on ethical comportment, Benner et al. (2008) speak about formation and quote M. E. Mohrmann (2006):

> One forms . . . the moral content of the practices—the obligations entailed, the demands imposed—and thus to the moral formation of the practitioners. Moreover, it is generally the case that one is formed toward something, some telos, some ideal shape or condition. . . . A better metaphor [for being true to form] is dance: having and displaying integrity is more a matter of being able to move in ways that are consistent with the originating and developing themes of our lives. Teachers, guides, and practice make us better dancers because they help us listen more carefully and follow the music we hear more confidently. We learn which movements fit the rhythms and which do not. (Mohrmann, 2006, pp. 93, 95)

One's guides are sometimes one's leaders, who are caught within systems where they are often choosing between self-interest (keeping their position) or carefully selecting their battles (maintaining their position to improve the environment) or drawing a line in the sand and acting altruistically, knowing the costs. The ANA *Code of Ethics for Nurses* (2015) sites in Provision 6.3, Responsibility for the Healthcare Environment, that "[n]urse executives have a particular responsibility to ensure that employees are treated fairly and justly, and that nurses are involved in decisions related to their practice and working conditions" (p. 24). The code also clarifies that violations must be addressed, yet never held over a nurse as an obligation if their efforts remain unaddressed; "by remaining in such an environment . . . nurses risk becoming complicit in ethically unacceptable practices" (p. 25).

How leadership responds ripples out into the environment. The staff quickly learns "which movements fit the rhythms, and which do not" of the institution—but the opportunity of ongoing formation of those nurses impacted by the leader's response can reinforce moral formation, contrasted to ethical silencing or even the abandonment of their profession. Voicelessness must be attended to by all within the institution, but the nurse leader is especially accountable in creating an environment of skillful and effective voicing of ethical concerns.

Creative Responding: Voice Lessons

If one turns the challenge of voicelessness around and sees the opportunities that voice can have within an institution, conceivably there may be a new way to begin to frame a robust ethical environment. But how that voice is used is critical, and like voice lessons—the combination of understanding music theory, how to read music, technique (open throat, jaw dropped, deep 360-degree breathing, chest up) and practice—can culminate in accomplished singing. In her book on corporate ethics, Gentile asserts that individuals often react to ethical conflicts with a deer-in-the-headlights approach, essentially imagining that they are not up to the task, followed by an emotional decompensation and panic. She advocates for training that in a sense desensitizes one to the fear, allowing one to respond clearly and effectively (Gentile, 2010). Pianalto (2012) also addresses this element of fear or anger, attributing the act of confronting another moral agent as an act of moral courage. Increasing confidence was noted in nurses after the experience of speaking up in an ethical situation (Wurzbach, 1999). The nature of ethics in healthcare is similar to that of corporations; addressing an ethical issue often means addressing those in power, this is especially true for nurses. This produces anxiety and generally an avoidance, until the stakes are too high to continue to ignore the issue. Questioning ethical issues is often interpreted by the other as blame or criticism of their ethical competence, so the ethical discussion is met with defensiveness or justification, and the much-needed ethical dialogue is shut down. This can occur at all levels throughout the organization; however, in the hierarchy of power, clinical nurses who experience significant ethical intensity due to their proximity and time spent with patients, who are silencing or avoiding, will often only speak when they reach a tipping point. Then they tend to speak emotionally, with frustration, anger, and accusations, while those with power dismiss the blows. Or they remain silent, disengaged, and hopeless. If we utilize the analogy of voice lessons, understanding theory (philosophy and principles) is critical, as is reading a new language and learning a new vocabulary; learning techniques (skills of self-awareness, ethical analysis, communication) and having the opportunity to *practice* will provide effective moral agency. Gentile's work promotes practicing the expression of one's values. Wisely, she suggests this be done "not as coming from a place of self-righteousness—something few of us can truly claim and a stance that rarely wins followers—but as coming from a place of competence and conviction" (Gentile 2010, p. xiv). Normalizing ethics dialogue throughout the institution can begin with ethical awareness through education programs that not only inform, but also send a clear message that ethics is valued within the organization. A lecture series that brings a multidisciplinary audience and administration together is one simple way to begin the process. Grady reported the poor presence of ethics education among nurses, with roughly 22.7% having had none (Grady et al., 2008). Given this lack of ethics education, specialty education for clinical nurses and nursing leadership is also critical and provides knowledge and moral space to acknowledge and process their lived experiences.

While the intense ethical dilemmas may provoke attention, there are other ethical concerns that may go unrecognized and yet have daily impacts for nurses, for example determining daily patient assignments, in the context of which patient will get the strongest nurse, or combating the unintended consequences of the opioid crisis, where chronic pain patients are not receiving adequate pain management, or implicit biases being played out in determining quality of life. These occurrences of microethics, the ethics of everyday clinical practice, benefit from education as well (Hoskins et al., 2018).

Dialogue and Education

Offering intensive programs for nurses requires significant resources yet provides another avenue of building ethics expertise and supports from the ground up, for instance localized ethics champions and potential nursing representatives on ethics committees (Totochaud et al., 2018). In the Clinical Ethics Residency for Nurses (CERN) program, essays demonstrated that the participants felt prepared to empower their colleagues in ethical deliberation (Lee et al., 2020; Robinson et al., 2014).

While competition among medical centers for both staff and patients has become the business norm, collaborative education can achieve improved programs that meet the needs of both the individual institution and the greater community. Ethics of Caring achieved this 30 years ago, when nursing ethics leaders in the community reached out to their CNOs to support a collective effort that no individual institution could provide as well. That support has now grown into the National Nursing Ethics Conference. Collaboration is an ethical path, whether within teams or in communities. For nurse leaders, that means broadening the view and outreach and moving beyond competition (Davidson et al., 2020).

Working on the tertiary level, "a prevention framework included emphasizing education and policy development, identifying at-risk populations, targeting early risk reduction interventions, and creating cohesive, organization-wide, and multi-segment intervention programs" (Pavlish et al., 2013a, p. 274) is vital. An example of this is encouraging interdisciplinary voice by building ethics dialogue into routine clinical care. The use of an electronic medical record (EMR) tool to prompt ethics assessment was built upon evidence-based early indicators and risk factors for ethical conflict. Tested in six ICUs at three large academic medical centers and used daily, the protocol prompted scoring and interventions and team discussion of ethical concerns during daily rounds. With the use of the tool, increased family conferencing and chaplain referrals were significantly higher; congruently, palliative care consults, code discussions, and ethics consults increased over the six-month period. The protocol also impacted clinicians, demonstrating increased perceptions of both the ethical climate and the effectiveness of dealing with ethical issues (Pavlish et al., 2020). In this same study, while the nurses' moral distress decreased, the doctors' moral distress frequency subscale was trending upward, perhaps indicating a higher degree of the awareness of ethical issues for physicians through daily dialogue and assessment (Pavlish et al., 2021).

These examples demonstrate a variety of ways to integrate ethics resources; they are also highly visible, generating awareness that leadership is appreciating the concerns and needs, is actively engaged, and is committed to change.

Further actions are required to enhance the formal mechanisms to address clinical ethical interests. The Joint Commission on Accreditation of Healthcare has requirements for organizational ethics mandating that the hospital operates according to a code of ethical behavior, and that code addresses marketing, admission, transfer, discharge, and billing, as well as relationships to other healthcare providers, educational institutions, and payers (RI.4, RI.4.1, RI.4.2). The bar it sets for responding to ethical concerns, however, only requires *a mechanism for addressing ethical issues* (The Joint Commission, 2022).

There are clearly far greater benchmarks that organizations should hold themselves to, and the needs and responses deserve careful evaluation, planning (that includes all stakeholders), and funding.

Ethics Committees and Ethics Consults

Ethics committees can provide a litmus test for the health of the ethical climate in an institution. They function in diverse ways across the country with too few requirements, given their power. There is often little oversight, evaluation, or quality-improvement efforts, let alone robust education of its members (Fox et al., 2021; Kelly et al., 2018; May, 2001; Tarzian et al., 2015). There is a need for a fine balance of the administrative presence, so that both the issues being discussed and the functioning of the committee are viewed in real time, yet not such a heavy presence that it is perceived as hierarchical. Having year-long membership appointments which are rotated through the top leadership serves not only informational purposes—that is, what is going on in the institution—it also allows for a natural ethical influence on these leaders, which advances their consideration of ethical practices within their own spheres. Committee representation requires an avoidance of homogeneity, seeking inclusion of the many professions, racial, ethnic, religious, age, and gender diversity, and community representation. There should also be an avoidance of nepotism in the choice of members and an effort to obtain a group with diverse views. All institutions live within one overarching silo, providing the benefit of finding convergence over mission and values; however, that also naturally provokes "group think."

The ethics committee can become one of the silos where "group think" shrinks the possibility of adept analysis, honest exploration of biases, and the provision of just recommendations. Additionally, those who take on leadership roles in ethics (committee chairs or consultants) within the institution are not only given the mantle of being ethics experts, but also carry auras of virtuosity. With the mandate of confidentiality and a closed loop system, there is little opportunity for discussion outside of the silo, and without evaluation, practices can become sloppy even with good intentions.

Nursing leadership should be actively involved and knowledgeable about the ethics processes, for those cases that come before the committee for appraisal and ethical recommendations are the most vulnerable populations. These are frequently the unrepresented or those families who disagree with end-of-life decisions deemed to be non-beneficial (many of whom who have suffered health inequities, lack trust, and who look very different than the committee they are facing) and maybe perceived as verdicts without a representative jury. A nurse leader should know the structure of the committee:

1. In the organizational chart, to whom does the ethics committee report? Is it one-dimensional in the organizational chart (i.e., a medical staff committee), or is it representational (a multidisciplinary executive committee or board)? The movement has been toward the latter (Courtwright & Jurchak, 2016).
2. What are the bylaws?
3. Chair leadership: are there restrictions perhaps by discipline, and if so, why? Who appoints the chair, and are there term limits?
4. How is membership chosen or appointed? What are the requirements for members?
5. What is the committee's work? If they are consulting, how many consults are referred a year? Does it include policy development and review, and if so, what is the focus and how are they determining needs for development?
6. What resources/budget is dedicated to ethics?

Finally, the appointing of nurses to the ethics committee is critical and extraordinarily difficult. It requires nurses who not only are educated and practiced in ethics, but they must also be nurses who are not intimidated, yet measured, and who have good skills in analytical and critical thinking and communication. They will hopefully bring the ethic of care perspective to the table, knowing the principle-based language which they will balance with the narrative and the psycho-social components. Walker (1993) describes this skill as moving, "from thinking about morality as a theory applied to cases, to thinking about morality as a medium of progressive acknowledgment and adjustment among people in (or in search of) a common and habitable moral world" (p. 35). If a family or patient is coming to the committee, the nurse can provide a measure of empathy and comfort. Lastly, they must have the time and passion to devote. Most good committees do policy work that requires reading and reviewing, as well as committee consults that often come at inconvenient times. Staff nurses, clinical nurse specialists, and nursing administrators should be present in good measure, providing a balanced representation of clinicians with a nurse always at the table.

Just as important as the ethics committee are the ethics consults themselves. While many institutions still have the committees doing consults, there are concerns with this approach. In one national study, consults were found to be done primarily by physicians and nurses, with only 41% having formal training (Fox et al., 2007). In recent studies examining ethics consults, they averaged less than a case a week (Kaps & Kopf, 2020; Wasson et al., 2016). A robust ethics consult service is often receiving 4 to 7 consults a week, and there is value in having clinical ethicists with advanced degrees in ethics (Cederquist et al., 2021; Harris et al., 2021). There is often a gap in knowledge that these services exist within an institution; in a recent survey at an academic center, 25%–33% of the physicians, advanced practice providers (APPs), and registered nurses (RNs) were unaware of the availability of ethics consults (Cederquist et al., 2021). Education and awareness increase nurses' utilization of these services (Bartlett & Finder, 2018). Walker (1993) helps one to understand why ethicists can transform ethical conflict, "The moral expertise of clinical ethicists is not a question of mastering codelike theories and lawlike principles. Rather, ethicists are architects of moral space within the health care setting, as well as mediators in the conversations taking place within that space" (p. 33). This, like so many of the other actions presented, sends a message that the institution values ethics and is not depending upon volunteers to do the work. While ethics is a component of all healthcare professionals' practice, an expertise in ethics is quite different and raises the bar immensely, not only in having highly competent experts for the consulting, but also for teaching and policy development.

Guiding Ethics Through Policy

Policies, first and foremost, promote quality and safety by creating consistency and standards within the institution. They also tend to have their eye on risk management and in "dotting every i" and because of this they are not always valued and can be viewed as cumbersome. Policies are rarely written to inspire others, and frequently are not read at all until there is a crisis. An overview of policies for nurse leaders includes an appreciation that:

1. Some policies explicitly address ethical issues, and nurses should be in-volved in the formation and dissemination of these policies;
2. There are many additional policies that could benefit from being examined through an ethical lens;
3. There are policies which must be repeatedly reinforced/revisited because of their potential impact on the moral climate of the institution and the moral distress of the clinicians.

Policies are often created from the top down, without adequate input from clinical nurses. Sometimes nurses take the risk of ignoring them in favor of pro-viding good care; an example of this was the adoption of the Centers for Disease Control and Prevention's 30-minute rule for timely delivery of medication, well-intentioned but compromising care (Davidson et al., 2020). Another example is a policy (and decision) of employing a new technology, using video monitoring versus the presence of sitter. While seemingly cost-saving and effective by preventing harm (i.e., falls), Jurchak and Eagan-Bengston (2012) point out how the policy lost sight of the ethical variables, such as respect for the patient and compassionate humanity. Often policies specific to ethics (consent, surrogate decision-making, etc.) are developed or reviewed by those involved in ethics, yet many other policies could benefit from appraisal through an ethics lens.

Especially important to nursing are well developed policies that address con-scientious objection (CO). Studies have found that nursing CO issues involving a wide swath of clinical issues, including refusal of treatment, abortion, mandated referrals for euthanasia (Canada), refusal of blood transfusions, and undermanaged pain, especially in neonates (Ford & Austin, 2018; Lamb et al., 2019; Toro-Flores et al., 2019). Moral concerns over care are not infrequent. A study surveyed intensive care nurses and physicians, finding that in a 24-hour period, 27% recounted concerns about the appropriateness of treatment that went against their beliefs, either personally or professionally. Most of these re-lated to over-treatment (Piers et al., 2011).

At times these CO policies are developed by the human resources (HR) departments with a focus on managing employees, rather than ethical aspects. Nurses especially in ICUs feel the frustration of not being included in policy de-velopment and deem those policies addressing over-treatment or non-beneficial treatment as not strong enough to establish appropriate limits. Honoring an egal-itarian process, many institutions' ethics consultation policies make it clear that anyone involved in clinical care can request a consult. Others restrict who can call, or they require the permission of the attending physician, leading to a hier-archical obstruction that dismisses the need for ethics contributions for ethical exploration and advice. If this is the case, nurse leaders should be addressing the policy. There will also be a great need to tackle the underlying power structure, reconfiguring a request so that it is seen as a natural process given the nature of ethical challenges.

Attending physicians sometimes underutilize or are unaware of policies related to specific patient-care situations. This tends to undermine the use of policies and can create systems where written policies only exist on a shelf, or that rely upon nurses to advocate for a relevant policy. One such an example is an underutilized policy that clarifies the physician's responsibility to determine efficacy of resuscitation when a patient is imminently dying, where resuscitation would not achieve the goals of care, causing great suffering and/or harm. Given the proximity of death, the policy needs to be judicious, yet efficient, with built-in protections such as a second opinion, prior documented family meetings (assuring they understand the medical recommendations), and a formal ethics consult. If the withholding of resuscitation is deemed to be ethically appropriate, then families would be informed that the plan of care would not include resuscitation. This fair process-based mechanism could be instituted quickly, yet nurses found physicians not utilizing the policy for a variety of reasons, for example, wanting to avoid further conflict or having concerns of harming the family, while dismissing the harm to the patient. One can imagine the nurses' powerlessness and moral angst of having to code a dying patient, when maleficence could have been prevented by using the institution's policy. These are the policies that need to be revisited and reinforced, with multidisciplinary moral dialogues and the support of clinical ethicists, and appreciation for the differing perspectives that can inform practice and provide good outcomes. Davidson et al. (2020) reminds leaders, "The obligation to monitor the impact of policies and standards rests on nurse leaders who have the duty to advocate when policies fail. Nurses providing direct care are beholden to report failed policies" (p. 43). Often this duty will be neglected unless nurse leaders recognize the impact on patient care, the disruption in interdisciplinary relationships, and appreciate the repercussions of moral distress.

Ethical Financial Tensions

Healthcare budgets are created annually in an effort to divide the resource pie, one that never has enough to feed all the needs and no magic wands to make additional slices. The administrators focus on numbers and the demands of chronic shortages and growing requirements. Investments in technology and innovative equipment can be seductive, and patient satisfaction necessitates that hospitals look and act more like hotels. When budget decisions are being made, the voices grow louder to protect one's turf, and almost all managers play the game so that there are no annual leftovers, for fear one's next budget will be cut. Those who are careful stewards present well thought-out budgets, only to be asked to cut them, and then are chastised when they go over budget to cover essential expenses of staffing, and so on. At the bottom of all these requests and competing needs are those who do the work, sometimes protected by unions, laws, or established standards (i.e., set ratios), or in academic centers, the broader university's policies and benefits. Nursing leaders, like legislators, understand that there are plenty of lobbyists and they must be willing to negotiate to keep peace. Ultimately those leaders build allegiances, and something is likely sacrificed. If that leader does not understand the true needs at the bedside or how to balance their commitment first to patients and then to the larger institution, frequently nursing values will be negatively impacted. The greater the distance from the demand, the easier it is to deny the appeal. Nurse leaders who make a commitment to spend time with their nurses and to listen carefully to their challenges will find it far more difficult determining how that pie should be divided. They will almost certainly be more closely aligned with the highest needs for patient care and will be in the position to defend those necessities.

Ironically, as though the juggling of budget, quality improvement, safety, efficiencies, and the myriad of other needs is not taxing enough, the business model has created a culture of incentivizing. While funding is denied as the institution justifies the lack of resources, in many institutions, leadership has linked performance to bonuses. Those performance reviews are often related to keeping costs down. In some institutions the bonus program has only been available for administration; in others, bonuses may reach across all employees. Those in administration, typically making the highest salaries, also often have a higher percentage tied to the bonuses, essentially having an exponential effect resulting in significant financial incentives. Initially these performance incentives were tied to financial performance. Now, fortunately, at least in part due to insurance companies connecting reimbursements to hospitals for quality and safety performance, they address these as well (Healthcare Business & Technology, 2014).

While financial incentives do sometimes work, they are fraught with ethical issues. One question that arises is: Why in healthcare does incentivization not rely upon employees' commitment to caring for the vulnerable and the sick and furthering the mission statement of the institution? While business skills are needed, especially in complex health systems, injustices remain; for example, compensations of $7.3 million and $6.7 million were paid to two CEOs (Mount Sinai Health System in New York City and McLaren Health Care Corp., respectively), mocking the rank and file who need resources for patient care (Kacik, 2019). How is it ethically justifiable to not reallocate some healthy portion of these moneys into the healthcare system challenged to care for the sick? Second, is it not an unjust system that rewards those with the highest salaries in the institution a performance bonus at a higher percentage, contrasted to those with lower salaries and lower percentages? Furthermore, numerous studies point to concerns of motivation of unethical behavior with payment tied to performance goals (Sauer et al., 2018; Stout, 2014). Just as worrisome, when the leader has created performance goals linked to their bonus, they are incentivized to ig- nore immediate and important issues that surface unexpectedly during the year. Paying attention to pressing and immediate needs will cost one significantly, meaning that most individuals will keep their eye on the financial gains. The conflict of interest for the nursing leader is significant; they are well aware of the consequences when budgets are cut to provide for bonuses.

Human Resources (HR)

The 2020 pandemic has brought to light what nurses have known all along—it is not the number of beds. The most precious resources in the institution are competent nurses. Keeping those nurses in the profession is a moral obligation of *every* institution and nurse leader. While nursing internships now appreciate the support and mentorship needed at the beginning of nurses' careers, there is a dearth of efforts to address healthy work environments, wellness programs, and moral distress prevention and healing programs. Integrating ethics into the re- cruitment and orientation process deserves serious consideration. When there is a robust ethics program in the institution, it is a valuable recruitment tool, espe- cially for experienced nurses who have come from institutions without capable ethics resources. Interviews can ask questions, utilize case examples, or role-play scenarios that elicit ethical sensibilities and give a window into the potential of the individual's ethical critical thinking. Orientation provides an opportunity to see how ethics is valued within the institution and what resources are available.

HR can also be educated as to practices of justice; for example, are there discrepancies in the approach to a violation of privacy or a medical error? Nurses have often been seen as disposable and without the same level of power and therefore may experience far harsher consequences, may be expected to take the blame, or may be used as "the example" to send a warning to others.

Evaluations are an opportunity not only to inform staff of areas that need improvement, but also to acknowledge the good in one's practice. This rarely extends to ethical competency. The ANA *Code of Ethics for Nurses'* nine provisions (2015) could provide a launching pad for an annual assessment and acknowledgment of advancing skills by addressing one provision annually and requiring brief narratives to demonstrate competency of both staff and nurse leaders. Finally, there are times while ethical issues are being addressed yet a nurse leader is not able to share that information with staff for privacy reasons, or it is premature to make announcements of solutions. This gap can cause tremendous frustration or can be the source of speculation and misinformation. To control rumors, keep cynicism at bay, and enhance trust, it is imperative that nurse leaders work with HR to develop approaches and communication so that individuals and teams feel that they are being heard.

Consideration of a New Model: A Nursing Ethics Leader

The foregoing has been an overview of the challenges that nurse leaders face integrating the multifaceted ethical issues into their responsibilities, as well as providing some examples of success. As mentioned earlier, the perspective of ethics not as an expertise, but as something that anyone can do, is troubling. While ethics needs to be incorporated into everyone's practice, whether clinical or administrative, relying upon volunteers for ethics consultation and education is no longer adequate given the complexities of ethical issues and the time it takes to address both clinical and organizational ethics. Nurse leaders have competing demands, and ethics' concealed nature (until issues erupt) means that ethics pieces are often neglected. Even within the educational systems, reports on nursing education have stressed the need for improved curriculums on ethics (Hoskins et al., 2018), yet it is often a faculty member without training in ethics who takes on the added responsibility. Clinical ethics research is yet another challenge, neglected, with limited research funds mostly directed to the ethical aspects of research, not the clinical concerns. Ethics, whether committees or programs, has generally not been given the recognition nor the resources to do the important work (Hamric & Wocial, 2016).

Appreciating these obstacles provides an opportunity to think about how to move forward. Mindful of the needs and stewardship, the sharing of resources can make it manageable. Having a doctorally prepared nurse in bioethics can open many doors and vastly enrich ethics programs and teaching. A joint appointment at a school of nursing and a clinical appointment within a medical center provide a consummate nurse to both areas in need. The appointee, being part of a clinical consultation team, provides direct access to staff for mentoring and informal education with each exposure. In turn, this will inform the nurse ethicist's academic teaching, making it relevant through current, rich clinical experience. Additionally, this ethics nurse leader, being close to the clinical work, will be able to address relevant research and to include nurses, which exposes them to the power of research, an antidote to powerlessness, and moves evidence-based practice forward. Staff education becomes embedded in this holistic approach. This appointment would also provide the resources to address the system issues that are often the root cause of moral distress. Given the cost of moral distress for nurses, the institution, our profession, and society, this position is inestimable. The presence of an ethics nurse leader on an ethics committee will endow mentorship of the nurses joining the committee. Having a nurse with ethics expertise join in leadership meetings brings a perspective that has long been missing, bringing an expertise and preventive view. The institutional investment is not for this individual to carry ethics for everyone, but to offer expertise and, like a contagion factor, it will proliferate ethics awareness and discourse. Fortunately, this specialty and programs for education are on the rise; what is now needed are nurse leaders who recognize their value and create and support these positions.

Closing

Many of the ethical challenges and concerns that nurse leaders face have been addressed in this chapter. In closing, we return to the nurse leaders and explore key elements that will help them integrate an ethics of care to enhance their resiliency. Beneficially, there is a greater appreciation of effectiveness for the leader who starts with a relational process, both with themselves and others. The mantra repeated over and over in healthcare is "I have no time." Many leaders, overwhelmed with relentless demands and competing priorities, lose sight of what matters most. As one looks over one's shoulder of the journey of leadership, values may have been misplaced along the way when one attempted to "do it all" with immediacy.

Once a year, stepping out of the chaos as one is setting goals, perhaps the question at the top of the page should come from Mary Oliver's 1990 poem, "The Summer Day": "Tell me, what is it you plan to do with your one wild and precious life?" (p. 60). What that simple, stunning question asks of us is: What really matters? Becoming a professional nurse hopefully arose from a place of deep caring and compassion for the sick, mixed with a love of science and a willful determination to make things better. The etymology of the word "profession" stems from the Latin *profiteri*, meaning to declare aloud, to profess (*Oxford English and Spanish Dictionary*, n.d.). What is it that a nurse leader should be professing out loud? How can holding the lens of ethics help define that professing? Most importantly, that lens is enlightening others as to what nursing is, what values are core and honored to guide in the caring for others, especially the vulnerable and, just as importantly, what nursing is not. At the end of one's serving their vocation, what will be remembered is who that nurse was, not the list of endless tasks accomplished. How one related to others, how one had courage to stand the ground when it mattered, how one took that same courage to "en-courage" others. To have courage requires a passionate heart of moral muscle, balanced with the head's wisdom. That wisdom must include boundary setting, placing limits so that one is able to remain creative, engaged, and flourishing. While the world seems to move at lightning speed, ethics rooted in ancient virtues, diverse values, and dynamic complex environments does not deliver with neat efficient fixes. Patience and persistence and the ability to continue to see both what has been accomplished and what remains ahead are the task at hand. For nurse leaders to uphold a vision for the future of healthcare that creates the inclusive and responsive moral community, they must remember always the crucible and the many so in need of light.

Acknowledgment

The author would like to thank Marilyn Shirk for her thoughtful comments.

References

American Nurses Association. (2015). *Code of ethics for nurses, with interpretive statements.* https://www.nursingworld.org/practice-policy/nursing-excellence/ethics/code-of-ethics-for-nurses/.

American Organization for Nursing Leadership. (2020). *Nursing leadership COVID-19 survey.* https://www.aonl.org/resources/nursing-leadership-covid-19-survey.

American Organization of Nurse Executives. (2015). *AONE nurse executive competencies.* http://www.aone.org/resources/nurse-leader-competencies.shtml.

Anderson, J. (2018). The ethics of silence: Does conflict of interest explain employee silence? *Healthcare Management Forum, 31*(2), 66–68.

Azoulay, E., Timsit, J. F., Sprung, C. L., Soares, M., Rusinová, K., Lafabrie, A., Abizanda, R., Svantesson, M., Rubulotta, F., Ricou, B., Benoit, D., Heyland, D., Joynt, G., Français, A., Azeivedo-Maia, P., Owczuk, R., Benbenishty, J., de Vita, M., Valentin, A., . . . Schlemmer, B. (2009). Prevalence and factors of intensive care unit conflicts: The conflicus study. *American Journal of Respiratory and Critical Care Medicine, 180*(9), 853–860.

Barkhordari-Sharifabad, M., Ashktorab, T., & Atashzadeh-Shoorideh, F. (2018). Ethical competency of nurse leaders: A qualitative study. *Nursing Ethics, 25*(1), 20–36.

Bartlett, V. L., & Finder, S. G. (2018). Lessons learned from nurses' requests for ethics consultation: Why did they call and what did they value? *Nursing Ethics, 25*(5), 601–617.

Benner, P., Sutphen, M., Leonard-Kahn, V., & Day, L. (2008). Formation and everyday ethical comportment. *American Journal of Critical Care, 17*(5), 473–476.

Brown, M. T. (1990). *Working ethics.* Jossey-Bass.

Cathcart, E. B. (2008). The role of the chief nursing officer in leading the practice: Lessons from the Benner tradition. *Nursing Administration Quarterly, 32*(2), 87–91.

Catlin, A., Armigo, C., Volat, D., Vale, E., Hadley, M. A., Gong, W., Bassir, R., & Anderson, K. (2008). Conscientious objection: A potential neonatal nursing response to care orders that cause suffering at the end of life? Study of a concept. *Neonatal Network, 27*(2), 101–108.

Cederquist, L. C., LaBuzetta, J., Cachay, E., Friedman, L., & Zhang, Y. (2021). Identifying disincentives to ethics consultation requests among physicians, advance practice providers, and nurses. *BMC Medical Ethics, 22*(1), 44.

Connor, J. (2020). *A competency framework: Professional moral courage and nurse executive competency.* Springer.

Courtwright, A., & Jurchak, M. (2016). The evolution of American hospital ethics committees: A systematic review. *The Journal of Clinical Ethics, 27*(4), 322–340.

Davidson, J. E., Marshall, M. F., & Watanabe, J. H. (2020). Policy impact: When policy fails. *Nursing Forum, 55*(1), 37–44.

Ford, N. J., & Austin, W. (2018). Conflicts of conscience in the neonatal intensive care unit: Perspectives of Alberta. *Nursing Ethics, 25*(8), 992–1003.

Fox, E., Danis, M., Tarzian, A. J., & Duke, C. C. (2021). Ethics consultation in U.S. hospitals: A national follow-up study. *The American Journal of Bioethics, 22*(4), 5–18.

Fox, E., Myers, S., & Pearlman, R. A. (2007). Ethics consultation in United States hospitals: A national survey. *The American Journal of Bioethics, 7*(2), 13–25.

Garon, M. (2012). Speaking up, being heard: Registered nurses' perceptions of workplace communication. *Journal of Nursing Management, 20*(3), 361–371.

Gaudine, A. P., & Beaton, M. R. (2002). Employed to go against one's values: Nurse managers' accounts of ethical conflict with their organizations. *The Canadian Journal of Nursing Research, 34*(2), 17–34.

Gentile, M. C. (2010) *Giving voice to values: How to speak your mind when you know what's right.* Yale University Press.

Grady, C., Danis, M., Soeken, K. L., O'Donnell, P., Taylor, C., Farrar, A., & Ulrich, C. M. (2008). Does ethics education influence the moral action of practicing nurses and social workers? *The American Journal of Bioethics, 8*(4), 4–11.

Grossman, S. C., & Valiga, M. (2020). *The new leadership challenge: Creating the future of nursing* (6th ed.). F. A. Davis.

Hakimi, H., Joolaee, S., Ashghali Farahani, M., Rodney, P., & Ranjbar, H. (2020). Moral neutralization: Nurses' evolution in unethical climate workplaces. *BMC Medical Ethics, 21*(1), 114.

Hamric, A. B. (2000). Moral distress in everyday ethics. *Nursing Outlook, 48*(5), 199–201.

Hamric, A. B., & Epstein, E. G. (2017). A health system-wide moral distress consultation service: Development and evaluation. *HEC Forum, 29*(2), 127–143.

Hamric, A. B., & Wocial, L. D. (2016). Institutional ethics resources: Creating moral spaces. *Hastings Center Report Supplement, 46*(Suppl 1), S22–27.

Harris, K. W., Cunningham, T. V., Hester, D. M., Armstrong, K., Kim, A., Harrell, F. E., & Fanning, J. B. (2021). Comparison is not a zero-sum game: Exploring advanced measures of healthcare ethics consultation. *AJOB Empirical Bioethics, 12*(2), 123–136.

Healthcare Business & Technology. (2014). *Pay incentives tied to performance: A new trend for hospital administrators.* https://www.healthcarebusinesstech.com/administrators-incenti ves-tied-performance/.

Hoskins, K., Grady, C., Ulrich, C. M., (2018). Ethics education in nursing: Instruction for future generations of nurses. *OJIN: The Online Journal of Issues in Nursing, 23*(1), 1–4.

Jurchak, M., & Eagan-Bengston, E. (2012). 12.3 The inquiry of ethics rounds. In M. Hickey & P. B. Kritek (Eds.), *Change leadership in nursing: How change occurs in a complex hospital system* (pp. 164–172). Springer.

Kacik, A. (2019, June 22). Highest-paid not-for-profit health system executives earn 33% raise in 2017. *Modern Healthcare.* https://bettersolutionsforhealthcare.org/news-modern-hea lthcare-health-executives-raise/.

Kalshoven, K., Den Hartog, D., & De Hoogh, A. (2011). Ethical leadership at work questionnaire (ELW): Development and validation of a multidimensional measure. *The Leadership Quarterly, 22*(1) 51–69.

Kalshoven, K., Den Hartog, D., & De Hoogh, A. (2013). Ethical leadership and follower helping and courtesy: Moral awareness and empathic concern as moderators. *Applied Psychology, 62*(2), 211–235.

Kambhampati, A. K., O'Halloran, A. C., Whitaker, M., Magill, S. S., Chea, N., Chai, S. J., Kirley, P. D., Herlihy, R. K., Kawasaki, B., Meek, J., Yousey-Hindes, K., Anderson, E. J., Openo, K. P., Monroe, M. L., Ryan, P. A., Kim, S., Reeg, L., Como-Sabetti, K., Danila, R., ... Kim, L. (2020, October 30). Covid-19-associated hospitalizations among healthcare personnel: Covid-net,

13 states, March 1–May 31, 2020. *Morbidity and Mortality Weekly Report, 69*(43), 1576–1583.

Kaps, B., & Kopf, G. (2022). Functions, operations and policy of a volunteer ethics committee: A quantitative and qualitative analysis of ethics consultations from 2013 to 2018. *HEC Forum, 34*(1), 55–71.

Kelly, P., & Porr, C., (2018). Ethical nursing care versus cost containment: Considerations to enhance RN practice. *Online Journal of Issues in Nursing, 23*(1).

Kish-Gephart, J. J., Harrison, D. A., & Treviño, L. K. (2010). Bad apples, bad cases, and bad barrels: Meta-analytic evidence about sources of unethical decisions at work. *The Journal of Applied Psychology, 95*(1), 1–31.

Lamb, C., Evans, M., Babenko-Mould, Y., Wong, C., & Kirkwood, K. (2019). Nurses' use of conscientious objection and the implications for conscience. *Journal of Advanced Nursing, 75*(3), 594–602.

Lee, S., Robinson, E. M., Grace, P. J., Zollfrank, A., & Jurchak, M. (2020). Developing a moral compass: Themes from the Clinical Ethics Residency for Nurses' final essays. *Nursing Ethics, 27*(1), 28–39.

Leuter, C., Petrucci, C., & Lancia, L. (2013). Request for ethics support in healthcare practices. Reasons and characteristics of Ethics Consultation Service users. *Annali di Igiene: Medicina Preventiva e di Comunita, 25*(6), 539–552.

Ludwick, R., & Silva, M. C. (2003). Errors, the nursing shortage and ethics: Survey results. *Online Journal of Issues in Nursing, 8*(3).

May, T. (2001) The breadth of bioethics: Core areas of bioethics education for hospital ethics committees, *Journal of Medicine and Philosophy, 26*(1), 101–118.

McAndrew, N. S., & Hardin, J. B. (2020). Giving nurses a voice during ethical conflict in the intensive care unit. *Nursing Ethics, 27*(8), 1631–1644.

McCarthy, J., & Gastmans, C. (2015). Moral distress: A review of the argument-based nursing ethics literature. *Nursing Ethics, 22*(1), 131–152.

McKenna, J., & Jeske, D. (2021). Ethical leadership and decision authority effects on nurses' engagement, exhaustion, and turnover intention. *Journal of Advanced Nursing, 77*(1), 198–206.

Meyer-Zehnder, B., Barandun Schäfer, U., Wesch, C., Reiter-Theil, S., & Pargger, H. (2021). Weekly internal ethical case discussions in an ICU: Results based on 9 years of experience with a highly structured approach. *Critical Care Explorations, 3*(3).

Mohrmann, M. E. (2006). On being true to form. In C. Taylor & R. Dell'Oro (Eds.), *Health and human flourishing, religion, medicine, and moral anthropology* (pp. 90–102). Georgetown University Press.

Moss, M., Good, V. S., Gozal, D., Kleinpell, R., & Sessler, C. N. (2016). An official critical care societies collaborative statement: Burnout syndrome in critical care healthcare professionals: A call for action. *Critical Care Medicine, 44*(7), 1414–1421.

Newton, L., Storch, J. L., Makaroff, K. S., & Pauly, B. (2012). "Stop the noise!": From voice to silence. *Nursing Leadership, 25*(1), 90–104.

Oliver, M. (1990). The summer day. In *House of light* (p. 60). Beacon Press.

Olson, L. L. (1998). Hospital nurses' perceptions of the ethical climate of their work setting. *Image: The Journal of Nursing Scholarship, 30*(4), 345–349.

Oxford English and Spanish Dictionary. (n.d.). Crucible. In LEXICO. Retrieved July 20, 2020, from https://www.lexico.com/en/definition/crucible.

Oxford English and Spanish Dictionary. (n.d.). Profess. In LEXICO. Retrieved November 20, 2020, from https://www.lexico.com/en/definition/profess.

The Joint Commission on Accreditation of Healthcare Organizations. (2022). *Comprehensive accreditation manual.* Joint Commission Resources.

Pavlish, C. L., Brown-Saltzman, K., Dirksen, K. M., & Fine, A. (2015a). Physicians' perspectives on ethically challenging situations: Early identification and action. *American Journal of Bioethics, 6*(3), 28–40.

Pavlish, C. L., Brown-Saltzman, K., Fine, A., & Jakel, P. (2013a). Making the call: A proactive ethics framework. *HEC Forum, 25*(3), 269–283. https://doi.org/10.1007/s10730-013-9213-5.

Pavlish, C. L., Brown-Saltzman, K., Fine, A., & Jakel, P. (2015b). A culture of avoidance: Voices from inside ethically difficult clinical situations. *Clinical Journal of Oncology Nursing, 19*(2), 159–165.

Pavlish, C. L., Brown-Saltzman, K., Hersh, M., Shirk, M., & Nudelman, O. (2011a). Early indicators and risk factors for ethical issues in clinical practice. *Journal of Nursing Scholarship, 43*(1), 13–21.

Pavlish, C. L., Brown-Saltzman, K., Hersh, M., Shirk, M., & Rounkle, A. M. (2011b). Nursing priorities, actions, and regrets for ethical situations in clinical practice. *Journal of Nursing Scholarship, 43*(4), 385–395.

Pavlish, C. L., Brown-Saltzman, K., Jakel, P., & Fine, A. (2014). The nature of ethical conflicts and the meaning of moral community in oncology practice. *Oncology Nursing Forum, 41*(2), 130–140.

Pavlish, C. L., Brown-Saltzman, K., Jakel, P., & Rounkle, A. M. (2012). Nurses' responses to ethical challenges in oncology practice: An ethnographic study. *Clinical Journal of Oncology Nursing, 16*(6), 592–600.

Pavlish, C. L., Brown-Saltzman, K., Raho, J. A., & Chen, B. (2019). A national survey on moral obligations in critical care. *American Journal of Critical Care, 28*(3), 183–192.

Pavlish, C. L., Brown-Saltzman, K., Robinson, E. M., Henriksen, J., Warda, U. S., Farra, C., Chen, B., & Jakel, P. (2021). An ethics early action protocol to promote teamwork and ethics efficacy. *Dimensions of Critical Care Nursing, 40*(4), 226–236.

Pavlish, C. L., Brown-Saltzman, K., So, L., Heers, A., & Iorillo, N. (2015c). Avenues of action in ethically complex situations: A critical incident study. *The Journal of Nursing Administration, 45*(6), 311–318.

Pavlish, C. L., Brown-Saltzman, K., So, L., & Wong, J. (2016). SUPPORT: An evidence-based model for leaders addressing moral distress. *The Journal of Nursing Administration, 46*(6), 313–320.

Pavlish, C. L., Hellyer, J. H., Brown-Saltzman, K., Miers, A. G., & Squire, K. (2013b). Barriers to innovation: Nurses' risk appraisal in using a new ethics screening and early intervention tool. *Advances in Nursing Science, 36*(4), 304–319.

Pavlish, C. L., Hellyer, J. H., Brown-Saltzman, K., Miers, A. G., & Squire, K. (2015d). Screening situations for risk of ethical conflicts: A pilot study. *American Journal of Critical Care, 24*(3), 248–256.

Pavlish, C. L., Henriksen, J., Brown-Saltzman, K., Robinson, E. M., Warda, U. S., Farra, C., Chen, B., & Jakel, P. (2020). A team-based early action protocol to address ethical concerns in the intensive care unit. *American Journal of Critical Care, 29*(1), 49–61.

Peter, E., Lunardi, V. L., Macfarlane, A. (2004). Nursing resistance as ethical action: Literature review. *Journal of Advanced Nursing, 46*(4), 403–416.

Pianalto, M. (2012) Moral courage and facing others, *International Journal of Philosophical Studies, 20*(2), 165–184.

Piers, R. D., Azoulay, E., Ricou, B., Dekeyser Ganz, F., Decruyenaere, J., Max, A., Michalsen, A., Maia, P. A., Owczuk, R., Rubulotta, F., Depuydt, P., Meert, A. P., Reyners, A. K., Aquilina, A., Bekaert, M., Van den Noortgate, N. J., Schrauwen, W. J., Benoit, D. D., & APPROPRICUS Study Group of the Ethics Section of the ESICM. (2011). Perceptions of appropriateness of care among European and Israeli intensive care unit nurses and physicians. *JAMA, 306*(24), 2694–2703.

Reinhart, R. J. (2020, January 6). Nurses continue to rate highest in honesty, ethics. *Gallup.* https://news.gallup.com/poll/274673/nurses-continue-rate-highest-honesty-ethics.aspx.

Robinson, E. M., Lee, S. M., Zollfrank, A., Jurchak, M., Frost, D., & Grace, P. (2014). Enhancing moral agency: Clinical ethics residency for nurses. *The Hastings Center Report, 44*(5), 12–20.

Roy, A. (2004, November 4). *Peace and the new corporate liberation theology* [Speech, The 2004 City of Sydney Peace Prize Lecture]. The Sydney Peace Foundation. https://sydneypeacefou ndation.org.au/peace-prize-recipients/2004-arundhati-roy/.

Rushton, C. H., Caldwell, M., & Kurtz, M. (2016). Moral distress: A catalyst in building moral resilience. *American Journal of Nursing, 116*(7), 40–49.

Sauer, S. J., Rodgers, M. S., & Becker, W. J. (2018). The effects of goals and pay structure on managerial reporting dishonesty. *Journal of Accounting, Ethics & Public Policy, 19*(3), 377–418.

Scherer, A., Alt-Epping, B., Nauck, F., & Marx, G. (2019). Team members perspectives on conflicts in clinical ethics committees. *Nursing Ethics, 26*(7–8), 2098–2112.

Schick-Makaroff, K., & Storch, J. L. (2019). Guidance for ethical leadership in nursing codes of ethics: An integrative review. *Nursing Leadership, 32*(1), 60–73.

Simha, A., & Pandey, J. (2020). Trust, ethical climate and nurses' turnover intention. *Nursing Ethics, 28*(5), 714–722.

Stout, L. A., (2014) Killing conscience: The unintended behavioral consequences of pay for performance. *Journal of Corporation Law, 39*(3) 525–561. https://scholarship.law.cornell. edu/cgi/viewcontent.cgi?article=2526&context=facpub.

Swetz, K. M., Crowley, M. E., Hook, C., & Mueller, P. S. (2007). Report of 255 clinical ethics consultations and review of the literature. *Mayo Clinic Proceedings, 82*(6), 686–691.

Tangirala, S., Kamdar, D., Venkataramani, V., & Parke, M. R. (2013). Doing right versus getting ahead: The effects of duty and achievement orientations on employees' voice. *The Journal of Applied Psychology, 98*(6), 1040–1050.

Tarzian, A. J., Wocial, L. D., & The ASBH Clinical Ethics Consultation Affairs Committee. (2015). A code of ethics for health care ethics consultants: Journey to the present and implications for the field. *The American Journal of Bioethics, 15*(5), 38–51.

Toro-Flores, R., Bravo-Agüi, P., Catalán-Gómez, M. V., González-Hernando, M., Guijarro-Cenisergue, M. J., Moreno-Vázquez, M., Roch-Hamelin, I., & Velasco-Sanz, T. R. (2019). Opinions of nurses regarding conscientious objection. *Nursing Ethics, 26*(4), 1027–1038.

Trotochaud, K., Fitzgerald, H., & Knackstedt, A. D. (2018). Ethics champion programs. *The American Journal of Nursing, 118*(7), 46–54.

U.S. Department of Veterans Affairs. (2020, May 13). *VHA directive 1005: Informed consent for long-term opioid therapy for pain.* https://www.ethics.va.gov/docs/policy/VHA_Handbook _1005_Opioid_Therapy_IC.pdf

Van den Bulcke, B., Metaxa, V., Reyners, A. K., Rusinova, K., Jensen, H. I., Malmgren, J., Darmon, M., Talmor, D., Meert, A. P., Cancelliere, L., Zubek, L., Maia, P., Michalsen, A., Kompanje, E., Vlerick, P., Roels, J., Vansteelandt, S., Decruyenaere, J., Azoulay, E., & Vanheule, S. (2020). Ethical climate and intention to leave among critical care clinicians: An observational study in 68 intensive care units across Europe and the United States. *Intensive Care Medicine, 46*(1), 46–56.

Victor, B., & Cullen, J. B. (1987). A theory and measure of ethical climate in organizations. In W. C. Frederick & L. Preston (Eds.), *Research in corporate social performance and policy* (Vol. 9, pp. 51–71). JAI Press.

Vincent, H., Jones, D. J., & Engebretson, J. (2020). Moral distress perspectives among interprofessional intensive care unit team members. *Nursing Ethics, 27*(6), 1450–1460.

Walker, M. U. (1993). Keeping moral space open: New images of ethics consulting. *The Hastings Center Report, 23*(2), 33–40.

Wasson, K., Anderson, E., Hagstrom, E., McCarthy, M., Parsi, K., & Kuczewski, M. (2016). What ethical issues really arise in practice at an academic medical center? A quantitative and qualitative analysis of clinical ethics consultations from 2008 to 2013. *HEC Forum, 28*(3), 217–228.

Wurzbach, M. E. (1999) Acute care nurses' experiences of moral certainty. *Journal of Advanced Nursing, 30*(2), 287–293.

9

Conceptions of Vulnerability Within the Context of Clinical Research

Michael J. Deem and Judith A. Erlen

Introduction

Clinical research aims to produce new knowledge, understanding, and therapeutics to advance the care and treatment of patients, thereby improving health outcomes. Achieving these goals typically involves recruitment of patient populations that meet the inclusion criteria for a particular study, and these patients are asked individually to volunteer as participants in clinical research. While their participation is often necessary and essential to this goal, their participation is not without some risk of harm, even when Institutional Review Boards (IRBs) conclude that a given study involves no more than a minimal risk. IRBs are, after all, fallible guides to the protection of human research subjects, often relying on the presence of specific, boilerplate language in research protocols for indications of standard protections for research participants generally, and "vulnerable" subjects in particular. But the discernment of risk of a study should not fall exclusively within the purview of the IRB. It seems that it is especially incumbent upon investigators themselves to identify which factors within their research programs present risk of harm to participants and to establish measures that, where practical and probable in effect, mitigate the risk of harming or wronging those participants. Because clinical research involving human subjects presents *some* risk of harm, all research participants are vulnerable by virtue of their participation, including those who might appear to be healthy, decisionally capable, and participating on a voluntary basis. But, if it is the case that all (or nearly all) participants in clinical research are vulnerable to harm or being wronged, then we should examine the customary ways that nursing ethics discourse traditionally characterizes "vulnerable populations" as groups of individuals in need of *special* protections.

Despite the nearly ubiquitous presence of the term *vulnerable populations* in discourse about nursing education, care, and research, it is not clear that such discourse consistently picks out the same referent when using the term. To be sure, ethicists, researchers, and international ethics commissions have recognized that certain individuals and groups require special considerations and greater protections when invited to participate in research. We tend to label such individuals or groups as "vulnerable," because we suppose—rightly or wrongly— that they are *more* susceptible to harms or violations of their interests than is the "typical" research subject or "general" population. Populations frequently labeled as "vulnerable" in the nursing ethics literature include incarcerated individuals, children, pregnant women, human fetuses, patients with particular health conditions such as HIV, individuals with mental health challenges, persons in residential facilities, persons who have cognitive impairment, individuals who are not fluent in the language of the study, people who are socially and economically disadvantaged, and racial and ethnic minorities (among many others) (Gehlert & Mozersky, 2018; National Commission, 1979; Wilson & Neville, 2009). However, there have been several criticisms of this "labeling" approach to identifying groups that are vulnerable. One common criticism is that the list of "vulnerable populations" seems to be ever-expanding, potentially locating *any* prospective research participant under one or more groups at any given time. But if each prospective participant could plausibly be grouped into one or more vulnerable populations on our list, it becomes unclear precisely what rationale should be used to classify an individual or group as "vulnerable" and accordingly in need of special protections (Bracken-Roche et al., 2017a, 2017b). Moreover, as this list of groups expands, the use of the label "vulnerable" in research contexts might become so diluted that it no longer specifies which participants might need enhanced protections and what those protections should be (Hurst, 2008; Rogers, 2014; Schroeder & Gefenas, 2009; Wendler, 2017).

Another criticism is that the labeling approach fails to account for not only what circumstances give rise to vulnerability—be they physiological, psychological, socioeconomic, geographic, and so on—but also how these circumstances form "layers" of vulnerability that may interact, compound, and shape one another (Guidry-Grimes & Victor, 2012; Luna, 2009). For example, understanding and responding to the vulnerability of a research participant who is a child, whose family lives below a defined poverty line, and who has a rare genetic condition is not a matter of simply affixing to the participant the label "vulnerable" according to a group on our prespecified list of "vulnerable populations." Rather, it seems that we should also recognize that various circumstances give rise to different levels, or layers, of vulnerability that potentially entrench or reinforce one another.

A third common criticism of this labeling approach is that it threatens to stereotype or falsely categorize an individual as "vulnerable." For instance, classifying too rigidly a group as "vulnerable" for research purposes carries the potential to wrongly and condescendingly infer that *all* such individuals stand in need of enhanced protection in research. Might not this result in projecting and imposing vulnerability on some individuals (Heaslip & Ryden, 2013)?

This is not to suggest that there are no such groups that should be recognized as marginalized and disenfranchised within society, and whose members are more susceptible to risk of harm when enrolled in studies because of particular characteristics or positionality. However, as the foregoing considerations show, researchers should be cautious not to assume that a potential research participant is vulnerable *solely on the basis* of group identification constructed by researchers or international ethics bodies. All individuals within the specified group are not the same, although they may share a common characteristic, such as an identified disease. Thus, the assumptions about vulnerability and susceptibility to harms do not apply in the same way to all individuals (e.g., incarcerated individuals, human fetuses, adult patients with dementia), even within a specified "vulnerable population." Additionally, the degree to which an individual is vulnerable is influenced by both internal/individual and external/situational factors (Bracken-Roche et al., 2017a, 2017b). Whether a research participant is vulnerable in the relevant sense of needing additional protections within research requires a more measured and nuanced consideration than the typical labeling approach accomplishes.

In this chapter, we bring together two styles of bioethical inquiry to begin rethinking aspects of vulnerability in research. The following section begins with mapping the conceptual terrain of vulnerability in the context of clinical research, particularly as it has developed over the past decade in philosophical bioethics. Because the concept of vulnerability is central to much of the work of nurse researchers and nurse ethicists, it is important in our view that nursing ethics be attentive to these conceptual developments and contribute to this broader conversation in bioethics. The next section complements this conceptual mapping with a narrative bioethical account of vulnerability. One of us (JAE) reflects on her own research experience with two different study populations—one with patients with HIV and the other with kin or kin-like caregivers of community-dwelling persons with memory loss—to illustrate ethical issues in situations involving vulnerability. Finally, we discuss ethical and practical insights gained from combining these conceptual and narrative approaches to vulnerability and suggest that a labeling approach to vulnerability in research can be useful in a limited sense when researchers bear in mind certain qualifications regarding to what and to whom the term *vulnerable* refers.

Vulnerability: Mapping Some of the Conceptual Terrain

Within the clinical and bioethical literatures, one encounters various conceptions of vulnerability. In this section, we aim to clarify and disentangle some of the more commonly utilized conceptions. Then, following a taxonomy developed and modified over the last decade by Wendy Rogers, Catriona Mackenzie, and Susan Dodds, we map some of these conceptions to arrive at a clearer notion of vulnerability in research and why clinicians and researchers often have the intuition that those research participants who are particularly vulnerable deserve special protections. Put another way, we wish to understand why researchers have special moral obligations to protect especially vulnerable research participants, before we later explore what those obligations might be.

Fundamental Elements of the Concept of Vulnerability

For most, the concept of vulnerability carries some negative connotation, and rightly so, given the etymology of the term. The Latin term *vulnus*, from which we derive the English term *vulnerable*, refers to a wound or harm that one undergoes. Hence, in the clinical and bioethical literatures, vulnerability is frequently defined in terms of susceptibility to harm or exploitation by others. In his classic philosophical study of vulnerability, Robert Goodin characterizes vulnerability as "a matter of being under threat of harm" (Goodin, 1985, p. 110). More recently, Joel Anderson defines vulnerability as the condition of being unable to "prevent occurrences that would undermine what [one] takes to be important to [one]" (Anderson, 2014, p. 135). Florencia Luna (2009) characterizes vulnerability as something from which one *suffers*, while Doris Shroeder and Eugenijus Gefenas provide a risk-based definition of vulnerability as the "significant probability of incurring an identifiable harm while substantially lacking ability and/or means to protect oneself" (2009, p. 117). While these are nonequivalent definitions of vulnerability, a common thread through them is that each highlights a *negative* experience or condition for the one who is vulnerable. Some philosophers and bioethicists, however, have argued that when this negative aspect of vulnerability becomes too focal, it fuels the notion that *invulnerability* is a more valued or prized state of being. This could account, at least in part, for the tendency for some researchers to frame vulnerability—and the related concept of dependency—as antithetical to autonomy and independence, leading to an overemphasis on protections surrounding *consent* for research or identifying vulnerable populations primarily as those whose *ability to consent* is compromised (at the expense of protections from other potential harms or violations of interests in research).

The concept of dependency, which likewise is often taken to be a condition that negatively affects one's autonomy, is closely linked to the concept of vulnerability. Philosophers such as Dodds, Rogers, Erinn Gilson, and Alasdair MacIntyre have independently challenged the notion that vulnerability is necessarily opposed to autonomy (Dodds, 2014; Gilson, 2014; MacIntyre, 1999;

Rogers, 2014). Gilson addresses what she sees as a "reductively negative understanding of vulnerability" in ethical theory and bioethics that leads us to overlook its other neutral, perhaps even positive, aspects (Gilson, 2014, p. 5). Insofar as vulnerability is understood as something undesirable and to be prevented, Gilson argues that we might find ourselves in a futile enterprise of pursuing a state of unachievable safety from harm, given that vulnerability is an unavoidable aspect of human life. As a corrective, she proposes that vulnerability be thought of as "an openness to all experience, negative, positive, and ambiguous" and as a "specific, fundamental mode of passivity, which can be thought in terms of reciprocity rather than simply as susceptibility" (Gilson, 2014, pp. 24, 133, 134). On Gilson's view, vulnerability grounds dependency and corresponding obligations of care and concern. She suggests that vulnerability should not be viewed as hindering autonomy and independence, but rather as making them possible in the first place. Dodds, in contrast, identifies dependency as a *form* of vulnerability that "requires the support of a specific person (or people)—that is, care" (Dodds, 2014, pp. 182–183). On Dodds's account, being in a state of dependency and receiving care—be it in familial, social, or institutional contexts— need not be a hindrance to one's agency and sense of independence, but rather can be a condition in which they are fostered.

These accounts of dependency provide important insights into basic conceptual elements of vulnerability. We agree with Gilson that vulnerability is not necessarily a state or condition from which one *suffers*, but rather it is, at least in part, a state in which one is opened to being affected by one's natural and social environments. Moreover, recognizing ourselves as vulnerable—and being recognized by and responded to appropriately by others given our vulnerability— typically enables social relationships such as filial and erotic love to flourish. Indeed, in the context of loving relationships in which one embraces and does not deny one's own vulnerability, one might feel oneself to be most recognized, most cared-for, and most self-possessed (Straehle, 2017). Still, something seems to have been lost in Gilson's account of vulnerability; namely, the difference between, on the one hand, being open and receptive to these environments in a variety of ways, and, on the other hand, our susceptibility to being injured, afflicted, and wronged within these environments. Lest it be so emptied of content that it either reduces to or can no longer be distinguished from the broad concepts of experiential passivity and receptivity, we should understand the concept of vulnerability as including the possibility of being *wounded* and as picking out the condition of being at risk of being harmed, exploited, or afflicted within particular relational, environmental, or institutional contexts. Indeed, one can consistently maintain both that many of the basic and secondary human conditions that render us susceptible to harm—for example, embodiment, dependency, cognitive and physiological traits, social situatedness—also open opportunities for enhancing our well-being and agency through relationships of care, respect, and cooperation. But this means, in contrast to Dodds, that we do not take vulnerability to be a form or species of dependency, insofar as it is *grounded in* and *consequential to* dependency (or other basic and secondary human conditions). Vulnerability, moreover, seems to be a *normative* dimension of such basic and relational properties of the human condition (Deem, 2017). Our embodiment, relations of dependency and trust, and social and environmental situatedness are basic to vulnerability (cf. MacIntyre, 1999).

As we discuss below, there are multiple and overlapping conditions that give rise to vulnerability and that have implications for how researchers should understand their obligations to protect individuals whose risk of harm is heightened through their participation in research. But first, it is important to distinguish different kinds of vulnerability, particularly if we are to address questions about when and which protections for research participants are appropriate.

Vulnerability: Inherent, Special, and Pathogenic

We all are acquainted with our own experiences of being susceptible to physical injury, illness, psychological harm, and dysphoric emotional experiences. And many of us are well-acquainted with others' experiences of vulnerability, particularly in the context of our familial and social relationships. In virtue of our embodiment, we find that we are always "at risk" of not only such physiological and psychological discomfort, pain, affliction, and loss, but also of facing external constraints on meeting our basic needs and developing those fundamental capabilities that are integral to a decent human life (Hoffmaster, 2006; Mackenzie, 2014; Nussbaum, 2011; Rogers, 2014). Our inherent vulnerability need not, however, be viewed as a *negative* condition that we ought to seek to minimize or eliminate, even if it opens us to the risk of harm, disease, injury, and exploitation. Rather, inherent vulnerability is a "background condition" of human life, constituted by the limitations, fragility, and dependence that mark our universal, embodied nature (Straehle, 2016). However, it is this background condition of inherent vulnerability that makes possible those situations in which we or others face a heightened risk of harm that may be viewed as morally problematic and as generating moral obligations to respond in ways that eliminate, mitigate, or compensate for that risk.

Recent philosophical and bioethical accounts of vulnerability have drawn an important distinction between vulnerability understood as an inherent condition of human life and vulnerability that strikes us as morally problematic and as calling for some kind of response on the part of others to address, mitigate, or eliminate its sources (Guidry-Grimes & Victor, 2012; Hurst, 2008; Martin et al.,

2014; Rogers et al., 2012). It is this *special*, or *situational* vulnerability that seems to generate the kind of moral and social concern that nursing ethics has traditionally associated with care and research involving vulnerable populations. In contrast to inherent vulnerability, which is a universal and constant feature of human life, special vulnerability arises in situations and circumstances where an individual faces significantly increased risk of being harmed (hence, the bioethics literature tends to use *special vulnerability* and *situational vulnerability* interchangeability). The situations in which an individual experiences or is placed at heightened risk of harm are manifold, capable of arising from physiological and psychological conditions (e.g., chronic or acute illness; mental illness) and socioeconomic contexts (e.g., disparity in access to healthcare; economic status; oppressive political and legal structures).[1] Not only are the sources of situational vulnerability variable, then, but also are its duration and iterations; special vulnerability can be intermittent, brief, enduring, or permanent (Mackenzie, 2014). Insofar as situational vulnerability is morally problematic, the situations and circumstances in which it arises are important for determining who is responsible for addressing it, be it other individuals, associations, or political authorities. For instance, it may be appropriate for local or regional governments to intervene with policy and protections for individuals or populations whose health risks are exacerbated by industries that release toxic chemicals into groundwater and air. Or, a staff nurse might have an obligation to advocate for a patient suffering from a chronic illness who has historically felt that her preferences and concerns have been ignored or dismissed by attending physicians.

However, responses to special vulnerability can sometimes have the effect of perpetuating, exacerbating, and even generating new vulnerabilities for the individuals or groups we aim to help through action or policy. In their rich, threefold taxonomy of the degrees of vulnerability, Rogers, Mackenzie, and Dodds (2012) characterize such outcomes as *pathogenic* forms of vulnerability. Laws or public policy can be causes of pathogenic vulnerability. For example, we can think of laws aimed at reducing the distribution of harmful substances within a community that result in increased incarceration and poverty for the members of that community, or policies that aim to curb unemployment through reduction of social programs and food support but which result in exacerbating child hunger. Within healthcare, policies and perspectives that may

---

[1]   In contrast to Heaslip & Ryden (2013) and Scammell & Thomas (2013), we avoid characterizing vulnerability solely in terms of one's social environment. While some vulnerabilities have their sources in social arrangements and institutions, this strong social constructivist view of vulnerability may underestimate both the physiological and psychological sources of situational vulnerability and the reliability of associations that individuals make between their own vulnerability and these sources. As Tom Shakespeare similarly notes with respect to what he calls "cultural disability studies" (Shakespeare, 2014), strong social constructivist views of vulnerability may risk unjustified neglect of the material realities that give rise to feeling and being situationally vulnerable.

be buttressed by good intentions and genuine social concern can produce pathogenic vulnerabilities. For instance, in the care of elderly patients with dementia, a nurse may use terms of endearment, such as "pops" or "sweetie," with the intention of communicating compassionately and clearly about a patient's preferences. However, the nurse might not realize that he may be infantilizing this patient and further hindering the patient's agency with such terms. *Pathogenic* vulnerability should be understood as a kind of *situational* vulnerability, given that it is an exacerbated or emergent risk of harm or wronging (Rogers et al., 2012).

Vulnerability thus needs to be considered within the context of time, place, and particular relationships. This suggests that, within the contexts of healthcare and clinical research, vulnerability should not be primarily attributed to individuals on the basis of their belonging to one or more identified "vulnerable" populations (Gordon, 2020; Tallman et al., 2019; Wendler, 2017). If one only considers group identification to determine vulnerability, then the significance of the context, time, place, and study may be diminished or ignored (Bracken-Roche et al., 2017a, 2017b); indeed, one would be abstracting from the specific features that might render one situationally vulnerable. Given this, an individual's vulnerability when engaged in research participation may exist on a continuum—minimal or low vulnerability to maximal or high vulnerability—which may not be evident to researchers who rely primarily on a labeling approach to identify "vulnerable populations." Considering vulnerability situationally and as a continuum points to the dynamic nature of this concept and asks under what circumstances are special protections truly demanded for individuals (Schroeder & Gefenas, 2009). Understanding different degrees of vulnerability—inherent, special, and pathogenic—and its manifold sources can provide nurse researchers with a clearer picture of when a research participant's vulnerability should be a focus of moral concern. A taxonomy, like that which Rogers, Mackenzie, and Dodds provide, is thus a useful tool for facilitating this understanding and developing acceptable protections for research participants who are at heightened risk of harm.

While every prospective research participant is inherently vulnerable, it is a subject's situational vulnerabilities that precede, arise as a result of, or are exacerbated by participation in research that engender duties on the part of researchers to prevent or mitigate compounding that risk of harm or wronging, as well to work to ensure that new risks of harm associated with that research are not generated. In the following section, we provide a narrative account of how participants' vulnerabilities arose in the context of two research studies conducted with adult populations. This account sets the stage for reflecting on how both the conceptual taxonomy of vulnerability we sketch here and the actual experience of individuals within research can clarify the particular protections that researchers owe to research participants.

Illustrative Research Scenarios

One of us (JAE) has conducted both descriptive and intervention studies with patients with HIV infection, a traditionally defined "vulnerable population" using a disease category. The intervention studies with patients with HIV infection were conducted over two decades, 1990–2010, a time when these individuals were frequently shunned or stigmatized. Thus, establishing trust and addressing concerns related to privacy, confidentiality, and anonymity were foremost when recruiting and enrolling patients with HIV into these medication-adherence studies. Peer advisors provided guidance on participant recruitment, as well as advice on the study's protocol. Peer advisors were members of the HIV community and were familiar with ways to engage this patient population. Patients were recruited through HIV clinics with the assistance of a clinical liaison and a peer mentor. Individuals who were interested in participating were provided with information about the study and were asked to speak with or call the researcher to learn more about the study and what would be expected of them. These conversations were held in private conference rooms or by telephone in order to protect the patient's privacy. Once informed consent was obtained, measures were put in place in regard to placing the intervention phone calls, leaving any phone messages, or sending material by mail. Although all participants in JAE's studies were adults who were decisionally capable, their existing special vulnerabilities and the possible exacerbation of that vulnerability had to be considered and addressed throughout the length of each study. Thus, the research protocol and potential risks were reviewed periodically with participants during these studies; they were given the opportunity to ask questions and to withdraw from the study if it had become too burdensome. These measures helped to promote respect for the individual and trust between the patient and the research team, which were paramount to success in these studies as patients participated for 18–24 months.

Likewise, JAE conducted descriptive and intervention studies with caregivers and patients with memory loss. The intervention study enrolling caregivers of patients with memory loss included individuals who were often the patient's spouse or son or daughter and not necessarily from one of the identified vulnerable groups. In this study the research team obtained informed consent from the caregiver and from the person with memory loss when possible, or proxy consent from the person's caregiver. The study continued only if both individuals agreed to participate. In the caregiver study, an intervention trial that occurred from 2008 to 2014, individuals self-identified that they met the inclusion criteria. Flyers were strategically placed in the community with information to call the research team if they were interested in obtaining more information. Also, an advisory committee was used to assist with recruitment. This group offered names of key individuals from the community who were able to serve as liaisons with the study population and assist with recruitment. Websites that possible participants might frequent, such as Craigslist, were also used. The research team purchased names and addresses from subscriber lists to caregiver publications in order to send brochures with information about the study, including contact information if the person wanted to learn more about the study and their prospective role. The first visit to prospective participants' homes provided an opportunity to explain the study in more detail and obtain informed consent for enrollment in the study.

During the recruitment of volunteers for these intervention studies, we explained that all participants would receive a small amount of monetary compensation. The team was aware that completing the questionnaire booklets took considerable time, and that participants were asked to do this multiple times throughout these studies, which varied in length from 6 to 24 months. Regardless of the study arm to which participants were randomly assigned, they were only compensated for completing the questionnaires; no one was compensated for completing the intervention. The team recognized that any compensation needed to occur after each set of questionnaires was completed so as not to influence unduly individuals to enroll in or continue in the studies.

For both studies, the research team was able to recruit the sample size identified in the protocol. However, while the sample size was reached or exceeded, the issue was that the sample was not necessarily representative of the population, thereby limiting the generalizability of the findings and underscoring the difficulties in recruiting members from vulnerable populations. Fear of research and lack of trust may have influenced decisions of some prospective participants to dismiss the invitation to consider enrolling in the study. The extra time that was required to complete the intervention, phone calls, and home visits may have also deterred people from volunteering. Possibly, the time required to enroll and participate in the study was an obstacle for socioeconomically disadvantaged caregivers who were not able to take time away from paid work to be in the study. Moreover, study participation might have highlighted that they or their family members were living with a health issue that carried social stigma, such as HIV or dementia. In the end, these studies demonstrated that conducting research with individuals facing special vulnerabilities required sensitivity to the many ways in which participants were individually at heightened risk of harm or being wronged both prior to enrolling and through the duration of the studies.

The process that JAE's research team used to obtain informed consent focused on demonstrating respect and building trust between the researcher and the potential participant. The goal was more than securing the person's signature on the consent document; rather, the goal was enabling understanding of the study. The informed consent process included a clear, unambiguous explanation in everyday language about the study, the participant's role, and the possible risks and benefits. The process was not rushed, and time was provided to allow a fair exchange of information through words, graphics, or other visual aids between the researcher and the potential participant (Beauchamp, 2011). The goal was for consent to be informed, understood, and voluntary. Potential participants were educated about the study rather than just given information (Ingelinger, 1972). Pressure was not exerted on the person to sign the consent document (Henderson et al., 2007). During this process, JAE's research team ascertained that the individual being recruited understood the study, what would happen to them and what was expected of them, as well as that person's expectations of the study. Because these studies were clinical trials, the research team provided a clear presentation of what it meant to be randomized to a study arm. Since they were blinded studies, the research team was careful not to mislead potential participants that being in the study would benefit them personally or give these volunteers a sense of false hope about the outcome. Additionally, the consent process continued throughout the study to assure that participants understood the study and their role and wanted to continue. In each of these studies, some participants did withdraw from the study because of the time commitment or because the patient's health deteriorated; however, no one suffered adverse effects from study participation or was treated differently as a result of their withdrawal. The research team respected the decisions that were made.

In general, the research team explained that the benefits derived from the planned study were for future patients. However, some participants in these randomized controlled trials may have hoped that they would be in the experimental arm and receive the medication-management or problem-solving intervention. Participants may have believed or expected that they would benefit; they may have expressed a sense of optimism because they were in a clinical trial and might receive the intervention. Even though the study may seem to offer individuals randomized to the experimental arm a sense of hope, the research team cautioned that this hope or expectation may be unrealistic (Wiles et al., 2008). The research team guarded against the therapeutic misconception by not giving potential participants a sense of false hope leading them to believe that they would be receiving treatment (Appelbaum et al., 1982; Lidz & Applebaum, 2002). The research team was clear that the goal of the study was generalizable knowledge, rather than a treatment specific to the patient. Actually, in JAE's studies, the control group as well as the treatment group demonstrated some benefit; their medication-management behavior improved. Quite possibly being in a study and having their medication behavior monitored, even though they did not receive the intervention, changed the behavior of the control group and possibly led to this behavior change.

Protecting the rights and interests of participants is paramount throughout the research process. Vulnerable groups may perceive that they are being exploited or are being used or treated unfairly when asked to participate in research. In some respects, one could argue that all research participants are "used" in research given that without participants, human subjects research cannot occur. The question for potential participants is whether they perceive that they have a free choice regarding their study participation. Have their questions about the study protocol, risks, and benefits been answered to their satisfaction? Will they receive the standard treatment if they are in the control arm? Can they withdraw from the study at any time without repercussion? Are they being influenced by the promise that they will receive a reward for participation? The undue influence of a reward can be a reason that people lie about issues in their background so that they can be considered eligible for a study, ignore the study's risks or their own values, or make poor decisions about study participation (Williams & Walter, 2015). In JAE's studies the same monetary rewards were provided at the completion of each data collection to both the experimental and control group participants. No one had to wait until the end of the study to receive compensation for their participation. If the compensation had been offered only at the end of completing all aspects of the study, participants could have viewed the study as being coercive. The research team justified the decision to offer a small monetary incentive after each data collection on the basis that completing the questionnaires took time and that the participants' time was valuable.

The orientation of the research staff was critically important and included a discussion of not only the study protocol but also research ethics. Role-play was used to prepare staff to obtain informed consent, conduct interviews, and collect data. One of the goals of the intensive orientation was to boost the trust of individuals, whether patients with HIV or caregivers of patients with memory loss, which might have weakened when inquiring about or when they were invited to participate in research. Research staff were prepared so that they could establish an atmosphere of mutual respect beginning with the initial telephone or in-person contact. Individuals were not treated differently because of age, gender, health condition, or some other defining characteristic. One aspect of mutual respect required the research team to examine any biases or prejudices that they might have toward the study population given that explicit and implicit bias can hinder the development of a trusting relationship.

When JAE conducted her studies with HIV patients, recruitment was an ongoing issue. Some patients refused because they were participating in other studies. Others refused because they were frequently shunned by society and were afraid that being in the study would further stigmatize them. These individuals had experienced discrimination or were discredited for multiple reasons, including their disease, sexual orientation, and illicit drug use. They had what Goffman (1963), a sociologist, called a "spoiled identity." Society exhibited fear toward these patients. For them, employment was an issue. Patients were concerned that their privacy would not be protected and that their family members or friends who were not aware of the diagnosis might inadvertently learn this information because of study participation. Therefore, the research team only used contact information specifically given by research participants. Any messages that were left did not mention the study. Study questionnaires were sent in plain envelopes. The title of the study did not include HIV or AIDS; we instead called it "Managing Medications" as we were interested in testing an intervention to improve medication adherence.

As JAE's studies demonstrate, the ethical issues that may occur in clinical research are heightened when an investigator is recruiting from individuals who face or experience situational vulnerabilities. Yet, the inclusion of these individuals in studies is crucial. Their participation allows researchers to investigate questions specific to these populations and to gain a clearer understanding of the relevance of the findings to these groups, thereby decreasing disparities. Moreover, their exclusion from research due to overly paternalistic policies can have the effect of generating pathogenic vulnerabilities, including missed opportunities to tailor interventions for these groups, or signaling a lack of regard or respect for them in clinical research. What is paramount is that investigators must recognize that additional protections and safeguards may be necessary so that these populations are not exploited.

Ongoing Considerations When Conducting Research With Vulnerable Participants

Researchers are typically familiar with many of morally relevant interests of research participants. Common lists of such interests include the scientific integrity of the study, probable social benefits of the study, fairness in recruiting prospective research subjects, adequate acquisition of informed by the research subjects (or their surrogates), and acceptable levels of risk imposed by the study (Hurst, 2017). More recently, it has become clear that particular socially and economically disadvantaged populations or subsets of the general population are underrepresented or have a disproportionately low representation in research. There is currently a sense of urgency to include these groups (Shepherd, 2016). From a justice perspective, this underrepresentation of certain populations in research produces its own unique set of challenges and pathogenic vulnerabilities (e.g., unreliable generalizations about intervention effectiveness or safety).[2]

However, there are additional challenges that remain for researchers whose studies enroll individuals who are recognized as feeling vulnerable or as facing increased risk of harm (i.e., special vulnerability),[3] which are not commonly discussed within nursing ethics. Much attention has been given to discussions of ensuring that adequate informed consent for research is obtained, especially for participants who lack decisional capacity or whose agency is compromised (e.g., young children; patients living with dementia). And this is not surprising, given that familiar international and national guidelines for research, such as the *Declaration of Helsinki* and the "Belmont Report," strongly emphasize the importance of informed and voluntary participation in research. Less common in the nursing ethics literature—though not entirely absent—are discussions about situational vulnerabilities that persist and pathogenic vulnerabilities that arise over the duration of a study and after its conclusion. Reflecting on the conceptual taxonomy of vulnerability and the narrative account of JAE's studies above, we identify two additional sources of vulnerabilities that should be included within nursing ethics discourse.

Epistemic Dependence and Trust

When approached by a researcher about study participation, prospective research participants who already feel vulnerable or are situated at increased risk of harm may experience a sense of powerlessness. Research may be a new experience for them, or they may have heard of or read about studies where participants

---

[2] Underrepresented populations are frequently smaller and thus create issues for recruitment (Ballinger, 2018). Researchers will need to plan on a longer time for recruitment and consider using multiple sites for recruitment. Barriers to recruitment exist because underrepresented individuals may have limited access to healthcare facilities where research flyers are posted. Thus, individuals from socially disadvantaged groups may not see or receive announcements about research (Gehlert & Mozersky, 2018). These difficulties may mean that persons from underrepresented groups are not provided with the opportunity to participate in studies. Without their inclusion in research, findings may be skewed and ungeneralizable to these populations. Individuals from populations that have historically been labeled as "vulnerable" may be reluctant to participate in a study; they fear being set apart or being treated differently; they may be suspicious of research and researchers. These fears can occur because of prior personal experience, hearsay, or published accounts of unethical research practices. On the other hand, participants from vulnerable groups may be pleased that they are now being included. It is possible that they believe that their group has been overlooked or undervalued by investigators and deserves the attention that they are now receiving. Regardless of the reason for participation or nonparticipation, researchers need to be certain that they are not exploiting a particular group for the researcher's own ends.

[3] Our conceptions of feeling or experiencing vulnerability and facing increased risk of harm or wronging roughly correspond to the *etic* vulnerability and *emic* vulnerability distinction deployed by some nurses and ethicists (e.g., Heaslip & Ryden, 2013; Mackenzie, 2014).

who were situationally vulnerable due to political, social, or personal forces were historically exploited, taken advantage of, or deceived. They may be intimidated by the credentials of the investigator, the language used to describe the study, and the reason they are being asked to participate. They may feel helpless and think that they do not have a choice. In many respects, the researcher-participant relationship is not unlike that of the healthcare provider-patient relationship; there is a perceived or perhaps an actual power imbalance, with the patient often seen in a more subordinate role than as an equal (Racine & Bracken-Roche, 2019). This sort of power differential can undermine the agency of a prospective research participant, especially in cases of clinical research where the individual's healthcare provider is also the principal investigator or a member of the research team.[4] But, as one of us (MJD) has argued elsewhere, the imbalance may not only be one of power or prestige, but also of knowledge and expertise (Deem, 2017).

The researcher, who possesses knowledge about the rationale, methods, aims, and scientific integrity, stands in a position of power toward prospective research participants, particularly those who may be situationally vulnerable due to social and educative factors, or who may lack decisional capacity. The prospective research subject is thus in a position of significant reliance on the researchers' competence, ability, and willingness to present and elucidate information about the rationale, risks, and aims of a study. This *epistemic* dependence engenders a form of situational vulnerability where the research participant is opened to the risk of being disappointed, betrayed, or exploited. While care might be taken in explaining these elements of the study in consent processes, consent documents are frequently lengthy and difficult to understand. Have participants received information in a language or in a manner such as the use of visual aids that they can understand? Do they comprehend the goals of the study and its procedures as will be applied to them? Do they understand the potential risks? And have they had an opportunity to ask questions? Can one say unequivocally that the consenting adult participant fully understands why they have been asked to participate and what the study entails? Participants may not know which questions to ask, even though they have an opportunity and are encouraged to ask questions of the researcher. The explanations that the researcher provides may not be very clear and may only add to the participant's confusion. Also, researchers are testing one or more hypotheses in their study; however, until the study is completed, they do not know what they will find. The study has been designed based on current knowledge and understanding with the goal to build on that knowledge and develop new theories, treatments,

---

[4] Researchers need to be cautious that they do not instill the idea of the therapeutic misconception in the mind of the participant such that the individual believes that being in the study will be of personal benefit (Appelbaum et al., 1982; Lidz & Applebaum, 2002).

and therapies. Much of this information, therefore, remains opaque to research participants. An additional concern is whether the health literacy of the potential participant has been considered during the consent process, which would be a situational vulnerability that could be exacerbated in the context of the study. Even consenting, decisionally capable adults may not fully understand what the study entails, even though their questions seem to have been answered and they have provided documented informed consent. Signed, IRB-approved consent forms, after all, do not alone render the process ethical.

Insofar as this epistemic gulf cannot be fully bridged in clinical research, epistemic dependence remains a source of situational vulnerability throughout the duration of participation in the study. Researchers, then, have a duty to safeguard the *trust* that is placed in them by research participants. Trust—a second source of vulnerability for research participants—involves an attitude of optimism on the part of one who trusts toward the competence of the one trusted to perform the expected task or fulfill the expected role (Jones, 1996; McLeod, 2002). Trust also involves an expectation that the trusted one is committed to fulfilling that role (Hawley, 2014). As JAE's studies show, fostering and honoring research subjects' trust requires far more from researchers than conducting appropriate consenting procedures. Appropriate moral response to the situational vulnerability engendered by epistemic dependence would not terminate in a properly conducted consent process, but rather extends through the duration of the study—including safeguarding the participant's trust that their prerogative to continue in or withdraw from the study will be honored. Thus, virtually *all* research participants are rendered situationally vulnerable with respect to the relation of trust formed with the research team, and that degree of vulnerability may vary according to the degree to which each participant is layered with other forms of vulnerability.

Continuing to Label Populations as "Vulnerable"

Throughout this chapter, we have intentionally characterized vulnerability in research as a condition that primarily affects individuals, rather than populations. We might ask: What are we then to make of nursing ethics' propensity to use the language of "vulnerable populations"? Should we jettison the term from nursing ethics discourse?

Even the most stalwart advocate of retaining the term *vulnerable populations* would admit that the individuals who fall within a pre-established vulnerable group are not necessarily experiencing or facing the same degree or even the same forms of situational vulnerabilities when compared to each other. For example, while King Charles III of the United Kingdom might be grouped among a pre-specified population of "elderly men," few would be under the illusion that he likely faces the same vulnerabilities (at the time of writing this chapter) as other male septuagenarians, let alone the same degree of vulnerability attached to, say, socioeconomic conditions.[5] So, the mere labeling of certain groups as "vulnerable"—such as young children, individuals with dementia or other agency-compromising conditions, human fetuses, historically marginalized communities—provides very little by way of ethical *guidance* to researchers for responding to the situational vulnerabilities of prospective research participants. Moreover, because situational vulnerability is context dependent and comparative, individuals who are members of a traditionally or newly identified category of vulnerable population cannot plausibly be taken to be in need of the same across-the-board protections. Even those who may have the same health condition—for example, the participants in JAE's study involving patients with HIV—were not affected by that condition in the same way. Painting all in a "vulnerable population" with the same brush could distract researchers from individual differences in the degrees and forms of situational vulnerabilities affecting each individual.

Given this comparative factor, one could argue that some persons within a specific group are even more vulnerable than others. One way to circumvent this issue would be to change our terminology from "vulnerable" populations to "special," "diverse," "distinct," "disparate," or "unique" populations. Using a different term has the potential to alter the traditional thinking away from notions of helplessness and defenselessness when considering vulnerable populations. On the other hand, using new terminology would require crystallization of adequate definitions and their widespread acceptance, potentially leading to similar misunderstandings to those which the label "vulnerable populations" generates. Additionally, any of these alternative terms might face similar scrutiny and be viewed as being too narrow and possibly discriminatory. Thus, as noted above, a challenge for researchers is to clearly and specifically define their understanding of "vulnerability" within their proposed study to avoid confusion and misinterpretation, and to use the term in a consistent and clear manner from the study's inception to its dissemination. Ultimately, it is individuals, not populations, who experience and face vulnerability due to a multitude of individual and social factors. Speaking strictly in terms of "vulnerable populations" not only ignores these nuances, but also may inadvertently result in stereotyping individuals, thereby engendering new, pathogenic vulnerabilities within research.

An additional, related concern is that discourse about "vulnerable populations" in nursing ethics education and nursing research tends to rigidify

---

[5] This is a variation on Heaslip's (2013) Queen Elizabeth II example.

the term, which might result in thinking about "vulnerable populations" as facing similar or the same kinds of risks. The conditions under which, say, a human fetus or a young child is vulnerable in an immunization clinical trial are not the same as those conditions that render an adult with decisional capacity vulnerable in a genomic research study or a decisionally incapacitated patient vulnerable in a hospice intervention trial. Moreover, labeling populations "vulnerable" without discriminating among individual differences could adversely affect both an individual's self-conception and how that individual is viewed and treated by clinicians and researchers. So, even if we correctly identify an individual as situationally vulnerable, the labeling approach can elevate that vulnerability to pathogenic levels.

Despite these concerns, we do not think that the term *vulnerable populations* should be altogether jettisoned from research ethics discourse. A qualified use of the label "vulnerable" for populations can still be useful in research contexts. From a pragmatic viewpoint, its use can be effective shorthand for noting that certain individuals from (sub)populations may be at a higher risk of harm or having their interests violated and therefore might *need* additional safeguards from risk. This would not replace the careful attention to individual variation in the degrees and forms of vulnerability, which the narrative accounts of JAE's research studies aim to illustrate. The moral response demanded of researchers who encounter vulnerability *qua* researchers, then, seems to be ensuring as far as possible that a research study does not exacerbate or generate additional risks of harm. Labeling groups as "vulnerable," we conclude, is convenient shorthand for flagging this risk, which might arise from any number of sources—inherent, situational, institutional. But labeling by itself is insufficient for determining an appropriate moral response to an individual's situational vulnerability. At best, it raises researchers' attention to an individual's circumstances and the possible effects of participation on well-being. Further, professional nursing associations are increasingly emphasizing the importance of research outcomes for ameliorating health inequities across populations. Recognizing situational vulnerabilities of prospective research participants can aid in the development of research aims and dissemination of findings with an eye toward reducing such disparities through evidence-based interventions and policies. However, as we have argued, rigid applications of the label "vulnerable populations" in nursing education and research can result in condescendingly stereotyping some individuals and imposing protections they do not need or may not want. The label "vulnerable populations" thus should be used with caution lest it become a source of pathogenic vulnerability for individuals. It is the *individual*, ultimately, who may need the protection.

Conclusion

While the goal of rigorous clinical research is to improve patient outcomes and the health and well-being of patients, researchers are challenged when designing and implementing studies that include and focus on vulnerable populations as participants. Vulnerable populations are critical to research. Therefore, investigators should not back away from groups that they deem to be "vulnerable," for without their participation and studies focusing on these groups, findings might have limited relevance for them. Researchers instead need to design carefully their studies, keeping in mind the special needs and protections that the *indivdiuals* of an identified "vulnerable population" may require. In so doing, there will be better odds that trust will be established, consent will be informed and voluntary, rights will be protected, and harms will be reduced or prevented.

Acknowledgments

Small parts of this chapter contain revised material that originally appeared in Deem (2017). MJD is grateful to Routledge for permission to include that material in this chapter.

References

Anderson, J. (2014). Autonomy and vulnerability entwined. In C. Mackenzie, W. Rogers, & S. Dodds (Eds.), *Vulnerability: New essays in ethics and feminist philosophy* (pp. 134–161). Oxford University Press.

Appelbaum, P. S., Roth, L. H., & Lidz, C. W. (1982). The therapeutic misconception: Informed consent in psychiatric research. *International Journal of Law and Psychiatry, 5*, 319–329.

Ballinger, T. (2018). Studying underrepresented groups. *Observer.* Retrieved October 27, 2020, from https://www.psychologicalscience.org/observer/studying-underrepresented-groups.

Beauchamp, T. L. (2011). Informed consent: Its history, meaning, and present challenges. *Cambridge Quarterly of Healthcare Ethics, 20*(4), 515–523.

Bracken-Roche, D., Bell, E., Macdonald, M. E., & Racine, E. (2017a). The concept of "vulnerability" in research ethics: An in-depth analysis of policies and guidelines. *Research Policy and Systems, 15*(1), 8.

Bracken-Roche, D., Bell, E., Macdonald, M. E., & Racine, E. (2017b). Erratum to: The concept of "vulnerability" in research ethics: An in-depth analysis of policies and guidelines. *Research Policy and Systems, 15*(1), 29.

Deem, M. J. (2017). Vulnerability in genetic counseling and the ground of nondirectiveness. In C. Straehle (Ed.), *Vulnerability, autonomy, and applied ethics* (pp. 138–156). Routledge.

Dodds, S. (2014). Dependence, care, and vulnerability. In C. Mackenzie, W. Rodgers, and S. Dodds (Eds.), *Vulnerability: New essays in ethics and feminist philosophy* (pp. 181–203). Oxford University Press.

Gehlert, S., & Mozersky, J. (2018). Seeing beyond the margins: Challenges to informed inclusion of vulnerable populations in research. *Journal of Law, Medicine and Ethics*, 46(1), 30–43.

Gilson, E. C. (2014). *The ethics of vulnerability: A feminist analysis of social life and practice*. Routeldge.

Goffman, E. (1963). *Stigma: Notes on the management of a spoiled identity*. Prentice Hall.

Goodin, R. E. (1985). *Protecting the vulnerable: A re-analysis of our social responsibilities*. University of Chicago Press.

Gordon, B. G. (2020). Vulnerability in research: Basic ethical concepts and general approach to review. *Ochsner Journal*, 20, 34–38.

Guidry-Grimes, L., & Victor, E. (2012). Vulnerabilities compounded by social institutions. *International Journal of Feminist Approaches to Bioethics*, 5(2), 126–146.

Hawley, K. (2014). Trust, distrust, and commitment. *Noûs*, 48(1), 1–20.

Heaslip, V. (2013). Understanding vulnerability. In V. Heaslip and J. Ryden (Eds.), *Understanding vulnerability: A nursing and healthcare approach* (pp. 6–27). Wiley-Blackwell.

Heaslip, V., & Ryden, J. (2013). Introduction. In V. Heaslip & J. Ryden (Eds.), *Understanding vulnerability: A nursing and healthcare approach* (pp. 1–5). Wiley-Blackwell.

Henderson, G. E., Churchill, L. R., Davis, A. M., Easter, M. M., Grady, C., Joffe, S., Kass, N., King, N. M. P., Lidz, C. W., Miller, F. G., Nelson, D. K., Peppercorn, J., Rothschild, B. B., Sankar, P., Wilfond, B. S., & Zimmer, C. R. (2007). Clinical health trials and medical care: Defining the therapeutic misconception. *PLOS Medicine*, 4(11), 1735–1738.

Hoffmaster, B. (2006). What does vulnerability mean? *Hastings Center Report*, 36(2), 38–45.

Hurst, S. A. (2008). Vulnerability in research and health care: Describing the elephant in the room? *Bioethics*, 22(4), 191–202.

Hurst, S. A. (2017). The most vulnerable patients in health care. In C. Straehle (Ed.), *Vulnerability, autonomy, and applied ethics* (pp. 123–137). Routledge.

Ingelfinger, F. J. (1972). Informed (but uneducated) consent. *New England Journal of Medicine*, 287(9), 465–466.

Jones, K. (1996). Trust as an affective attitude. *Ethics*, 107, 4–25.

Lidz, C. W., & Applebaum, P. S. (2002). The therapeutic misconception: Problems & solutions. *Medical Care*, 40 (9 Suppl.), v55–63.

Luna, F. (2009). Elucidating the concept of vulnerability: Layers not labels. *International Journal of Feminist Approaches to Bioethics*, 2(1), 121–139.

MacIntyre, A. (1999). *Dependent rational animals: Why human beings need the virtues*. Open Court.

Mackenzie, C. (2014). The importance of relational autonomy and capabilities for an ethics of vulnerability. In C. Mackenzie, W. Rogers, & S. Dodds (Eds.), *Vulnerability: New essays in ethics and feminist philosophy* (pp. 33–59). Oxford University Press.

Martin, A. K., Tavaglione, N., & Hurst, S. (2014). Resolving the conflict: Clarifying "vulnerability" in health care ethics." *Kennedy Institute of Ethics Journal*, 24(1), 51–72.

McLeod, C. (2002). *Self-trust and reproductive autonomy*. MIT Press.

National Commission for the Protection of Human Subjects of Biomedical and Behavioral Research. (1979). *The Belmont report: Ethical principles and guidelines for the protection of human subjects of research*. Retrieved from https://www.hhs.gov/ohrp/regulations-and-pol icy/belmont-report/read-the-belmont-report/index.html.

Nussbaum, M. C. (2011). *Creating capabilities: The human development approach*. Belknap Press.

Racine, E., & Bracken-Roche, D. (2019). Enriching the concept of vulnerability in research ethics: An integrative and functional account. *Bioethics*, 33(1), 19–34.

Rogers, W. (2014). Vulnerability and bioethics. In C. Mackenzie, W. Rogers, and S. Dodds (Eds.), *Vulnerability: New essays in ethics and feminist philosophy* (pp. 134–161). New Oxford University Press.

Rogers, W., MacKenzie, C., & Dodds, S. (2012). Why bioethics needs a concept of vulnerability. *International Journal of Feminist Approaches to Bioethics, 5*(2), 11–38.

Scammell, J., & Thomas, G. C. (2013). The social construction of vulnerability. In V. Heaslip & J. Ryden (Eds.), *Understanding vulnerability: A nursing and healthcare approach* (pp. 111–131). Wiley-Blackwell.

Schroeder, D., & Gefenas, E. (2009). Vulnerability: Too vague and too broad? *Cambridge Quarterly of Healthcare Ethics, 18,* 113–121.

Shakespeare, T. (2014). *Disability rights and wrongs revisited* (2nd ed.). Routledge.

Shepherd, V. (2016). Research involving adults lacking capacity to consent: The impact of research regulation on "evidence biased" medicine. *BMC Medical Ethics, 17,* 55.

Straehle, C. (2016). Vulnerability, health agency and capability to health. *Bioethics, 30*(1), 34–40.

Straehle, C. (2017). Vulnerability, autonomy and self-respect. In C. Straehle (Ed.), *Vulnerability, autonomy, and applied ethics* (pp. 33–48). Routledge.

Tallman, P. S., Valdés-Velásquez, A., Salmón-Mulanovich, G., Lee, G. O., Riley-Powell, A. R., Blanco-Villafuerte, L., Hartinger, S. M, & Paz-Soldán, V. A. (2019). A "cookbook" for vulnerability research. *Frontiers of Public Health, 7,* 353.

Wendler, D. (2017). A pragmatic analysis of vulnerability in clinical research. *Bioethics, 31*(7), 515–525.

Wiles, R., Cott, C., & Gibson, B. E. (2008). Hope, expectations and recovery from illness: A narrative synthesis of qualitative research. *Journal of Advanced Nursing, 64*(6), 564–573. doi.org/10.1111/j.1365-2648.2008.04815.x.

Williams, E. P., & Walter, J. K. (2015). When does the amount we pay research participants become "undue influence"? *American Medical Association Journal of Ethics, 17*(12), 1116–1121.

Wilson, D., & Neville, S. J. (2009). Culturally safe research with vulnerable populations. *Contemporary Nurse: A Journal for the Australian Nursing Profession, 33*(1), 69–79.

PART II

EMERGING ETHICAL ISSUES IN CLINICAL PRACTICE

10

A Matter of Trust

Balancing Ethical Duties and Legal Obligations in the Nursing Care of Pregnant Women With Substance Use Disorder

Liz Stokes

Substance Use Disorder

Year after year, nurses are voted by the public as the most honest and ethical professionals, over physicians, bankers, and members of other critical professions (Reinhart, 2020). People trust nurses with their health, personal medical information, and, most importantly, with their lives. Nurses are pivotal in advocating for patients, especially in situations of ethical and legal dilemmas that arise within their care. Nurses play a unique role in the delivery of care and advocacy for people with substance use disorder (SUD), which is defined by the *Diagnostic and Statistical Manual of Mental Disorders*, fifth edition (DSM-5), as the recurrent use of alcohol and/or drugs that causes clinical and functional impairment, such as health problems, disability, and failure to meet major responsibilities at work, school, or home (Substance Abuse and Mental Health Services Administration, 2019). SUDs include alcohol, tobacco, cannabis, stimulant, hallucinogen, and opioid use disorders (Substance Abuse and Mental Health Services Administration, 2019). SUD includes addiction, defined as the "continuous compulsive use of mood-altering, addictive substances" (Bettinardi-Angres et al., 2012, p. 16).

Nurses provide direct care to patients with SUD, but are also involved in all stages of SUD prevention, intervention, and recovery. Nurses also serve as champions for SUD outreach and prevention through research, legislative advocacy, innovative technology interventions, and education. Nurses may be the first and last healthcare professionals to interact with a patient with SUD during admission or discharge from a healthcare institution. An estimated 20.3 million people aged 12 and older in the United States identify as having an SUD relating to either alcohol use disorder (AUD) or illicit drug use disorder (Lipari & Park-Lee, 2018). Approximately 14.8 million people in the United States have AUD, and 8.1 million have an illicit drug use disorder, with the most commonly used illicit drug identified as marijuana (Lipari & Park-Lee, 2018). Approximately 2 million people have an opioid use disorder (OUD), with the majority of use identified as prescription pain relievers (Lipari & Park-Lee, 2018). It is important to note that an estimated 9.2 million people aged 18 or older in the United States have a co-occurring mental illness and at least one SUD (Lipari & Park-Lee, 2018). The high prevalence of SUD suggests that nurses across all practice settings will encounter affected individuals and must be prepared to deal with the clinical, legal, and ethical challenges that arise. Nurses have a critical role in the advocacy and treatment for pregnant people with SUD. Nurses must be prepared to recognize and respond to the complex ethical dilemmas that arise when caring for this population. SUD can often be stigmatized as a moral failing, rather than a clinical disease. As a result, legal consequences often negatively affect people with SUD and can exacerbate rather than treat the disease. This chapter will discuss moral perspectives regarding SUD and will address the legal and ethical considerations that a nurse must be prepared to encounter when caring for people with SUD. This chapter asserts that in response to the ethical and legal considerations raised herein, nurses and other healthcare professionals should advocate for policy for people with SUD that is evidence-based and socially just, and that addresses the true health needs of underrepresented populations.

Why Is SUD Controversial?

The ethical, legal, and social implications associated with SUD can pose numerous challenges for patients, families, communities, and clinicians delivering care. SUD is a polarizing issue within society and, by extension, within healthcare. The prevailing view within the science and healthcare community considers SUD as a public health issue and condition that must be treated clinically with compassion and understanding (Adams & Volkow, 2020; Volkow et al., 2017). The behaviors associated with SUD can include reluctance, impulsiveness, and refusal of care based on clinical symptoms of addiction, including lack of self-control, enhanced incentive for using substances, and increased stress reactivity (Nicolini et al., 2018). Underlying these behaviors is an intention to satisfy the addiction related to the SUD. Under this biomedical perspective, these behaviors are considered to represent symptoms of the disease, and not as actions that define the character of a person with SUD. However, an outdated socially constructed perspective views SUD as a voluntary act associated with neglect and willful conduct. Individuals with this view consider SUD as a "moral failing" (Jain et al., 2018, p. 374) and many laws still support the criminalization of people with SUD, who are perceived as a societal "nuisance" (Hines et al., 2020, p. 2).

Owing to the pervasiveness of this second view within society and the criminal justice system, the legal and social consequences for people with SUD can be profound. Despite research demonstrating widespread understanding of the neurobiological factors associated with SUD and mental illness, social stigma continues to create obstacles for people with SUD, such as restrictions on access to housing, food, education, and employment (Wogen & Restrepo, 2020). Unintentional structural stigma include institutional policies that restrict opportunities and infringe on the civil and liberty rights of people with SUD (National Academies of Sciences & Medicine, 2016). A disproportionate amount of people with SUD are in the criminal justice system, which is both a consequence and source of stigma against this population (National Academies of Sciences & Medicine, 2016). The collateral legal consequences from SUD, including drug convictions and imprisonment, result in widespread social issues such as poverty, inability to secure financial aid for education, and lack of employment opportunities (Vearrier, 2019). Research demonstrates that Black and Latinx communities are disproportionately affected by SUD policies, and individuals are incarcerated for drug convictions at a higher rate than white populations (Vearrier, 2019). Black Americans make up 12% of the U.S. population, but represent 62% of state prisoners incarcerated for drug offenses (Coyne & Hall, 2017). Black men are sent to prison on drug charges at 13 times the rate of white men, despite data showing that whites are just as, if not more, likely to use and sell illicit substances (Coyne & Hall, 2017; O'Neill, 2020). For example, research indicates that white populations are more likely to report lifetime cocaine use, and Black populations are more likely to use crack than powder cocaine in comparison (James & Jordan, 2018). Yet, disparate criminal sentencing patterns show that crack possession sentences are 18 times longer than those for possession of powder cocaine (James & Jordan, 2018). The overrepresentation of Black and Latinx individuals in drug offenses in the criminal justice system has implications on education and future earnings. One single conviction for drug possession may result in ineligibility for federal student aid for higher education (Coyne & Hall, 2017). As a result, minority individuals are more likely to be arrested for drug-related offenses, and they are more likely to be denied financial assistance for higher education, which can cripple future earning potential (Coyne & Hall, 2017).

In addition, the cyclical nature of poverty and SUD is evident from research that shows twice as many people who are unemployed struggle with SUD (O'Neill, 2020). Poverty and SUD perpetuate each other, as people with SUD may misuse substances as a way to cope with financial stress, and alternatively, poverty can be a result of a chronic and expensive habit that leads to overwhelming debt (O'Neill, 2020). SUD is associated with greater poverty because it results in lower productivity, reduced earnings, and lower educational attainment (O'Neill, 2020). The following anonymous story demonstrates the trajectory of harm that is associated with the criminalization of SUD.

Nicole (pseudonym) was separated from her three young children, including her breastfeeding newborn. When the baby visited Nicole in jail, she could not hear her mother's voice or feel her touch because there was thick glass between them. Nicole finally accepted a deal from the prosecutor: she would do seven months in prison in exchange for a guilty plea for the 0.01 grams of heroin found in the baggie, and he would dismiss the straw charge. She would return to her children later that year, but as a "felon" and "drug offender." As a result, Nicole said she would lose her student financial aid and have to give up pursuit of a degree in business administration. She would have trouble finding a job and would not be able to have her name on the lease for the home she shared with her husband. She would no longer qualify for the food stamps she had relied on to help feed her children. As she told us, she would end up punished for the rest of her life (Human Rights Watch, 2016, p. 1).

Nicole's story highlights life-altering challenges that people with SUD face, especially if they are pregnant or breastfeeding. Women with SUD face particular challenges such as gender-based violence and economic displacement. Women with SUD are vulnerable to domestic violence, homelessness, and are regularly denied access to necessary healthcare services and social support (Kontautaite et al., 2018). Women with SUD are more prone to mental health conditions and are likely already socially disadvantaged from lower employment and income levels (Kontautaite et al., 2018). As a result, women with SUD may be unhoused or at risk of homelessness. A study of women in Canada who were without a home found that 82% had at least one type of SUD (Torchalla et al., 2012). In the United States, an estimated 20% of unhoused women are admitted to SUD treatment facilities each year (Finfgeld-Connett et al., 2011). It is critical for nurses treating pregnant people with SUD to have an ethical awareness of competing obligations for both mother and fetus, in addition to having appropriate screening tools for identifying SUD and advocating for this population.

Effects of SUD on the Pregnant Person and the Unborn Child

SUD among pregnant people has risen in the United States and globally since the 1990s (Hand et al., 2017). In a study conducted in the United States, 50% of pregnant women consumed alcohol, 20% consumed tobacco, and 13% consumed illicit substances (Tabatabaei et al., 2018). This is a significant public health issue. SUD, specifically OUD and AUD, can have devastating and permanent effects on a newborn. AUD is the leading known preventable cause of intellectual and developmental disabilities (Roszel, 2015). Research demonstrates that alcohol use, even at low levels, can result in negative effects to a fetus (Esper & Furtado, 2019). Sporadic use or misuse of alcohol while pregnant can result in miscarriage, stillbirth, and fetal alcohol spectrum disorders (FASDs) (Bailey & Sokol, 2011; Crawford-Williams et al., 2015). FASD includes a host of physical features, behavioral problems, functional deficits, and cognitive conditions (Zoorob et al., 2014). Children with exposure to alcohol commonly exhibit diminished intellectual capacity, cognitive deficits, attention deficits, and problems with social interactions (Roszel, 2015).

Another devastating effect on infants born to mothers with SUD is neonatal abstinence syndrome (NAS). NAS is the result of exposure to opioids in utero and is characterized by signs and symptoms in the central nervous system of the newborn that include hyper-irritability, agitation, jitteriness, tremors, inconsolable crying, sleep difficulty, tachypnea, nasal flaring, and nasal stuffiness (Kocherlakota, 2014). NAS may be a result of the use or misuse of morphine, heroin, methadone, buprenorphine, prescription opioid analgesics, antidepressants, anxiolytics, and/or other substances by the mother (Artigas, 2014). Infants with NAS may require long, complex hospitalizations for complications such as respiratory diagnosis, low birth weight, sepsis, feeding problems, and seizures (Patrick et al., 2015). Research shows that infants with NAS are 2.5 times more likely to require readmission within 30 days of their birth (Patrick et al., 2015).

SUD in pregnant people can also cause stillbirth, which results in an entirely different set of moral emotions and perspectives from patients and healthcare professionals. For example, tobacco use alone is associated with a nearly 3 times greater risk of stillbirth (Varner et al., 2014). Even passive exposure to tobacco, such as secondhand smoke, doubles the risk of stillbirth. Risk of stillbirth with marijuana use is 2.3 times greater (Varner et al., 2014). Prescription pain medication, which is often overlooked and often not thought of as a drug that can be misused—simply because it is prescribed—can increase the risk of stillbirth by 2.2 (Varner et al., 2014). The potential risk of not only harm, but in this case, death of the fetus creates a deep moral divide among many healthcare professionals. The complexity is reflected in the need to assess the interests of the pregnant person and the fetus. Pregnancy does not necessarily diminish a person's capacity to make decisions for themself and their fetus (Kaye, 2021). However, some nurses may view the fetus as the more vulnerable of the two parties, which may fuel negative and unproductive attitudes toward mothers. Once a nurse determines that a mother's decisions are deemed risky and potentially harmful to the fetus, then clinicians may blame the mother or consider her a "bad actor," thus dehumanizing care delivery.

History of Criminalization

Most U.S. states have public policies to address the use of substances while pregnant (Roberts et al., 2019). Policy scholars have categorized these laws, rules, and regulations as either supportive or punitive measures. Supportive policies prioritize treatment, gathering data for public health research, and prohibitions of sanctions or criminal prosecution (Roberts et al., 2019). Some states, however, have laws that criminally punish pregnant people with SUD, citing harm to the child. These punitive measures use coercion to compel a change in behaviors associated with addiction through civil commitment or defining SUD during pregnancy as abuse or neglect (Roberts et al., 2019). However, a moral distinction that is often overlooked is the risk of fetal harm from the genetic father. A man's substance use or misuse, which can also contribute to fetal outcomes, is not screened or criminalized in the same way as the same actions by pregnant people, thus resulting in discrimination (Day et al., 2016). It is difficult to connect paternal substance use to adverse fetal outcomes, which results in a disparate effect of blame and consequences between women and men. A recent study highlights the association of preconception paternal alcohol consumption with increased fetal birth defects, but overall, research of preconception paternal SUD risks is scant (Zhou et al., 2021).

Punitive measures against pregnant and breastfeeding people have been enforced in the United States since the 1970s, with over 1,000 women prosecuted for substance misuse while pregnant (Jessup et al., 2019). There is a critical legal distinction in these situations. Most laws criminalize drug possession and not drug use. For the general population, drug use itself has not been criminalized and it is typically not a crime to test positive for an illicit substance (Bridges, 2020). Therefore, when pregnant people are arrested and charged after a positive drug screen or self-admittance of substance use, it is because pregnancy has transformed otherwise legal behavior into a crime (Bridges, 2020).

For example, in 2014, Tammy Loertscher stopped using illicit drugs when she discovered she was pregnant (Cohen, 2017). She had previously been using methamphetamine and marijuana as a self-coping mechanism for depression secondary to hypothyroidism. Tammy was transparent with her providers and notified them of her prior use and cessation. Tammy tested positive for illicit drugs and was threatened with the possibility that her baby would be taken away from her upon birth (Cohen, 2017). Tammy was charged under a Wisconsin state law for harm to an unborn child and was incarcerated. She was only allowed to be released from jail if she agreed to participate in a drug treatment program, which she refused to attend, based on the fact that she had already stopped using illicit drugs. Tammy spent 18 days in jail, during which time she suffered complications due to the stress and was initially denied the right to a physician and placed in solitary confinement (Cohen, 2017). The Department of Human Services in Wisconsin determined that Tammy had committed "child mistreatment," but a Wisconsin district court ruled that this law was unconstitutional.

Significant racial disparities exist for Black mothers resulting in discriminatory criminalization. Black pregnant people have faced years of states' efforts to criminalize a woman's reproduction (Goodwin, 2020). A notable case in 2001 involved a Black pregnant woman with a developmental disability named Regina McKnight. Regina began to use drugs in 1998 to cope with her pain after her mother was killed in a hit-and-run accident (Page, 2002). Within two years after her mother's accident, Regina was dependent on drugs, homeless, and pregnant (Page, 2002). When Regina arrived at Conway Hospital in South Carolina to deliver her baby, she suffered a stillbirth (Page, 2002). Five months later, Regina was arrested on charges of homicide by child abuse, despite an autopsy that was inconclusive as to the cause of death (Page, 2002). During her stay at Conway Hospital, a test for substances was done without her consent and the positive result was disclosed to the police (Page, 2002). Regina was eventually exonerated, but remained incarcerated for 10 years after several court cases and appeals (Page, 2002). In a similar case, Rennie Gibbs, a 16-year-old Black mother, was charged with depraved-heart murder when her pregnancy resulted in a stillbirth whose blood showed traces of cocaine byproduct, despite her pregnancy being a product of statutory rape given her age (Goodwin, 2017). Murder charges were finally dropped in 2014 after more than seven years of legal entanglements, but charges were dismissed with the possibility to be re-filed (Stone, 2015).

This discrimination against pregnant people with SUD has become a policy initiative for many organizations that emphasize the social and racial injustices against pregnant people (American College of Obstetricians and Gynecologists, 2011; American Nurses Association, 2017; Jessup et al., 2019). Coercion and other threats of criminal prosecution may affect a person's decision to obtain prenatal care, perpetuating the stigma associated with SUD and contributing to increasing maternal mortality rates (Goodwin, 2017).

Nurses' Role and Responsibility in Addressing SUD Policy

Nurses represent the single largest body of healthcare professionals. The depth of a nurse's interaction with patients often results in the nurse being privy to the patient's innermost thoughts and feelings, not only in relation to their illness, but the impact the illness may have on their life and family. A nurse frequently makes decisions that may result in benefit or harm to patients. It is imperative that nurses have the opportunity to consider their own integrity and personal value systems, in addition to the obligation to practice and contribute to the provision of healthcare, in an ethical and legal manner.

The science of addiction and the chemical disorders associated with SUD must be understood by nurses. The *Code of Ethics for Nurses with Interpretive Statements* outlines professional ethical obligations for nurses, stating: "Respect for patient decisions does not require that the nurse agree with or support all patient choices. When patient choices are risky or self-destructive, nurses have an obligation to address the behavior and to offer opportunities and resources to modify the behavior or to eradicate the risk" (American Nurses Association, 2015, p. 1). This does not suggest that the respect for autonomy of the pregnant person always outweighs other ethical obligations, such as the obligation of non-maleficence to the fetus. Some scholars consider this situation as a maternal-fetal conflict where the moral obligations of the mother appear to conflict with those owed to the fetus (Harris, 2000). However, an appropriate relational and equality-based moral theory should be considered for these situations. Nurses are often placed in challenging situations that test their personal and professional integrity. In the majority of cases involving the prosecution of pregnant people, information regarding misuse has come from healthcare professionals—intentionally or not—and was given to law enforcement officials without the patient's consent (Goodwin, 2017). Nurses are placed in these difficult situations because of mandatory reporting laws or organizational policies obligating them to do so. Mandatory reporting is a legal exception covered under the Health Insurance and Accountability Act (HIPAA) that allows disclosure of private health information to a health oversight agency for purposes of civil and criminal investigations (U.S. Department of Health and Human Services, 2000). These laws are not supportive of people with SUD, but are generally created solely for the protection of the unborn child.

Pregnant people who are prosecuted and incarcerated face significant health disparities. Prison systems are not designed to care for pregnant people, and a majority lack access to maternal education, Lamaze preparation classes, breastfeeding support services, maternity clothes, and basics such as toilets, mattresses, and pillows (Ferszt & Clarke, 2012; Van den Bergh et al., 2011). The denial of these necessities for comfort and support violates human dignity and do not foster a nurturing environment for the mother who is preparing for delivery, in addition to the potential separation from her child. The rate of miscarriage for incarcerated pregnant people is higher than the normal rate due to insufficient prenatal care, lack of access to drug treatment programs, and the general stress of incarceration (Ferszt & Clarke, 2012). Therefore, attempts to protect the child by placing the pregnant people in jail or prison could actually harm the child by putting the pregnant person in a situation associated with poorer maternal and fetal outcomes (Goodwin, 2017).

Ethical and Legal Considerations

Some states have mandatory reporting laws that require nurses to report positive substance use results to law enforcement agencies (Guttmacher Institute, 2020). Yet, nurses have an ethical obligation of veracity in healthcare which refers to truthful, accurate, objective communication of information (American Nurses Association, 2015). This leaves nurses in a compromising situation, balancing transparency with trust, which is a hallmark of the nurse-patient relationship (American Nurses Association, 2017).

In 1973, the *International Code of Ethics for Nurses* provided the impetus for other nursing professional ethics codes (Stievano & Tschudin, 2019). Currently, the American Nurses Association (ANA) publishes the *Code of Ethics for Nurses with Interpretive Statements*, which fundamentally directs the ethical practice of nursing. The *Code of Ethics for Nurses* places a strong emphasis on the realized trust necessary in the nurse-patient relationship (American Nurses Association, 2015). This trust can easily be broken due to disclosure of confidential patient information. Nurse-patient confidentiality is not absolute and does warrant some exceptions, including for patient and public safety and circumstances of mandatory disclosure for public health reasons.

Mandatory Reporting

It is the legal and fiduciary duty for nurses to report any suspicion of child abuse and neglect. All states require nurses to report child abuse, but only a few states require reporting of domestic violence (Institute of Medicine & National Research Council, 2014). The details regarding mandatory reporting of nurses can be found through the licensing board for nurses in every state. In addition, the nurse practice act of each state governs the practice of nursing. Every nurse should have a copy of their state's nurse practice act, regulations, and any other official documents governing nursing practice. Each of these documents defines the legal scope of nursing practice, and guides and protects nurses in performing their duties. To comply with federal law, all states have some form of regulation that requires health professionals to report child abuse/neglect to the appropriate agency. The goal of mandatory reporting of these abuses is to protect individuals who may not always be able to protect themselves.

In 2003, Congress passed an amendment to the Child Abuse Prevention and Treatment Act (CAPTA) requiring all states that receive federal grants to have policies in place to "address the needs of infants born and identified as being affected by illegal substance abuse or withdrawal symptoms resulting from prenatal exposure" (Keeping Children and Families Safe Act, 2003). In response

to this broad federal law, states use varying approaches to address this population. Twenty-three states and the District of Columbia consider substance use
during pregnancy to be child abuse, and three states consider it grounds for
civil commitment such as forced admission to an inpatient treatment program
(Guttmacher Institute, 2020). Twenty-five states and the District of Columbia
require nurses and other healthcare professionals to report suspected prenatal drug use, with eight states requiring testing for prenatal drug exposure
(Guttmacher Institute, 2020). States that have not yet passed laws are still required under CAPTA to have policies or procedures in place to address the
needs of infants exposed to substances, even if they are not regulations (Bridges,
2020). These laws and policies can place an undue burden on nurses and other
clinicians when attempting to care for this population in a nonjudgmental and
sensitive manner. A failure to file a mandatory report can subject nurses to criminal and civil liabilities. A nurse can also be subject to disciplinary charges by the
state board of nursing, as well as malpractice suits for failure to report. Nurses
should know the criminal and civil penalties for not reporting in their state of
employment. This legal requirement places nurses in an ethical dilemma, balancing a commitment to patient confidentiality, trust, non-maleficence, and fidelity to patients. In these situations, nurses must be compassionate, transparent,
and truthful when communicating the legal and ethical obligations with patients
(American Nurses Association, 2017).

Separation and Child Protection

There is a strong relationship between maternal substance use and involvement
with child protection (Canfield et al., 2017; Marcenko et al., 2011). Over half
of children in foster care originate from households with at least one parent
identified with SUD (Canfield et al., 2017; Fernandez & Lee, 2013). As a result,
pregnant people with SUD are incredibly fearful of detection. Those pregnant
people who fear detection avoid seeking prenatal care, thus risking an even
greater harm to themselves and their fetus. A recent study showed that 73% of
women reported were afraid of being identified as using substances because they
would lose custody of their children and face other criminal justice consequences
(Stone, 2015). Legally, states have taken different approaches in civil child protection cases involving prenatal substance exposure. Overall, state courts generally do not legally define a fetus in utero as a "child" (American Bar Association,
2021). For example, the Oklahoma Supreme Court ruled that the legislative intent of the Oklahoma Children's Code applied to human beings who have been
born and are under age 18 (*Unborn Child of Starks*, 2001). In this case, a mother
was arrested and incarcerated for possession of methamphetamine when she

was seven months pregnant, and the trial court took temporary emergency custody of the fetus based on a belief that potential harm could result if the mother was released from jail (*Unborn Child of Starks*, 2001). On appeal, the Oklahoma Supreme Court narrowed the interpretation of the Oklahoma Children's Code to clarify that it was not applicable to unborn children (*Unborn Child of Starks*, 2001). In states that allow state intervention after a child is born after being prenatally exposed, the evidence to support these claims varies (American Bar Association, 2021). Some states consider a positive drug screen from either mother or baby, or simply the mother's admittance of use, as sufficient evidence to establish abuse or neglect (American Bar Association, 2021).

In Colorado, the Court of Appeals held that despite the mother's denial of using or misusing substances and refusal to undergo drug testing, a baby's positive drug screen was sufficient to establish child abuse and neglect (*T.T.*, 2005). As a result, the state took custody of the child, therefore terminating parental rights under the child protection statute (*T.T.*, 2005). The Vermont Supreme Court decision in *M.M.* (2015) demonstrated that a child did not need to suffer "actual harm" that rises to the level of abuse or neglect. In this case, a pregnant woman with SUD enrolled in a medically monitored program for SUD later in her pregnancy but failed to comply (*M.M.*, 2015). The child was born with a dependence on opioids at birth and the court found that sufficient evidence existed that the child was without proper parental care necessary for their well-being and was "in need of services" in accordance with the state statute (*M.M.*, 2015).

It is important to note that not all children of mothers with SUD are removed from maternal care. The Supreme Court of New Jersey considered a case involving an infant diagnosed with neonatal abstinence syndrome as a result of the mother's treatment in a medically prescribed program to address her SUD during pregnancy which recommended that she not abruptly stop using opioids (*New Jersey Division of Child Protection & Permanency v. Y. N.*, 2014). The court found that the state statute determining abuse or neglect required proof that the mother unreasonably inflicted harm on her newborn. In this case, the mother's timely participation in a treatment program prescribed by a licensed healthcare professional was not an unreasonable infliction of harm, and the mother's parental rights were not terminated (*New Jersey Division of Child Protection & Permanency v. Y. N.*, 2014).

This highlights a critical aspect for nurses to consider when caring for this population. It should not be assumed that all mothers who use substances neglect their children or are in need of intervention to remove parental rights (Canfield et al., 2017). There are a host of other broader social factors that nurses should be aware of when assessing the needs of mothers with SUD. Research shows that mothers with lower socioeconomic status, criminal justice involvement, mental health comorbidity, lack of social support, and adverse childhood experiences all increase the risk of mothers who use substances to lose care or custody of their children (Canfield et al., 2017). These issues can contribute to existing stigma-associated barriers to treatment, as well as financial and access barriers (McKeever et al., 2014). Nurses should work with the interdisciplinary team to ensure that access to care for pregnant people with SUD is prioritized, including treatment for SUD, psychosocial support, and adequate monitoring of patient progress and complications (McKeever et al., 2014).

Systemic Factors of Substance Screening of Mothers and Infants

Pregnant people of color and low socioeconomic status have been particularly targeted for years for drug screening and even imprisonment (Ellsworth et al., 2010; *Ferguson v. City of Charleston*, 2001). Research shows that Black women and their newborns are 1.5 times more likely to be screened for illicit substance use (Kunins et al., 2007). Black newborns are more likely than white newborns to be reported to Child Protective Services (CPS) related to maternal substance use during pregnancy (Roberts et al., 2015). Similarly, clinicians serving patients with a lower socioeconomic status were less likely to test white women than Black women for cocaine use (Kerker et al., 2006). State-level interventions reveal that Black women are more likely to be screened for drug use during pregnancy and face legal consequences such as incarceration or losing parental rights (Harp & Bunting, 2020). Screening decisions for prenatal substance use occurs at the health-system level, and no federal mandates exist (Harp & Bunting, 2020). Clinicians often have discretion in determining which pregnant patients are screened, leaving a significant risk for bias and discrimination (Harp & Bunting, 2020), as illustrated by the following scenarios:

A patient is a Black woman whose partner came on the unit and smelled like marijuana. The healthcare team immediately decided to test the baby for illicit substances based on the assumption that if the partner was using marijuana, so was the mother. However, a white woman whose infant had obvious signs of withdrawal was not screened for illicit substance use because the healthcare team attributed the symptoms to the mother "accidentally" using opioids due to a chronic pain issue.

Different approaches to identifying pregnant people with SUD have been proposed through policy proposals for universal screening or assessing risk factors for SUD as a determination for drug screening. On the surface, this appears to be a just approach to identify pregnant people with SUD. Policy approaches to standardize clinician bias toward Black pregnant and postpartum people continue to result in inequitable care (Roberts et al., 2015).

Language Matters

A growing body of literature on SUD reveals that language frames social perceptions of people with SUD, as well as how these individuals perceive themselves and their ability to recover (Wogen & Restrepo, 2020). Disparaging or stigmatizing language is one of the key mechanisms that infringes on human dignity and negatively fuels bias against people with SUD (Wogen & Restrepo, 2020). SUD was previously referred to as "substance abuse." However, the term "abuse" has a negative connotation and suggests an intentional willingness to cause harm (Ashford et al., 2018). In 2016, the U.S. Substance Abuse and Mental Health Services Administration reclassified SUD in accordance with the DMS-5, which combined addictive disorders, such as substance dependence, and SUDs into one phrase, *substance use disorder* (Robinson & Adinoff, 2016). In addition, federal legislation was passed to encourage agencies to update all health policy language to reflect the clinical diagnosis of brain disorders and to reduce stigma (Office of National Drug Control Policy, 2017).

It is critical that appropriate and respectful language is used when referring to people with SUD. Nurses must implement person-first language (PFL), which emphasizes what a person "has" rather than who a person "is." PFL places the person before the disease (Robinson, 2017). PFL is intended to promote respect, dignity, and avoid dehumanization. The use of words and phrases such as "addict," "frequent flyer," "alcoholic," "smoker," and "pill popper" and other disparaging remarks perpetuate the stigma and bias against people with SUD and lead to discrimination and health disparities (Ashford et al., 2018; Wogen & Restrepo, 2020). As the largest workforce in healthcare, nurses are influential and have the opportunity to champion PFL to preserve dignity and respect for people with SUD and other conditions.

Medication-Assisted Treatment

Nurses' voices have the power to change the narrative and stigma associated with SUD to provide a compassionate and medically appropriate response to this disease. Nurses must assess the vulnerabilities of people with SUD and promote human dignity and respect as part of the nurse-patient relationship. Advanced practice nurses, such as nurse practitioners (NP), have a unique role in the treatment of people with SUD. In some states, NPs have prescribing authority for SUD treatment interventions such as medication-assisted therapy. Medication-assisted treatment (MAT), such as methadone, buprenorphine, and naltrexone, are well-documented effective interventions used to improve health and social outcomes for people with SUD, specifically for OUD (Brezel et al., 2019).

When considering treatment options, nurses should respect patient autonomy and utilize shared decision-making when treating people with SUD (Denis, 2019). A nurse's ethical and clinical deliberation includes discussing treatment preferences, history, and risk for treatment diversion, mental health, and psychosocial situations that could interfere with effective treatments (Denis, 2019). This reform must include nurses' advocacy for policy that is evidence-based, socially just, and addresses the true health needs of vulnerable populations such as pregnant people with SUD.

Advocacy and Reform for SUD

Nurses and other allied health professionals provide the majority of mental health and SUD services in the United States (Outlaw et al., 2020). A recent study of state strategies to address SUD in pregnant people found that most solutions focused on access to and coordination of quality services. States reported that clinicians had ethical concerns, yet very few programs addressed the ethical, legal, and social implications such as mandatory reporting, a mother's fear of separation from the child, screening, poverty, systemic factors, stigma, and mental health services (Kroelinger et al., 2019). This is a prime opportunity for nurses to fill this gap by influencing programs and policies to effect change for pregnant people with SUD. Nurses are able to draw upon their experiences caring for pregnant people with SUD, witnessing discriminatory screening practices and negative outcomes, being forced to lawfully report positive substance use, and navigating the challenges of a health system to better understand the gaps in law and clinical practice (Outlaw et al., 2020).

There are a number of promising practice models designed to support pregnant people and their families, including care that is a didactic family-based approach, support for positive parenting behavior, focus on physical and emotional wellness, early intervention, MAT, and the intervention of peer support (Larson et al., 2019). Research has shown that public health nurse-led approaches result in positive outcomes for pregnant people with SUD and strong professional advocacy to inform policy change (Stone, 2015). Pregnant people reported a benefit of wraparound care that included transportation to and from appointments, access to car seats, cribs, and other necessities, including childcare assistance (Stone, 2015). These nurses are critical in court cases and other legislative reform to attest to individual efforts to recover from SUD and focus on motherhood (Stone, 2015).

The discussion and arguments in this chapter point to actionable measures that nurses can take to effectuate their duties to people with SUD. These practical guidelines are placed in guideline format, which is a familiar delivery of recommendations in the field of nursing.

Guidelines for Nurses

- Nurses should join local and national advocacy initiatives to raise awareness of criminalizing approaches to treat SUD, provide research and education to legislators, and lead in research agendas to inform practice and policy (Outlaw et al., 2020).
- It is critical for nurses to effectively communicate with patients and provide explanation of boundaries and legal obligations of the profession, especially in states with mandatory reporting requirements. Pregnant people with SUD must be informed about potential punitive measures that could occur related to disclosure of use or misuse of substances.
- Regardless of a nurse's moral perspective about a pregnant person's substance use, nurses must provide compassionate and respectful care to all patients.
- Nurses should use person-first language to reduce the stigma and bias associated with caring for pregnant people with SUD.
- Nurses should participate in advocacy at the bedside, as well as at organizational, local, and national levels to abolish punitive laws and policies toward reform to support pregnant people with SUD.
- Nurses must be informed about relevant state and federal laws regarding mandatory reporting at all levels.
- Nurses must consider alternative approaches to treating pregnant people with SUD, including MAT, and comprehensive family-based initiatives to address patients' social needs.

Conclusion

Nursing advocacy for all patients, regardless of illness or diagnosis, is an ethical obligation outlined in the *Code of Ethics for Nurses*. Pregnant people with SUD face a myriad of challenges from diagnosis, intervention, and recovery. Nurses must have the requisite ethical guidance to address mandatory reporting issues, transparency, and veracity with patients, and to continue organizational advocacy to abolish punitive practices against pregnant people. Nurses must be sensitive to the stigma and bias associated with SUD. Pregnant people with SUD face unique challenges due to competing maternal and fetal interests. Treatment for SUD continues to be controversial, and initiatives come with divergent social acceptance, despite research outcomes. Advocacy exists on many levels, including at the bedside, organizationally, locally, and nationally. As the most trusted profession, nurses are uniquely positioned to deliver compassionate unbiased care, as well as advocate for nondiscriminatory treatment for pregnant people with SUD.

References

Adams, V. J. M., & Volkow, N. D. (2020). Ethical imperatives to overcome stigma against people with substance use disorders. *AMA Journal of Ethics, 22*(8), 702–708.

American Bar Association. (2021). *Key legal issues in civil child protection cases involving prenatal substance exposure.* Retrieved from https://www.americanbar.org/content/dam/aba/administrative/child_law/prenatal-substance-use-case-law-brief_full-508.pdf.

American College of Obstetricians and Gynecologists. (2011). *Health care for pregnant and postpartum incarcerated women and adolescent females.* Retrieved from https://www.acog.org/Clinical-Guidance-and-Publications/Committee-Opinions/Committee-on-Health-Care-for-Underserved-Women/Health-Care-for-Pregnant-and-Postpartum-Incarcerated-Women-and-Adolescent-Females?IsMobileSet=false.

American Nurses Association. (2015). *Code of ethics for nurses with interpretive statements.* American Nurses Association.

American Nurses Association. (2017). *Non-punitive treatment for pregnant and breast-feeding women with substance use disorders* [Position statement]. Retrieved from https://www.nursingworld.org/~4af078/globalassets/docs/ana/ethics/nonpunitivetreatment-pregnantbreastfeedingwomen-sud.pdf.

American Psychiatric Association. (2013). *Diagnostic and statistical manual of mental disorders* (5th ed.). APA.

Artigas, V. (2014). Management of neonatal abstinence syndrome in the newborn nursery. *Nursing for Women's Health, 18*(6), 509–514.

Ashford, R. D., Brown, A. M., & Curtis, B. (2018). Substance use, recovery, and linguistics: The impact of word choice on explicit and implicit bias. *Drug and Alcohol Dependence, 189*, 131–138.

Bailey, B. A., & Sokol, R. J. (2011). Prenatal alcohol exposure and miscarriage, stillbirth, preterm delivery, and sudden infant death syndrome. *Alcohol Research & Health, 34*(1), 86–91.

Bettinardi-Angres, K., Pickett, J., & Patrick, D. (2012). Substance use disorders and accessing alternative-to-discipline programs. *Journal of Nursing Regulation, 3*(2), 16–23.

Brezel, E. R., Powell, T., & Fox, A. D. (2019). An ethical analysis of medication treatment for opioid use disorder (MOUD) for persons who are incarcerated. *Substance Abuse, 41*(2), 1–5.

Bridges, K. M. (2020). Race, pregnancy, and the opioid epidemic: White privilege and the criminalization of opioid use during pregnancy. *Harvard Law Review, 133*(3), 770.

Canfield, M., Radcliffe, P., Marlow, S., Boreham, M., & Gilchrist, G. (2017). Maternal substance use and child protection: A rapid evidence assessment of factors associated with loss of child care. *Child Abuse & Neglect, 70*, 11–27.

Cohen, L. B. (2017). Informing consent: Medical malpractice and the criminalization of pregnancy. *Michigan Law Review, 116*, 1297–1316.

Coyne, C. J., & Hall, A. R. (2017). Four decades and counting: The continued failure of the war on drugs. *Cato Institute.* Retrieved from https://www.cato.org/sites/cato.org/files/pubs/pdf/pa-811-updated.pdf.

Crawford-Williams, F., Steen, M., Esterman, A., Fielder, A., & Mikocka-Walus, A. (2015). "If you can have one glass of wine now and then, why are you denying that to a woman with no evidence": Knowledge and practices of health professionals concerning alcohol consumption during pregnancy. *Women and Birth*, *28*(4), 329–335.

Day, J., Savani, S., Krempley, B. D., Nguyen, M., & Kitlinska, J. B. (2016). Influence of paternal preconception exposures on their offspring: Through epigenetics to phenotype. *American Journal of Stem Cells*, *5*(1), 11–18.

Denis, A. M. (2019). Managing opioid use disorder: The nurse practitioner addressing the challenge. *Journal of the Academy of Medical-Surgical Nurses*, *28*(5), 281–316.

Ellsworth, M. A., Stevens, T. P., & Angio, C. T. (2010). Infant race affects application of clinical guidelines when screening for drugs of abuse in newborns. *Pediatrics*, *125*(6), e1379.

Esper, L. H., & Furtado, E. F. (2019). Stressful life events and alcohol consumption in pregnant women: A cross-sectional survey. *Midwifery*, *71*, 27–32.

Ferguson v. City of Charleston, 532 U.S. 67, 71–72 (2001).

Fernandez, E., & Lee, J.-S. (2013). Accomplishing family reunification for children in care: An Australian study. *Children and Youth Services Review*, *35*(9), 1374–1384.

Ferszt, G. G., & Clarke, J. G. (2012). Health care of pregnant women in US state prisons. *Journal of Health Care for the Poor and Underserved*, *23*(2), 557–569.

Finfgeld-Connett, D., Bloom, T. L., & Johnson, E. D. (2011). Perceived competency and resolution of homelessness among women with substance abuse problems. *Qualitative Health Research*, *22*(3), 416–427.

Goodwin, M. (2017). How the criminalization of pregnancy robs women of reproductive autonomy. *Hastings Center Report*, *47*(S3), S19–S27.

Goodwin, M. (2020). *Policing the womb: Invisible women and the criminalization of motherhood*. Cambridge University Press.

Guttmacher Institute. (2020). *Substance use during pregnancy*. Retrieved from https://www.guttmacher.org/state-policy/explore/substance-use-during-pregnancy.

Hand, D. J., Short, V. L., & Abatemarco, D. J. (2017). Substance use, treatment, and demographic characteristics of pregnant women entering treatment for opioid use disorder differ by United States census region. *Journal of Substance Abuse Treatment*, *76*, 58–63.

Harp, K. L. H., & Bunting, A. M. (2020). The racialized nature of child welfare policies and the social control of Black bodies. *Social Politics*, *27*(2), 258–281.

Harris, L. H. (2000). Rethinking maternal-fetal conflict: Gender and equality in perinatal ethics. *Obstetrics & Gynecology*, *96*(5, Part 1), 786–791.

Hines, S., Carey, T. A., Hirvonen, T., Martin, K., & Cibich, M. (2020). Effectiveness and appropriateness of culturally adapted approaches to treating alcohol use disorders in Indigenous people: A mixed-methods systematic review protocol. *JBI Evidence Synthesis*, *18*(5), 1100–1107.

Human Rights Watch (2016, October 12). Every 25 seconds: The human toll of criminalizing drug use in the United States. https://www.hrw.org/report/2016/10/12/every-25-seconds/human-toll-criminalizing-drug-use-united-states

Institute of Medicine & National Research Council. (2014). *New directions in child abuse and neglect research*. National Academies Press.

Jain, A., Christopher, P., & Appelbaum, P. S. (2018). Civil commitment for opioid and other substance use disorders: Does it work? *Psychiatric Services*, *69*(4), 374–376.

James, K., & Jordan, A. (2018). The opioid crisis in Black communities. *Journal of Law, Medicine & Ethics*, *46*(2), 404–421.

Jessup, M. A., Oerther, S. E., Gance-Cleveland, B., Cleveland, L. M., Czubaruk, K. M., Byrne, M. W., D'Apolito, K., Adams, S. M., Braxter, B. J., & Martinez-Rogers, N (2019). Pregnant and parenting women with a substance use disorder: Actions and policy for enduring therapeutic practice. *Nursing Outlook*, *67*(2), 199–204.

Kaye, D. K. (2021). Lay persons' perception of the requirements for research in emergency obstetric and newborn care. *BMC Medical Ethics*, *22*(1), 1–13.

Keeping Children and Families Safe Act of 2003, 117 Stat. 800, 809 C.F.R. § § 114(b)(1)(B)(ii) (2003).

Kerker, B. D., Leventhal, J. M., Schlesinger, M., & Horwitz, S. M. (2006). Racial and ethnic disparities in medical history taking: Detecting substance use among low-income pregnant women. *Ethnicity and Disease, 16*(1), 28–34.

Kocherlakota, P. (2014). Neonatal abstinence syndrome. *Pediatrics, 134*(2), e547.

Kontautaite, A., Matyushina-Ocheret, D., Plotko, M., Golichenko, M., Kalvet, M., & Antonova, L. (2018). Study of human rights violations faced by women who use drugs in Estonia. *Harm Reduction Journal, 15*(54), 1–15.

Kroelinger, C. D., Rice, M. E., Cox, S., Hickner, H. R., Weber, M. K., Romero, L., Ko, J. Y., Addison, D., Mueller, T., Shapiro-Mendoza, C. & Fehrenbach, S. N. (2019). State strategies to address opioid use disorder among pregnant and postpartum women and infants prenatally exposed to substances, including infants with neonatal abstinence syndrome. *Morbidity & Mortality Weekly Report, 68*(36), 777–783. https://doi.org/10.15585/mmwr.mm6836a1.

Kunins, H. V., Bellin, E., Chazotte, C., Du, E., & Arnsten, J. H. (2007). The effect of race on provider decisions to test for illicit drug use in the peripartum setting. *Journal of Women's Health, 16*(2), 245–255.

Larson, J. J., Graham, D. L., Singer, L. T., Beckwith, A. M., Terplan, M., Davis, J. M., Martinez, J., & Bada, H. S. (2019). Cognitive and behavioral impact on children exposed to opioids during pregnancy. *Pediatrics, 144*(2), e20190514.

Lipari, R., & Park-Lee, E. (2018). Key substance use and mental health indicators in the United States: Results from the 2018 national survey on drug use and health. *SAMHSA*. Retrieved from https://store.samhsa.gov/system/files/pep19-5068.pdf.

M.M., No. 133 A.3d 379 ((Vt. 2015) 2015).

Marcenko, M. O., Lyons, S. J., & Courtney, M. (2011). Mothers' experiences, resources and needs: The context for reunification. *Children and Youth Services Review, 33*(3), 431–438.

McKeever, A. E., Spaeth-Brayton, S., & Sheerin, S. (2014). The role of nurses in comprehensive care management of pregnant women with drug addiction. *Nursing for Women's Health, 18*(4), 284–293.

National Academies of Sciences & Medicine. (2016). *Ending discrimination against people with mental and substance use disorders: The evidence for stigma change*. Retrieved from https://www.ncbi.nlm.nih.gov/books/NBK384915/.

New Jersey Division of Child Protection & Permanency v. Y. N., No. 104 A.3d 244 (N.J. 2014).

Nicolini, M., Vandenberghe, J., & Gastmans, C. (2018). Substance use disorder and compulsory commitment to care: A care-ethical decision-making framework. *Scandinavian Journal of Caring Sciences, 32*(3), 1237–1246.

O'Neill, T. (2020). *Incarceration and poverty in the United States*. Retrieved from https://www.americanactionforum.org/print/?url=https://www.americanactionforum.org/research/incarceration-and-poverty-in-the-united-states/.

Office of National Drug Control Policy. (2017). Memorandum to heads of executive departments and agencies. Retrieved from https://www.whitehouse.gov/sites/whitehouse.gov/files/images/Memo%20-%20Changing%20Federal%20Terminology%20Regrading%20Substance%20Use%20and%20Substance%20Use%20Disorders.pdf.

Outlaw, F. H., Coffey, J., Diehl, S. M., & Bradley, P. K. (2020). The unfulfilled promise of mental health and addiction parity. In D. J. Mason, G. A. Perez, M. R. McLemore, & E. L. Dickson (Eds.), *Policy & politics in nursing and health care-e-book* (p. 203). Elsevier.

Page, D. (2002). The homicide by child abuse conviction of Regina McKnight. *Howard Law Journal, 46*, 363.

Patrick, S. W., Burke, J. F., Biel, T. J., Auger, K. A., Goyal, N. K., & Cooper, W. O. (2015). Risk of hospital readmission among infants with neonatal abstinence syndrome. *Hospital Pediatrics, 5*(10), 513–519.

Reinhart, R. (2020, January 6). Nurses continue to rate highest in honesty, ethics. *Gallup*. Retrieved from https://news.gallup.com/poll/274673/nurses-continue-rate-highest-honesty-ethics.aspx.

Roberts, S. C. M., Mericle, A. A., Subbaraman, M. S., Thomas, S., Treffers, R. D., Delucchi, K. L., & Kerr, W. C. (2019). State policies targeting alcohol use during pregnancy and alcohol use among pregnant women 1985–2016: Evidence from the behavioral risk factor surveillance system. *Women's Health Issues, 29*(3), 213–221.

Roberts, S. C. M., Zahnd, E., Sufrin, C., & Armstrong, M. A. (2015). Does adopting a prenatal substance use protocol reduce racial disparities in CPS reporting related to maternal drug use? A California case study. *Journal of Perinatology, 35*(2), 146–150.

Robinson, S. M. (2017). "Alcoholic" or "person with alcohol use disorder"? Applying person-first diagnostic terminology in the clinical domain. *Substance Abuse, 38*(1), 9–14.

Robinson, S. M., & Adinoff, B. (2016). The classification of substance use disorders: Historical, contextual, and conceptual considerations. *Behavioral Sciences (Basel, Switzerland), 6*(3), 18.

Roszel, E. L. (2015). Central nervous system deficits in fetal alcohol spectrum disorder. The Nurse Practitioner, 40(4), 24–33.

Stievano, A., & Tschudin, V. (2019). The ICN code of ethics for nurses: A time for revision. *International Nursing Review, 66*(2), 154–156.

Stone, R. (2015). Pregnant women and substance use: Fear, stigma, and barriers to care. *Health & Justice, 3*(1), 2.

Substance Abuse and Mental Health Services Administration. (2019). *Substance use disorders.* Retrieved from https://www.samhsa.gov/find-help/disorders.

T.T., No. 128 P.3d 328 (Colo. Ct. App. 2005).

Tabatabaei, S. M., Behmanesh-Pour, F., Salimi-Khorashad, A., Zaboli, M., Sargazi-Moakhar, Z., & Shaare-Mollashahi, S. (2018). Substance abuse and its associated factors among pregnant women: A cross-sectional study in the southeast of Iran. *Addiction & Health, 10*(3), 162.

Torchalla, I., Strehlau, V., Li, K., Schuetz, C., & Krausz, M. (2012). The association between childhood maltreatment subtypes and current suicide risk among homeless men and women. *Child Maltreatment, 17*(2), 132–143.

U.S. Department of Health and Human Services. (2000). Uses and disclosures for which an opportunity to agree or object is not required. Pub. L. No. Title 45, Public Welfare, Part 164, Security and Privacy.

Unborn Child of Starks, 18 P.3d 342, 2001 OK 6 (Okla. 2001).

Van den Bergh, B. J., Gatherer, A., Fraser, A., & Moller, L. (2011). Imprisonment and women's health: Concerns about gender sensitivity, human rights and public health. *Bulletin of the World Health Organization, 89*(9), 689–694.

Varner, M. W., Silver, R. M., Rowland Hogue, C. J., Willinger, M., Parker, C. B., Thorsten, V. R., Goldenberg, R. L., Saade, G. R., Dudley, D. J., Coustan, D. & Stoll, B.; Human Development Stillbirth Collaborative Research. (2014). Association between stillbirth and illicit drug use and smoking during pregnancy. *Obstetrics and Gynecology, 123*(1), 113–125.

Vearrier, L. (2019). The value of harm reduction for injection drug use: A clinical and public health ethics analysis. *Disease-a-Month, 65*(5), 119–141.

Volkow, N. D., Poznyak, V., Saxena, S., Gerra, G., & Network, U.-W. I. I. S. (2017). Drug use disorders: Impact of a public health rather than a criminal justice approach. *World Psychiatry, 16*(2), 213–214.

Wogen, J., & Restrepo, M. T. (2020). Human rights, stigma, and substance use. *Health and Human Rights, 22*(1), 51–60.

Zhou, Q., Song, L., Chen, J., Wang, Q., Shen, H., Zhang, S., & Li, X. (2021). Association of preconception paternal alcohol consumption with increased fetal birth defect risk. *JAMA Pediatrics, 175*(7), 742–743.

Zoorob, R. J., Durkin, K. M., Gonzalez, S. J., & Adams, S. (2014). Training nurses and nursing students about prevention, diagnoses, and treatment of fetal alcohol spectrum disorders. *Nurse Education in Practice, 14*(4), 338–344.

11

The Ethical Rationale for Comprehensive Neonatal Intensive Care Unit Follow-Up

Angel C. Carter and Brian S. Carter

Ethical discussions regarding the limits of viability, the appropriate care of a fetal diagnosis, and care decisions in the neonatal intensive care unit (NICU) are more prevalent than ever before. Yet discussions regarding the ethical ramifications of the post-NICU follow-up care of the "products" of these early discussions—that is, the children we often refer to as "NICU graduates"—are still generally absent. These children may have several conditions at birth which may require long-term follow-up and special healthcare services. While nurses may play a crucial role in the deliberation of decision-making of the NICU, it is the nurse participating in the follow-up care of the NICU graduate who most confronts the care of these conditions and associated ethical issues.

The authors realize that this topic may represent somewhat of a novelty in clinical bioethics. As the care of these children requires interdisciplinary expertise, the joint efforts of nurses, advance practice nurses, and physicians together are aimed at the provision of comprehensive services designed to meet the many needs of NICU graduates and their families. Unlike the characteristic ethical dilemmas encountered in the NICU, those requiring attention in the outpatient clinics rarely revolve around life-and-death matters but attend to the significant ongoing needs of the most vulnerable patients, be they extremely premature or full-term yet critically ill.

The nursing perspective of ethical care has historical foundations arising from Florence Nightingale, the founder of modern nursing, whose belief was that the primary ethical responsibility of the nurse was the care of the patient (Nightingale, 1969). The Nightingale Pledge, a modified Hippocratic Oath inspired by the teachings of Florence Nightingale, became the basis for the current nursing code of ethics (Epstein & Turner, 2015). While many ethical discussions may highlight the work of Beauchamp and Childress (1979), and the principles of bioethics of respect for autonomy, non-maleficence, beneficence, and justice, we use the nursing codes as a way of illuminating the foundations of nursing as different from, and adjunctive to, what may be, arguably, the "medicalized" framework of bioethics (Fowler, 2017). These codes derived from the foundations of nursing as a "moral tradition" with a primary call to service, the belief that this call to service is not only for the patient but also in service to society, and that this service requires not just attention to the individual body but to the active participation in reformation of social injustices which impact the health of the patient, their families, and society (Fowler, 2017). Thus, the *Code of Ethics* of the American Nurses Association (ANA) and the *Fundamental Nursing Principles in Patient Care* developed by the National Association of Neonatal Nurses (NANN) serve as a framework as we discuss the issues surrounding follow-up of NICU graduates (American Nurses Association, 2015; National Association of Neonatal Nurses, n.d.). This chapter presents the nurse's role, acting within the professional codes, in the ethical issues of (a) care coordination, (b) liaising with community-based pediatric-specific resource capacity, (c) social determinants of health (SDH), and (d) the use of follow-up data to inform perinatal-neonatal counseling and the development of NICU best practices.

The NICU Graduate

Graduates of the NICU may require several specialty resources at discharge, or acquire the need following their discharge, and many develop chronic health conditions. These children are hereafter referred to as "children with special healthcare needs" (CSHCN). The designation of CSHCN was made when identifying a population of children with complex long-term needs and was defined by the Maternal Child Health Bureau (and later adopted by the AAP) as: "children with special healthcare needs are those who have or are at increased risk for a chronic physical, developmental, behavioral, or emotional condition and who also require health and related services of a type or amount beyond that required by children generally" (McPherson & Arango, 1998, p. 138). These include those who discharge home as "technology-dependent" (requiring mechanical ventilation, feeding tubes, or other medical equipment), infants with complex surgical interventions requiring follow-up, congenital heart disease, those with known severe neurodevelopmental impairment, many with genetic diagnoses, and the extremely premature/extremely low birth weight (ELBW) infant. To further distinguish CSHCN with such complex chronic conditions from CSHCN with chronic care needs arising from conditions such as asthma or diabetes, among others, the designation "children with medical complexity" (CMC) is given to former group (Turchi et al., 2014). Our primary focus in this chapter will be CMC.

Characteristics of CMC

Technology-Dependent

There are estimates that 600,000 children in the United States are "technology dependent" (e.g., requiring mechanical ventilation, feeding tubes, or dialysis) and live at home, with the number continuing to grow. Preterm and full-term infants with complex chronic conditions who are discharged home dependent on medical technology comprise approximately one-third of the population of technology-dependent children (Toly et al., 2016). Preparing home-caregivers to provide complex medical care for tracheostomies, tube-feedings, and equipment function is crucial in the transition to home, since adequate home nursing supports, and reimbursement for these, are not always present to help to prevent rehospitalization and mortality (Bowles et al, 2016).

Complex Surgical Needs

Studying the follow-up needs of post-surgical infants, Willard and colleagues (2018) identified conditions such as congenital diaphragmatic hernia, tracheoesophageal fistula, congenital gastrointestinal anomalies, and fetal repair of myelomeningocele, among others, as most often requiring additional post-discharge care (Willard et al., 2018). Many of these infants go home with feeding tubes, monitoring equipment, or surgical wounds needing additional management. Highlighted in this study is the realization that pediatric surgery is primarily available at limited, highly specialized centers, and families often must travel a great distance not only for the surgical care, but also for the required follow-up. Providing well-coordinated care is essential in preventing post-discharge complications and the provision of family-focused care.

Congenital Heart Disease

As the treatment and palliation of congenital heart disease has progressed, many more infants are discharging to home with complex healthcare follow-up needs (Lantin-Hermoso et al., 2017). Chief among these needs is communication with the primary care provider regarding diagnosis, home management and treatment requirements, prognosis, and future medical interventions, if any. Children with congenital heart disease are at risk for cardiopulmonary decompensation, growth challenges, and neurodevelopmental impairment. Guidelines for the follow-up of these infants were developed by the American Academy of

Pediatrics (AAP) and the American College of Cardiology and are designed to improve the care, and outcomes, for these complex conditions (Lantin-Hermoso et al., 2017).

Neurodevelopmental Impairment

Infants may discharge from the NICU with known, suspected, or substantial risk of neurodevelopmental impairment arising from perinatal brain injury, congenital malformation, or as a sequela of conditions associated with genetic diagnoses or prematurity. These infants may encounter feeding and growth challenges, seizures, and/or physical disabilities requiring assistive devices, medication, and intensive therapies. Numerous specialists may be involved in the care of these children, requiring many clinic appointments, therapies, and financial resources for their medical/equipment/nursing needs.

Genetics

Several genetic conditions result in the need for vigilant attention to long-term medical, psychological, and social concerns for the patient and family. These include diagnoses such as trisomy 21 (and other trisomies), brain malformations, cleft lip and palate, cystic fibrosis, and numerous other identified genetic disorders (currently, there are more than 6,000 identified disorders, not all resulting in disease or disability), and those for whom a known genetic cause has not yet been identified (estimated to be 30%–40% of CSHCN) (Lichstein et al., 2022; NIH National Human Genome Research Institute, 2013). Caring for these children may also involve complex systems for communication, coordination, and medical follow-up.

Premature, ELBW

Among the near fifty thousand preemies born in the United States annually, several conditions may continue past the NICU stay. These include cerebral palsy, cognitive impairment, chronic lung disease, hearing and/or vision impairment, poor growth, feeding difficulties, and developmental and behavioral challenges. Many of these will last long into adulthood and may or may not respond to specialized therapies and interventions.

Understanding these characteristics of CMC, one might well imagine certain ethical situations that can arise in the care of these children and their families. For example, the ethical precept of justice is of material interest in the manner in which care teams attend to care coordination, liaising with community resources, acknowledging and working through SDH, and the use of data acquired in the care of NICU graduates in shaping neonatal care and counseling.

Care Coordination

ANA #3: The nurse promotes, advocates for, and protects the rights, health, and safety of the patient.

NANN #4: Neonatal nurses will respect family autonomy and strive to ensure families have accurate, complete, and understandable information in order to make informed decisions.

Statements like these from the ANA broadly and NANN specifically convey the importance of a service orientation—that of caring, protecting, and advocating—of the nurse for their patients while respecting parental authority and what parents may determine to be in the family's best interests. While parents speak for their baby and must make decisions that are informed by reliable and understandable facts, they also are speaking for the interests of their family. The family unit has now grown and must adapt to the inclusion and needs of the baby, but still, in most instances, retains a veritable identity as a family that is distinct from all others. Whether in the NICU Follow-Up Clinic or the primary care clinician's office, his caregivers must respect and understand this. It will impact how his care is coordinated, accomplished, and evaluated. For many CSHCN and CMC, his caregivers must recognize that the family's home environment may well be negatively impacted by SDH that impede access to care, their receipt of knowledge, or their understanding and utilizing resources that could support and benefit them (Pankewicz et al., 2020).

Clinical Example

Baby B is born in a regional hospital at 27 weeks gestation. He requires mechanical ventilation and feedings through a nasogastric tube. At two weeks of age, he begins throwing up his feedings, his abdomen becomes distended, and he has concerning signs on his abdominal imaging. He is transferred to a pediatric specialty center two hundred miles from the parent's home. Upon arrival, his neonatologist notes that he has an intestinal perforation, and he is taken to surgery. His perforation is surgically repaired, and gradual, small feedings are attempted. Baby B spends several months in the specialty hospital with careful attempts to resume feedings by mouth. However, he ultimately requires a surgically placed feeding tube into his stomach (gastrostomy). He has spent the entire hospitalization with assisted ventilation and now requires continued oxygen therapy via nasal cannula. He has had screening exams for conditions that premature babies are at risk for and has a mild-moderate hemorrhage in his brain (now stable) and is at risk for retinopathy of prematurity requiring regular specialized eye exams. Upon discharge, he will need follow-up for his gastrostomy feedings, his oxygen therapy, continued eye exams, and close developmental follow-up. Dependent upon services in their area, these may require home nursing, early intervention, or specialty home-based therapists, and return visits to the specialty children's center. Routine primary care, infant immunizations, and sick-child care will all need to be incorporated into his follow-up, as well.

As these children transition to home with community-based primary care and specialty services, the need for well-coordinated care, across multiple systems and levels, becomes evident. Challenges to addressing these needs include the need for interdisciplinary training, improved access to appropriate support services, and reimbursement issues for the extended time and resources these children require (Turchi et al., 2014). With the development of the medical home model, these care needs were designed to be addressed by providing a local resource for preventive care, sick care, coordinated specialty services, and collaboration between primary and specialty teams (American Academy of Pediatrics, Medical Home Initiatives for Children with Special Needs Project Advisory Committee, 2002; U.S. Department of Health and Human Services, Health Resources and Services Administration, 2013).

In a survey of families with CSHCN, 72.2% were identified as needing help with care coordination, although only 55.2% were receiving the needed assistance, and this was higher among non-Hispanic white patients who had private insurance (Pankewicz et al., 2020).

To provide improved care for the NICU graduate and family at discharge, the role of "discharge planner" was developed. This often involved few or limited face-to-face contacts with the family, or follow-up clinicians, and focused on coordinating the most immediate needs following discharge (DME, initial nursing visits, and identification of a follow-up clinician) (Bowles et al., 2016). As these children were identified to be at risk for being chronic care patients, requiring coordinated long-term follow-up, the role of the discharge planner was updated to become the outpatient care coordinator (OCC) (Bowles et al., 2016).

To address the needs and challenges of the preterm infant more specifically as a subset of CMC, a system "redesign" was proposed (Kuo et al., 2017). This was in the context of continued efforts at healthcare reform throughout the United States and was based on the premise that the preemie should be given priority in the new system due to high level of healthcare needs, significant risk of rehospitalization, and long-term financial commitments to care (Kuo et al., 2017). In this redesign, the framework of care for the preterm would mirror the existing CCM but would be specific to the needs of the preterm infant (Bodenheimer et al., 2002). In the enhanced CCM, the NICU graduate would receive a specialty interdisciplinary team based on a population health model rather than individual problem-based systems (Kuo et al., 2017). This model would include decision support, linkages to resources, and alignment with evolving healthcare systemic changes. (Kuo et al., 2017; American Academy of Pediatrics, Committee on Fetus and Newborn 2008, reaffirmed 2019).

Nurses at all levels can facilitate care coordination, whether or not they are in a formal role. It is a crucial part of the NICU nurse's care process and framework—from the development of care plans to the discharge education provided to families regarding ongoing care needs. The ethical mandate of service to patient, families, and the community is fulfilled by a structured post-discharge process linking patients and families to long-term services, in collaboration with families.

Liaising With Community Resources

ANA #2.0: The nurse's primary commitment is to the patient, whether an individual, family, group, community, or population.

ANA #2.3.1 Collaboration: The complexity of healthcare delivery systems requires a multidisciplinary approach to the delivery of services that has the strong support and active participation of all the health professions. Nurses should actively promote the collaborative multidisciplinary planning required to ensure the availability and accessibility of quality health services to all persons who have needs for healthcare.

Here the ethical guidance is directed first toward helping the nurse identify their subject. Is the nurse trying to advocate for an individual baby? Liaising with resources through a governmental or private provider of nutrition support would require a prescription for formula or foods through the Women, Infant and Children's Program. But if the advocacy is for a broader subject—say a community in which there are nutritional deficiencies associated with a "food desert," or one in which infant formula, pharmaceuticals, or necessary medical device supplies are difficult to come by—advocacy takes on a different appearance. Advocacy may move from singular to more programmatic, public policy or even legislative levels. In either case, the ethical impetus for the nurse is the desire to see the patient benefit from some necessary service provision. The receipt of such provision(s) will help to care for the patient, see her benefit and thrive, mitigate harm or neglect, and demonstrate compassion, no matter who or what constitutes the particular subject of this ethical action.

As noted in the Clinical Example, Baby B will require many routine and specialty care follow-up appointments. Communication with community-based clinicians for the follow-up of the NICU graduate is considered to be a standard of care, but the access to locally based pediatric specialists is not often a requirement, nor is "bi-directional communication" a realized practice (American Academy of Pediatrics, Committee on Fetus and Newborn, 2008, reaffirmed 2019; Kuo et al., 2017). Establishing a NICU graduate medical home, while considered an ideal model for interdisciplinary, specialty follow-up, may still not address the long-distance, resource-limited family (Neufeld, 2012). Establishing a two-way communication pathway from family and pediatric practices, early intervention programs, and locally based allied health specialty services becomes essential.

Perhaps the most key role for the nurse in liaising with community resources is in the home-visiting program for NICU graduates and, more recently, in telehealth capabilities. Home health nursing began in the United States in the late 1800s and was aimed at providing care for those too sick to leave their homes, teaching the patient's family how to care for them, and preventing the spread of disease to the public (Kub et al., 2015). Home-visiting programs for the high-risk infant vary in scope from psycho-social services to facilitate parent-child bonding, physical assessments, the provision of nursing care for technology-dependent children, and lactation and breastfeeding support (Purdy et al., 2015). A study by Vohr et al. (2017) investigated the impact of intensive home-visiting supports on the rate of rehospitalization of NICU graduates. These supports included home nursing visits by a neonatal nurse practitioner (NNP) within the first week to provide assessments, education, and communication with medical team and support services for additional follow-up. Rates of rehospitalization for the infants receiving these supports decreased between year 1 and year 3 using a multipronged, multidisciplinary home-support model (Vohr et al., 2017).

Reaching families of NICU graduates discharged to rural areas has long been a challenge. With the advancement of telehealth capabilities, access to specialty follow-up may be improved. A model of supporting families of CMC using telephone only, or telephone with video, used advanced practice registered nurses (APRNs) to participate in discharge planning, to communicate with community resources, and to support and educate home caregivers (Cady et al., 2015).

By fulfilling the ethical responsibility of collaboration, the nurse can maintain the primary commitment to the patient.

Social Determinants of Health (SDH): Conditions in the Places Where People Live, Learn, Work, Play

ANA #1: The nurse, in all professional relationships, practices with compassion and respect for the inherent dignity, worth, and uniqueness of every individual, unrestricted by considerations of social or economic status, personal attributes, of the nature of health problems.

The primacy of the virtue of compassion is evident in this ANA directive. Similarly, the principle of respect of persons is upheld as the nurse practices to care for the infant or child without discrimination against their parents based upon social or economic status, personal attributes (e.g., age, skin art, body habitus), or abilities such as English-language usage and mobility. Further, recognizing human history and societal reactions to various epidemics (e.g., HIV/AIDS—and applicable even now amidst the COVID-19 pandemic), this superlative first statement in the ANA *Code of Ethics* directs the nurse to employ compassion in the care of all patients and families, whatever illness or condition they may be afflicted with. Such compassion must also be dispensed when attending to a child's complex needs that may arise out of, or be impacted by, any number of SDH—poverty, food or housing insecurity, poor education, lack of transportation—that impact the child directly, or her parents, or their ability to consistently adhere to prescribed plans of care.

As the complexity of these children's care increased, identification and management of challenges at home became crucial. Chief among these were the family stressors that may have already been present prior to the illness, or that were exacerbated by their duration, as more time, attention, and financial requirements became apparent for these CMC. Historically, the nursing profession has addressed the social, political, and economic status of the patient and their families, with awareness of the impact of health on the community. In the late 1800s the Settlement House movement sought to bridge the gap between the social classes which emerged due to population swells leading to urban "slums," lack of education, nonexistent healthcare, and subsequent disease spreading (Berry, 1986).

In subsequent years, many organizations recognized the "social roots" of healthcare and sought to address them with commissions, conferences, and calls to action (Bircher & Kuruvilla, 2014).

In 2005, the World Health Organization (WHO) established the Commission on Social Determinants of Health to "support countries and global partners in addressing the social factors leading to ill health and health inequities" (World Health Organization, 2020, n.p.). With data from leading health organizations indicating that SDH impact population health by as much at 75%, the National League for Nursing (NLN) called for the integration of education on the SDH into nursing undergraduate and graduate programs (National League for Nursing, 2019).

Investigations into the SDH of pregnancy outcomes and infant health indicate that access to healthcare, where a child lives, whether or where the family works, social support services, and racial and ethnic [status] play a large role in determining the health of the mother/child (U.S. Department of Health and Human Services, Office of Disease Prevention and Health Promotion, 2020). The physical and mental health of the parents also impacts infant health. The relationship of abuse, trauma, toxic stress, and poverty to child and later adult health was first studied by interviewing over 17,000 health maintenance organization (HMO) members via confidential surveys (Fellitti et al., 1998). The data revealed a strong link between exposure to adverse childhood events (ACEs) and multiple risk factors for early death later in life (Fellitti et al., 1998).

Subsequent studies on the impact of ACEs on the physical and mental health outcomes of children looked at the prevalence in pregnant women of a high ACE score as a marker for pregnancy outcome. In a study of 600 pregnant women, Nguyen et al. (2019) found that 67% had an ACE exposure of ≥ 1, with 19% ≥ 4. The relationship between indicators of social and/or psychological stressors and poor pregnancy outcomes is well established and continues to be of high public health concern (Hofheimer et al., 2020).

More recently, studies into the presence of elevated levels of stress induced by a NICU stay on both the patient and the caregivers have been published. While the effects of being born prematurely are well documented, there are now additional investigations into the physiological and psychological impact on the infant of the NICU environment itself (McGowan et al., 2020). Infant neurobehavioral studies indicate that the effects may be likened to the effects of trauma and that long-term stress responses of these infants may lead to lasting developmental and behavioral impairments (McConnico & Boynton-Jarrett, 2015). For the caregiver, the impact of having a critically ill infant is well studied. It has been suggested that "the mere absence of the parent creates toxic stress" in the typical NICU, and some have proposed that any pediatric hospitalization can precipitate toxic stress in the child as well as in the child's parent(s), particularly if the child and family lack support to buffer their experiences. Furthermore, the National Children's Traumatic Stress Network recently designated trauma during a childhood medical illness as an ACE (Sanders & Hall, 2018). Many programs are now developing and applying the principles of Trauma Informed Care within the NICU for home caregivers, as well as the NICU staff (Ashby et al., 2019).[1]

Nurses, at the bedside in the NICU, are often the first to identify families with existing, or developing, stressors which may impact the subsequent bonding and home care of the infant. The nurse who is motivated and moves with compassion, seeking to benefit her patient and mitigate harms, will learn about the presence and pertinence of SDH while the baby is in the NICU. Working with appropriate social work or psychology consultants, they may be capable of helping identify which resources might be anticipated to provide support for a mother and baby before discharge. When these things are conveyed through open discharge planning communication, the NICU follow-up nurse will be equipped to act upon them and actualize the desired model of ethical care—care that is motivated by compassion, informed by pertinent facts rather than biased assumptions, and consistent with the role of advocate for the patient and family's well-being.

Application of Data Acquired Through Follow-Up Care

ANA #7: The nurse, in all roles and settings, advances the profession through research and scholarly inquiry, professional standards development, and the generation of both nursing and health policy.

The importance of data, both global and local, has been noted in a review of local outcomes:

> The outcomes of premature infants, and of term infants born with conditions requiring an intensive care stay, have been widely reported and have impacted modern medical and nursing care throughout the world. Nonetheless, center specific reports that can inform local practices are often missing or reported as general matters such as survival to discharge, or the percent of survivors having any of a number of moderate to severe disabilities. These reports and the enumerated morbidities are arguably vague markers of the impact of prematurity, or the care received and may not portray an accurate "picture" of the center's outcome. (Carter et al., 2020, p. 1)

---

[1] Trauma Informed Care was developed by the Substance Abuse and Mental Health Services Administration to assist in recognizing and addressing the presence of trauma and subsequently mitigate any further or ongoing toxic effects (Sanders & Hall, 2018).

The National Association of Neonatal Nurses (NANN) issued a position statement on nurses' involvement in ethical decision-making processes (National Association of Neonatal Nurses, 1999, revised 2006, reviewed 2010). The statement puts forth that, as active caregivers for ICN patients, the "nurse is an essential contributor to the decision-making process surrounding the care of the critically ill neonate. (National Association of Neonatal Nurses, 2016, renewed 2021; p. 2). In her study of Pediatric ICU family conferences, Michelson found that nurses often not only participate in parental updates at the bedside, but at family conferences, and afterward, at times clarifying and expanding upon medical information given. (Michelson et al., 2011; The nurse is influential in the family adaptation and management of the ICN stay. To fulfill this role responsibly, the nurse must be knowledgeable of nursing care, implications of the medical state of the infant, and the prognosis and outcomes of infants receiving this care.

Using the knowledge of the prevalence of cerebral palsy (CP) as a marker of knowledge of outcomes, Janvier and colleagues (2007) reported that many nurses, and all groups of medical residents studied, frequently overestimated the occurrence of CP which led, in their experience, to more frequent ethical confrontations (Janvier et al., 2007). Additionally, to measure the accuracy of prenatal counseling, physicians, nurses, and nurse practitioners were asked to estimate survival and major disability in ELBW infants. Statistically significant underestimates of survival and overestimates of disability were reported in all groups (Blanco et al., 2005).

In literature on adult patients, comparable results can be found. Studying adult ICU staff, compared with a patients' own assessment, neither nurses nor doctors correctly predicted the patient or his/her family member's assessed quality of life. Generally, "false pessimistic and false optimistic appreciation was given" (Frick et al., 2003, p. 456.).

While Janvier indicated an overestimation of CP on the part of nurses and medical trainees, these clinicians did not take part in neonatal follow-up clinics, hence their projection of the outcome of CP was not fully informed. A manner of addressing this situation would be for all persons engaged in prognostication to be capable of reviewing the scholarly literature and empirical data while recognizing an ethical mandate to provide reasoned and reflective counseling to families.

Other scholarly pursuits that nurses should attend to include correlates of neonatal care and diagnoses with specific needs for community resource support to aid families in the care of their children with CMC. One of the most elaborate of such examples might include the care of home infant trach/vent patients. In these situations, nurses and nurse practitioners in the NICU who care for these patients and families should be able to collaborate with outpatient clinicians caring for these families to provide data-informed insights into care requirements, clinical complications, and psychosocial needs (Akangire et al., 2021).

Conclusion

For nurses and other clinicians desirous of seeing equitable access to post-NICU care, improved care coordination, and less disparate outcomes, an ethical mandate would be to first know the situation. NICU graduates need help and often benefit from care coordination across pediatric specialties, especially if they are living with chronic and complex conditions. Such care coordination needs to be available to all children, across all socioeconomic demographics, and will require advocacy for policy changes, improved payer programs, and extended services such as transportation—be it within urban centers or rural districts. Second, advocacy for these children and families will require creative liaisons with community services on behalf of children and families. Third, the ethically conscientious nurse will learn about the pertinent SDH that impact her patient population and engage in advocacy to mitigate those things that are remediable. Such engagement may include participation in outreach community-based clinics, efforts to improve resources for children, or advocating for policies that have the potential to improve the conditions where children live, play, and attend school. Finally, nurses who learn to incorporate scholarly and empirical data on NICU outcomes can more adeptly address with families the anticipated needs of their CMC in an ethically robust manner.

Ethics is about discerning, discussing, deciding, and doing the right thing. Ethical concerns for NICU graduates remain present in the months and years of follow-up after their discharge from the NICU. The rationale for attending to these matters might be simply to assure that all the gains in the NICU were not in vain. But beyond that, these are matters of respect for the babies and their families, a continuing promise to optimize clinical and socio-behavioral good and to minimize any potential for harm due to conditions treated in the NICU. Finally, they also bear attention in our collective efforts to secure equitable outcomes for all children.

References

Akangire, G., Begley, A., Lachica, C., Jensen, D. R., & Manimtim, W. (2021). Impact of the COVID-19 pandemic on children< 5 years of age with tracheostomy and home ventilator dependence. *Clinical Pediatrics*, *60*(14), 549–553.

American Academy of Pediatrics, Committee on Fetus and Newborn. (2008; reaffirmed 2019). Hospital discharge of the high-risk neonate. *Pediatrics*, *122*(5), 1119–1126.

American Academy of Pediatrics, Medical Home Initiatives for Children with Special Needs Project Advisory Committee. (2002). The medical home. *Pediatrics, 110*(1 Pt 1), 184–186.

American Nurses Association. (2015). *Code of ethics for nurses with interpretive statements.* Nursesbooks.org. Retrieved from https://www.nursingworld.org/practice-policy/nursing-excellence/ethics/code-of-ethics-for-nurses/coe-view-only.

Ashby, B. D., Ehmer, A. C., & Scott, S. M. (2019). Trauma-informed care in a patient-centered medical home for adolescent mothers and their children. *Psychological Services, 16*(1), 67–74. https://doi.org/10.1037/ser0000315

Beauchamp, T., & Childress, J. (1979). *Principles of biomedical ethics.* Oxford University Press.

Berry, M. (1986). *The settlement movement 1886–1986: One hundred years on urban frontiers.* United Neighborhood Centers of America. Retrieved from https://socialwelfare.library.vcu.edu.

Bircher, J., & Kuruvilla, S. (2014). Defining health by addressing individual, social, and environmental determinants: new opportunities for health care and public health. *Journal of Public Health Policy, 35*(3), 363–386.

Blanco, F., Suresh, G., Howard, D., & Soll, R. F. (2005). Ensuring accurate knowledge of prematurity outcomes for prenatal counseling. *Pediatrics, 115*(4), e478–e487.

Bodenheimer, T., Wagner, E. H., & Grumbach, K. (2002). Improving primary care for patients with chronic illness: The chronic care model, Part 2. *JAMA, 288*(15), 1909–1914.

Bowles, J. D., Jnah, A. J., Newberry, D. M., Hubbard, C. A., Roberston, T., & Forsythe, P. L. (2016). Infants with technology dependence. *Advances in Neonatal Care, 16*(6), 424–429.

Cady, R. G., Erickson, M., Lunos, S., Finkelstein, S. M., Looman, W., Celebreeze, M., & Garwick, A. (2015). Meeting the needs of children with medical complexity using a telehealth advanced practice registered nurse care coordination model. *Maternal and Child Health Journal, 19*(7), 1497–1506.

Carter, A., Knapitsch, A., Carter, B. S., Noel-Macdonnell, J., & Sheehan, M. (2020). Characteristics of ICN infants and special care outcomes (CISCO). Unpublished report.

Epstein, B., & Turner, M. (2015). The nursing code of ethics: Its value, its history. *The Online Journal of Issues in Nursing, 20*(2), 1–10.

Felitti, V. J., Anda, R. F., Nordenberg, D., Williamson, D. F., Spitz, A. M., Edwards, V., & Marks, J. S. (1998). Relationship of childhood abuse and household dysfunction to many of the leading causes of death in adults: The Adverse Childhood Experiences (ACE) Study. *American Journal of Preventive Medicine, 14*(4), 245–258.

Fowler, M. (2017). Why the history of nursing ethics matters. *Nursing Ethics, 24*(3), 292–304.

Frick, S., Uehlinger, D. E., & Zenklusen, R. M. Z. (2003). Medical futility: Predicting outcome of intensive care unit patients by nurses and doctors—a prospective comparative study. *Critical Care Medicine, 31*(2), 456–461.

Hofheimer, J. A., Smith, L. M., McGowan, E. C., O'Shea, T. M., Carter, B. S., Neal, C. R., Helderman, J. B., Pastyrnak, S. L., Soliman, A., Dansereau, L. M., DellaGrotta, S. A., & Lester, B. M. (2020). Psychosocial and medical adversity associated with neonatal neurobehavior in infants born before 30 weeks gestation. *Pediatric Research, 87*(4), 721–729.

Janvier, A., Nadeau, S., Deschenes, M., Couture, E., & Barrington, K. J. (2007). Moral distress in the neonatal intensive care unit: Caregiver's experience. *Journal of Perinatology, 27*(4), 203–208.

Kub, J., Kulbok, P. A., & Glick, D. (2015). Cornerstone documents, milestones, and policies: Shaping the direction of public health nursing 1890–1950. *Online Journal of Issues in Nursing, 20*(2), 3–3.

Kuo, D. Z., Lyle, R. E., Casey, P. H., & Stille, C. J. (2017). Care system redesign for preterm children after discharge from the NICU. *Pediatrics, 139*(4), e20162969. https://doi.org/10.1542/peds.2016-2969

Lantin-Hermoso, M. R., Berger, S., Bhatt, A. B., Richerson, J. E., Morrow, R., Freed, M. D., Beekman, R. H., Section on Cardiology: Cardiac Surgery, Minich, L. L., Ackerman, M. J., Jaquiss, R. D. B., Jenkins, K. J., Mahle, W. T., Marino, B. S., & Vincent, J. A. (2017). The care of children with congenital heart disease in their primary medical home. *Pediatrics, 140*(5), e20172607.

Lichstein J., Riley C., Keehn A., Lyon M., Maiese D., Sarkar D., & Scott J. (2022). Children with genetic conditions in the United States: Prevalence estimates from the 2016–2017 National Survey of Children's Health. *Genetics in Medicine, 24*(1), 170–178. https://doi.org/10.1016/j.gim.2021.09.004.

McConnico, N., & Boynton-Jarrett, R. (2015). Impacts of NICU stay on infant development and the child-parent relationship. *Therapeutic Parenting Journal.* Retrieved on December 21, 2022, from https://www.attachmenttraumanetwork.org/wp-content/uploads/2015AprilATNTherapeuticParentingJournal.pdf.

McGowan, E. C., Hofheimer, J. A., O'Shea, T. M., Carter, B. S., Helderman, J., Neal, C. R., Pastyrnak, S., Smith, L. M., Soliman, A., Dansereau, L. M., Della Grotta, S. A., & Lester, B. M. (2020). Sociodemographic and medical influences on neurobehavioral patterns in preterm infants: A multi-center study. *Early Human Development, 142*, 104954. https://doi.org/10.1016/j.earlhumdev.2020.104954

McPherson, M., & Arango, P. (1998). A new definition of children with special health care needs. *Pediatrics, 102*(1), 137–140. https://doi.org/10.1542/peds.102.1.137

Michelson, K. N., Emanuel, L., Carter, A., Brinkman, P., Clayman, M. L., & Frader, J. (2011). Pediatric intensive care unit family conferences: One mode of communication for discussing end-of-life care decisions. *Pediatric Critical Care Medicine, 12*(6), e336–e343.

National Association of Neonatal Nurses. (n.d.) *NANN code of ethics.* Retrieved February 19, 2019, from http://nann.org/about/code-of-ethics#:~:text=integrity%20and%20dignity.-,Fundamental%20Nursing%20Principles%20in%20Patient%20Care,or%20physical%20or%20mental%20challenges.

National Association of Neonatal Nurses. (2016 renewed 2021). *Position statement #3067: NICU nurse involvement in ethical decisions (treatment of critically ill newborns)* [Position statement]. NANN. https://nann.org/uploads/3067_NICU_Nurse_Involvement_in_Ethical_Decisions.pdf

National League for Nursing. (2019). A vision for integration of the social determinants of health into nursing education curricula. Living Document. NLN Vision Series.

Neufeld, M. (2012). The challenges of discharging an infant from a Neonatal Intensive Care Unit when home is far from specialized care. *Northwest Bulletin.* http://depts.washington.edu/nwbfch.

Nguyen, M. W., Heberlein, E., Covington-Kolb, S., Gerstner, A. M., Gaspard, A., & Eichelberger, K. Y. (2019). Assessing adverse childhood experiences during pregnancy: Evidence toward a best practice. *American Journal of Perinatology Reports, 9*(01), e54–e59.

Nightingale, Florence. 1969. *Notes on nursing: What it is, and what it is not.* Dover Publications.

NIH National Human Genome Research Institute. (2013). *Undiagnosed condition in a child: FAQ.* Retrieved from genome.gov/FAQ/Learning-About-an-Undiagnosed-Condition-in-a-Child.

Pankewicz, A., Davis, R. K., Kim, J., Antonelli, R., Rosenberg, H., Berhane, Z., & Turchi, R. M. (2020). Children with special needs: Social determinants of health and care coordination. *Clinical Pediatrics, 59*(13), 1161–1168.

Purdy, I. B., Craig, J. W., & Zeanah, P. (2015). NICU discharge planning and beyond: Recommendations for parent psychosocial support. *Journal of Perinatology, 35*(1), S24–S28.

Sanders, M. R., & Hall, S. L. (2018). Trauma-informed care in the newborn intensive care unit: Promoting safety, security and connectedness. *Journal of Perinatology, 38*(1), 3–10.

Toly, V. B., Musil, C. M., Bieda, A., Barnett, K., Dowling, D. A., Sattar, A., & Dowling, D. (2016). Neonates and infants discharged home dependent on medical technology. *Advances in Neonatal Care, 16*(5), 379–389.

Turchi, R. M., Antonelli, R., & Norwood, K. W. (2014). Council on Children with Disabilities and Medical Home Implementation Project Advisory Committee. Patient- and family-centered care coordination: A framework for integrating care for children and youth across multiple systems. *Pediatrics, 133*(5), e1451–e1460. https://doi.org/10.1542/peds.2014-0318

U.S. Department of Health and Human Services. (2013). *The National Survey of Children with Special Health Care Needs (NS-CSHCN) chartbook 2009–2010.* Rockville, MD: US Department of Health and Human Services, Health Resources and Services Administration, Maternal and Child Health Bureau. https://mchb.hrsa.gov/sites/default/files/mchb/data-research/nscsh-chartbook-06-2013.pdf

U.S. Department of Health and Human Services, Office of Disease Prevention and Health Promotion. (2020). *Maternal, infant and child health.* Retrieved January 2020 from https://www.healthypeople.gov/2020/topics-objectives/topic/maternal-infant-and-child-health#top.

Vohr, B., McGowan, E., Keszler, L., Alksninis, B., O'Donnell, M., Hawes, K., & Tucker, R. (2017). Impact of a transition home program on rehospitalization rates of preterm infants. *The Journal of Pediatrics, 181,* 86–92.

Willard, A., Brown, E., Masten, M., Brant, M., Pouppirt, N., Moran, K., Lioy, J., Chuo, J., & Meeker, T. M. (2018). Complex surgical infants benefit from post-discharge telemedicine visits. *Advances in Neonatal Care, 18*(1), 22–30.

World Health Organization. (2020). Commission on Social Determinants of Health, 2005–2008. Retrieved January 8, 2020, from https://www.who.int/social_determinants/thecommission/en/.

12

Empowering Parents for Better Decision-Making

A Distinct Role for Nursing Staff in Pediatric Clinical Care

Erica K. Salter

Parenting is difficult. In fact, it's often described as the most difficult job. Children enter the lives of their parents as intensely needy and demanding strangers, coaxing new parents into positions of sacrifice, vulnerability, and uncertainty. Sometimes babies cry, despite all attempts at feeding, swaddling, burping, and diaper changing; sometimes toddlers show willful defiance despite perfect applications of the latest discipline techniques; sometimes teenagers are withdrawn, sullen, and angst-ridden no matter how desperately you try to talk them through it. Slowly, though, through a constantly evolving process, most parents find their footing and mature into parenting roles that feel authentic to their values and appropriate for their children's needs. As circumstances and children change, parents will be tossed back into the torrents of uncertainty and strain, invited again and again to adjust their practices, their understanding of their children, and their understanding of themselves.

Among the most stressful and difficult experiences for a parent is parenting a child who is ill, in particular those with chronic illnesses requiring repeat hospitalizations. For reasons we will discuss later, these experiences don't merely disrupt typical parenting practices; they disorient and destabilize parenting roles, as well. When children are hospitalized, many of the most familiar and dependable practices of parenting are (or feel as though they are) subverted. No longer are parents the primary knowledge-bearers of their child; instead, crucial knowledge about the child's health and well-being belongs to a team of expert clinicians and is (often in-expertly) shared with the parent. No longer are parents the primary physical caregivers for their child; instead, a team of skilled nurses provide for their child's physical needs. And no longer do parents feel that they can protect their child; their child's disease or condition profoundly threatens their ability to defend them from harm. Families are forced out of the familiar territory of everyday life and tossed into a wilderness where nothing is familiar. Further, these situations often position nursing staff at the intersection of parent and child: a bedside nurse is now the child's "expert caregiver"; when all other clinicians have left, it is the nurse who is left by the parent's side, helping them make sense of their experience. It is frequently in the confidences of a nurse's steady presence that a parent will confide his or her darkest fears and uncertainties.

The field of pediatric clinical ethics has historically been centered around questions of decision-making: What does it mean to make decisions in a child's "best interest"? When can a parent's medical decision for his or her child be overridden by the state, and for what reasons? When is life-prolonging therapy no longer beneficial for a child? These questions draw our attention to *particular* medical decisions and how to make those decisions. Discussions about these questions are often fruitful and instructive, but their myopic focus on the content of the medical decision itself (benefits vs. burdens, satisfying a child's basic interests vs. best interests, etc.) often means that certain important aspects of the decision-making context are neglected. For example, we have learned that applying the "best interests standard" (BIS) to pediatric medical decision-making often confuses, rather than clarifies, the obligations of medical providers and parents because there are many different versions of the BIS, giving weight and priority to many diverse types of interests (Salter, 2012). Further, the most commonly appealed to version of the BIS traditionally emphasizes physiological and cognitive-developmental interests of the child, while minimizing the relational and social interests of both the child and family. Thus, we neglect the fact that when parents are placed in the decision-making role for ill children, they often engage with decision-making tasks from a place of disempowerment and disorientation regarding their role as parents. These realities mean that actual medical decisions are frequently made by parents that question how well they know their child, how well they can care for their child, whether they can protect their child from harm, and, perhaps most importantly, whether they are even a "good" parent anymore. Making decisions out of this sort of disempowered, insecure, and fearful parenting posture, I believe, is the root of more problems than we realize. This chapter encourages bioethicists, pediatric practitioners, and especially pediatric nurses to shift attention away from the particular medical decision at hand, and instead attend to the moral and relational context of the medical decision. The way in which parents engage in the decision-making tasks set before them depends largely on whether and how their parenting roles and practices have been cultivated in the bewildering and disorienting space of the hospital. Before describing the ways in which a hospitalization might disrupt parental roles and, in turn, influence decision-making, I will briefly turn to the work of Alasdair MacIntrye and Sara Ruddick (MacIntyre, 1999, 2007; Ruddick,

1989) to further illuminate what it might mean that parenting is a social practice with specific internal goods.

Parenting as a Social Practice

Building from Aristotle's *Nichomachean Ethics* as its primary normative foundation, Alasdair MacIntyre's *After Virtue* further advances the idea that central to a flourishing life—a life directed toward its proper telos—is the cultivation of a virtuous character (MacIntrye, 2007). For MacIntyre, however, the cultivation of virtue relies primarily on *embodied* and *social* practices, rather than individual practices. In this way, virtue becomes more widely accessible and the pursuit of flourishing becomes a shared community activity. MacIntyre defines a practice as:

> any coherent and complex form of socially established cooperative human activity through which goods internal to that form of activity are realized in the course of trying to achieve those standards of excellence which are appropriate to, and partially definitive of, that form of activity, with the result that human powers to achieve excellence and human conceptions of the ends and goods involved are systematically extended. (MacIntyre, 2007, p. 187)

MacIntyre goes on to explicitly mention "the making and sustaining of family life" as a social practice (p. 188). In his earlier book, *Dependent Rational Animals: Why Human Beings Need the Virtues* (1999), MacIntyre more explicitly addresses the social role of parenting, arguing even more explicitly that if children are to become independent practical reasoners in possession of the virtues, it is because of the care and education of parents (and others in relationship with the child). I will connect MacIntyre's specific reflections on the role of parents to the internal goods of parenting in later sections of the chapter. For now, and for the purposes of exploring parenting as a social practice and how that practice is disrupted or disoriented during a child's illness and hospitalization, I will focus on two aspects of parenting as a MacIntyrian practice: the internal and external goods of parenting (also called the "goods of excellence" and the "goods of effectiveness" in MacIntyre's later work) and the important distinction between practices and a set of technical skills.

I will begin by conceptualizing parenting as a social practice versus parenting as a set of technical "parenting" skills, an essential distinction for our purposes. MacIntyre (2007) is clear: social practices are never just a set of technical skills, and indeed, thinking of them as such can easily subvert the goods and goals of the practice itself. If parenting is understood simply as a set of technical "child-rearing techniques," which may describe a growing segment of modern, Western understandings of parenthood, the well-being, needs, or abilities of the child or children in question might be ignored, or worse, sacrificed in service to the appearance or actual achievement of technical "perfect parenting." Victoria Wynn Leonard claims that a "child rearing techniques" view (or a "strategic" view) of parenting is endemic in Western middle- and upper-class societies (Leonard, 1996). We might point to the proliferation of books, podcasts, social media sites, and parenting groups dedicated to mastering specific parenting techniques: the skill of feeding a child, the skill of toilet-training a child, the skill of disciplining a child, the skill of teaching a child to speak or read. This strategic view culminates in a child that perfectly conforms to these external standards of "being a good child" (a child who walks, talks, eats, toilets, and behaves in a certain way), which concomitantly results in the parental achievement of "being a good parent." Further, a strategic view of parenting means that the tasks of parenting are merely technical capacities that can be performed by anyone with the necessary skills, regardless of the relationship. "In strategic mothering, the child is not allowed to show up as a person but remains an object to be dealt with and manipulated" (Leonard, 1996, p. 127).

This distinction is essential to how we understand the roles of parent and nurse in the pediatric in-patient setting, where the tasks of caregiving for these roles might look very similar. Consider the early parenting tasks of a healthy newborn versus a critically ill newborn being treated in the neonatal intensive care unit (NICU). The healthy newborn will be taken into the home of a family, a family who will get to know that child over coming days, weeks, and months because of the considerable day-to-day, hour-to-hour caregiving demands of the family (primarily these demands are made of the mother, but not exclusively so, and this varies from family to family). Breastfeeding, bottle feeding, and/or pumping, diapering, swaddling and comforting, providing safe and comfortable opportunities for sleep are all required caregiving "tasks," but as the parents enjoy and get to know their child, these practices transcend the function of "technical skill" and become invitations into the intimate sphere of parenting as an embodied practice of a *particular* child. These practices of early parenting are not merely caregiving tasks; they are opportunities for parents to grow into the role of parent in a way that is authentic both to themselves and their child. These practices are slowly, through trial and error and through what might sometimes feel like an endless series of monotonous chores, forging adult caregivers into parents. It is precisely because of this extended intimate caregiving connection that a parent can mature into confidence in his or her role as mother or father.

Now consider the parents of the child in the NICU. Many of the same goals are present for this baby: effective feeding, comforting, diapering, and sleeping. However, the means of achieving these goals will be drastically different and will require advanced technology and special technical skills. Thus, most of these caregiving tasks—administering feeds, changing tubes, suctioning ventilators, clothing and diapering around clusters of wires and tubes—will be performed by a nurse; the special medical needs of the child demand a caregiver with special medical skills. This, of course, makes sense, and it is precisely this access to technology and skilled professionals that often make the hospital a "better" place for ill children. However, by dislocating the caregiving practices of parenthood (especially early parenthood) from the parental role itself, we should expect that many parents (especially first-time parents) will feel unsettled and unsure of their ability to fulfill that role. Further, we shouldn't be surprised when parents respond to this disorientation using behavior that we might find problematic or counterproductive, for example "micro-managing" care, resisting staff recommendations, or even retreating completely.

If parenting is, indeed, a social practice, then it has goods internal to it which develop the practitioner in a way that could not be developed outside of parenting. Internal goods are contrasted to "external goods," which are attached to the practice by "the accidents of social circumstance." The external goods of parenting might include such motivating benefits as tax advantages, social acceptability or inclusion, to "save" a failing marriage, or to secure a familial caregiver in old age. Many have argued that intimate relationships of varying kinds are essential to human flourishing, and these relationships come in various forms: romantic, sexual, close friendships, and close mentoring relationships. Insofar as the parenting relationship is a form of intimate relationship, many of the goods internal to the practice of parenting are also internal goods to other relational practices: being devoted to the well-being of another, listening toward the goal of understanding another person's experience, exercising verbal and nonverbal skills that communicate compassion and acceptance, sacrificing your own well-being for that of another. But many of the goods internal to parenting are *sui generis* (Brighouse & Swift, 2014), as they are the goods related to the *special* type of intimate, fiduciary relationship of parent and child. While an exhaustive account of all the conceivable internal goods of parenting is impossible, I argue that the list should include *at least* the three practices described by Sara Ruddick as "the demands" of motherhood. While Ruddick's work in *Maternal Thinking: Toward a Politics of Peace* is ultimately aimed at bringing mothering practices and virtues more deliberately into the public and political spheres, I will primarily rely on the first half of this text, where she elucidates an understanding of the practices of motherhood. While neither Ruddick nor MacIntyre cites the other in discussions of the virtues and practices of parenting, their approaches are compatible. For example, Ruddick describes the demands of mothering as both shaping and being shaped by "the metaphysical attitudes, cognitive capacities and identification of virtues that make up maternal thinking" (Ruddick, 1989,

p. 11). Ruddick's understanding of maternal practice emanates from two central maternal "visions," or recognitions: mothers must first see the biological vulnerability of their child as socially significant, and second, they must see this reality as one that demands the care of them as mothers. For Ruddick, the three basic demands that children present are: preservative love, nurturing growth, and training for social acceptability. I will explore each of these demands, or as I will call them, "central parenting practices," and how they might be disrupted or even dismantled by the powerful, although often unarticulated, cultural forces of the hospital itself.

The Internal Goods of Parenting: Parenting Practices

Before proceeding, I wish to make a note on my choice to address the hospital's influences on the *parenting* role versus *the mothering* role. It may feel mismatched to use Ruddick's *Maternal Thinking* to better illuminate the content of *parenting* practices and, indeed, the parent that is the most present in the hospital and is the most involved in medical decision-making is typically the child's mother. While Ruddick is explicit—she is addressing maternal practices, not paternal practices or parenting practices more generally—her concepts need not apply only to women. She says, for instance, that "men can be mothers," meaning that men and fathers can and perhaps should take up maternal work (Ruddick, 1989, p. 41). And while her understanding of the role of mother as a "person who takes on responsibility for children's lives and for whom providing childcare is a significant part of her or his working life" has historically been taken up by women, I believe this role is more increasingly taken up by both women and men, mothers and fathers, and I wish to acknowledge and affirm this shift. Where Ruddick was, in 1989, understandably more interested in recognizing and honoring the historical and cultural fact that most mothering has been done by women, and her political work was made more impactful by explicitly acknowledging the contributions of women (Ruddick, 1989), I believe my clinical aims will be more impactful if I use the broader term: "parent." With this term, I wish to affirm the (perhaps modest) movement we've made since 1989 toward truly shared maternal work, and I wish to explicitly affirm and include men and fathers in the work of bedside parenting.[1] Further, I wish to affirm and include a variety of family forms

---

[1] While I do not have space to engage it here, whether there exist distinct "fathering" practices, what those might be, and how they relate to mothering practices, specifically in the context of partnered parenting, are important related questions. I know of no philosophical works engaging these questions in a robust way, but the following references may be of interest to readers: W. H. Jeynes (2016), Meta-analysis on the roles of fathers in parenting: Are they unique? *Marriage and Family Review*, 52(7), 665–688; P. R. Amato (1998), More than money? Men's contributions to their children's lives, in A. Booth & A. Crouter (Eds.), *Men in families* (pp. 241–278). Lawrence Erlbaum

in the important work of parenting, including single-parent families, two-father families and two-mother families, foster families, and children being parented by extended relatives (grandparents, aunts, uncles, etc.). I believe the term "parent" more equitably captures the work of a range of invested caregivers. Further, clinical parlance speaks of "parental authority," "parenting decision-making," and "parental involvement"; by following suit, I strategically place my work here within those conversations.

Preservative Love

Ruddick (1989) describes the first mothering practice—"preserving the lives of children"—as "the central constitutive, invariant aim of maternal practice" and a mother's (or parent's) commitment to achieving this preservative aim is the "constitutive maternal act" (p. 19). This practice is an obvious central practice for parenting, as well: if nothing else, parents are tasked with the moral (and legal) responsibility of ensuring the survival and safety of their children. "In protective love, the natural is, before any moral judgment of it, what is given. The bodies of children are, in this sense, given." Especially in the early months of a child's life, this focus on bodily well-being is commanding: many of a parent's thoughts, feelings, and actions revolve around survival-based goals like successful feeding, safe sleep practices, cleanliness and diapering, monitoring body temperature and behavior for signs of illness, and so on. MacIntyre also speaks to this maternal practice, claiming that "If parents ... are to provide children with the security and recognition that they need, they have to make the object of their continuing care and their commitment *this* child, just because it is their child for whom and to whom they are uniquely responsible" (MacIntyre, 1999, p. 90). And while the threats from which a child must be protected evolve as the child ages, the centrality of a love that preserves and protects to the parenting role is undeniable.

It is easy to see how this primary role is disrupted in the context of a complex or chronically ill child: the very fact that a child needs to be hospitalized could be interpreted as direct evidence that a parent is "failing" or at least being fundamentally thwarted at achieving this most central parenting practice. Parents describe the experience of their child's illness as catastrophic: "Just the bottom drops out of your world. It's dreadful, it really is. You can't describe the shock" (Young et al., 2002, p. 1837). One mother of an adolescent with cancer reflected the concern that she should have been more vigilant, saying, "I still haven't come

Press.); S. E. Brotherson & J. M. White (2007), *Why fathers count: The importance of fathers and their involvement with children*, Men's Studies Press.

to terms with the fact that [she] is so ill after being so healthy, it just happened so quickly. I think, and you try and think back to perhaps you missed the warning signs" (Young et al., 2002, p. 1843). And as expected, research demonstrates that among the most defining experiences of mothers of a hospitalized child is a heightened significance of the roles of protection and responsibility (Young et al., 2002).

While the ability of a parent to enact the practice of preservative and protective love may be fundamentally thwarted by an unfavorable diagnosis, these abilities may be further exacerbated by parenting in a hospital setting through three common circumstances: (1) uncertainty about the quality of the child's care and prognosis, (2) the foreignness of the environment, and (3) the tendency for parental needs to go unarticulated and unmet.

First, emanating from an understanding of how to enact a preservative and protective love in the hospital setting, parents regularly express concern about the physical and emotional well-being of their child, and a desire to be physically close to their child as a way of establishing security (Coyne, 1995; Hallström et al., 2002; Young et al., 2002). Semi-structured interviews of 20 mothers of a child with cancer reveal that among the most defining experiences of these mothers is a heightened significance of the roles of protection and responsibility (Young et al., 2002). The desire to protect their children manifests in several behaviors that represented "areas where mothers felt they could reasonably exert some direct influence or control in protecting their children": concerns about the child's diet, avoiding infections, and maintaining close physical proximity to their child. Many mothers live full-time on the oncology ward with their child for weeks or even months after diagnosis, and of central importance are the tasks of "keeping watch over" and "comforting" their children (Young et al., 2002, p. 1837).

In addition, a commonly reported parental goal of hospitalized children is to establish rapport with the clinical team, which they expect would improve the quality of care their child received (Espezal & Canam, 2003). However, sometimes the desire to "fit in" with staff and the desire to assure the very best care for their child comes into conflict, as evidenced by this quote from a mother whose child experienced a negative incident during hospitalization:

> My husband was really upset and thought it was terrible and awful for the child. We never talked to the nurse about the incident. I was thinking about telling the nurse so it wouldn't happen again. But I never did and my husband did not.... You don't want to be a bother. (Hallström et al., 2002)

Second, the environment of the hospital—the people, the spaces, the technology, the language, the rhythms, the expectations—while intimately familiar to hospital staff, is a completely foreign world to most parents. Studies have found that parents regularly speak of inhabiting a "different" or "alien" world during periods of hospitalization: "I found it very distressing to start with . . . seeing lots of children . . . the noise at night . . . found it very hard to sleep . . . used to lie there and watch the clock go by . . . it was terrible just praying for morning to come" (Coyne, 1995).

Interviews with parents of children hospitalized for surgical interventions reveal that among the most important priorities of these parents is the need for re-establishing security in an unfamiliar environment (Kristensson- Hallström & Elander, 1997). This unfamiliar environment affects not only personal coping strategies of parents, but also the ways in which parents engage in medical decision-making with professionals.

Finally, parents experienced hospital stays to be very demanding, with many of their own basic needs, like eating, showering, and sleeping, regularly going unmet. Unmet maternal needs in the hospital setting naturally threaten a mother's ability to enact the level of protective care they expect from themselves, but parents are reticent to articulate these needs. "Clearly, in a world in which the role of mothers is constructed as being one of obligation and selflessness, it was difficult for them to give voice to their own needs" (Young et al., 2002, p. 1838). Mothers, especially, are used to sacrificing their own needs for the sake of preserving and protecting their children, but at a point, these sacrifices become self-defeating: a parent cannot care well for her child if she, herself, is unwell.

Fostering Growth

According to Ruddick, the second central maternal practice, to foster growth, is to "nurture a child's developing spirit—whatever is lively, purposive and responsive." This nurturing practice manifests primarily as daily decisions about how best to promote a child's "emotional, cognitive, sexual and social development," where development doesn't necessarily entail parental imposition, but instead is a "gradual unfolding" of the child's "possibilities" (Ruddick, 1989, p. 82). MacIntyre asserts that "what those who perform the role and function of a good parent achieve is to bring the child to the point at which it is educable, not only by them, but also by a variety of other different kinds of teachers" (MacIntyre, 1999, p. 91). While many others might be involved in the growth and nurturance of a child (teachers, coaches, neighbors, grandparents), typically the "mother assumes the primary task of maintaining conditions of growth: it is a mother who considers herself and is considered by others to be primarily responsible for arrested or defected growth" (Ruddick, 1989, p. 20). To enable this work of fostering growth, mothers must "practice her understanding of a child's mind."

First, I will focus on the epistemological component of "fostering growth": for a parent to discern which practices will best nurture their child's growth, they must first know their distinctive child and have at least some confidence in the content of that knowing. The fact of a child's hospitalization thwarts this essential knowing in two important ways: first, parents aren't always given complete information about their child's condition and treatment (Coyne, 1995; Meyer et al., 2006; Ygge & Arnetz, 2004); and second, a more insidious barrier is the tendency for clinical teams to devalue or dismiss parental knowledge in favor of clinical knowledge (Callery, 1997, pp. 27–34). "Unfortunately, some parents must work hard to get information: to ask the right questions, track down the right people and be at the bedside at the right time" (Meyer et al., 2006, p. 653). Regular access to desired information and to key clinical staff are associated with decreased parental anxiety and worry, and with increased confidence in parental decision-making (Pochard et al., 2001). One mother of a chronically ill child describes an incident that was common to parents in a parental interview study conducted by Ygge and Arnetz (2004):

> When I told the nurse that it is easier to put in an intravenous cannula in his left arm, the nurse said we always do it this way and we know what is right. Of course it failed and she could not put in the cannula in his right arm and had to finally take the left arm. But now my son was sad and crying. (p. 220)

Studies have demonstrated that empowering parents of ill children to adapt to the demands of the illness and continue parenting from a position of confidence requires that parents must be allowed to develop and deploy necessary knowledge, competence, and confidence (Gibson, 1995). Of particular importance to this process is the nature of parental interactions with the clinical team: interactions in which parents feel heard, encouraged, and supported are naturally associated with greater empowerment.

A second component of fostering growth is the actual physical and practical work of parental caregiving which, no matter the child's age, will be required if a child is hospitalized. Typically, nursing staff assumes primary responsibility for providing this type of care, but parents often wish to participate. Just as parents' knowledge is often dismissed in the hospital setting, parental caregiving can be similarly thwarted or devalued, and the level of parent participation (either too much or too little) can be a source of conflict between parents and staff (Ford & Turner, 2001). A central aspect of promoting parental caregiving is the parent's understanding of the control she does or does not have with respect to the technical work of hospital care (e.g., giving medications, suctioning, bathing, wound care, giving feeds). Many parents, especially those parents who had been providing nursing care at home, expect to provide some of their child's regular nursing care in the hospital. For example, a parent respondent in a semi-structured interview about parental participation in the hospital stated, "I basically do everything I do at home and I'd do it more if they let me 'cause he prefers it to come from me" (Coyne, 1995, p. 75). Another mother described her role the first week of her child's hospitalization as "pretty much a bystander . . . then when we can start to take care of some of the most basic needs we feel 'Okay, we're the parents'" (Heerman et al., 2005, p. 179). However, sometimes parents, especially parents of children who are newly diagnosed, are hesitant to participate in technical caregiving due to fear of harming their child, fear of being associated with the pain or discomfort of care, or discomfort with the actual tasks and environment of caregiving. As one parent shared, "I prefer to just be present for two reasons: first, if it involves pain, I don't want to be the one who hurts him; and second, as a rule I think it will hurt less if the staff do it" (Kristensson- Hallström & Elander, 1997, p. 364). Thus, the expectation that all parents will or desire to actively participate in technical caregiving is erroneous; instead, parents should be given control relative to how, when, and if they wish to provide this type of care at all. Further, even when parents are uncomfortable with providing their child with the technical care, the other, less obvious practices of parental caregiving (talking, listening, comforting, physical closeness, etc.) should be encouraged.

Training for Social Acceptability

The third and final parenting practice described by Ruddick is "training for social acceptability," in which parents shape a child's growth not primarily according to the child's needs, but instead based on the requirements of the various social groups or communities of which the child is a member. The parental practice of training is primarily associated with disciplining practices: how parents reinforce "good" or "acceptable" behavior and discourage "bad" or "unacceptable" behavior. Acceptability to particular social groups may not seem like an essential parenting practice, but we should remember that it is primarily by our membership in groups and communities (families, neighborhoods, religious communities, intellectual communities, schools, social groups, moral communities, or even "society" altogether) that we are able to ascribe language and meaning to our experiences. And it is through the resources of these communities that we identify our values and dominant explanatory narratives for life. This is, perhaps, the primary thrust of MacIntyre's text, *Dependent Rational Animals* (1999): the social relationships required by our (human beings') dependence and vulnerability are exactly what, in turn, cultivate the virtue required to act rightly as social beings in community. The hospital doesn't just interfere with a parent's ability to participate in her chosen communities; it thrusts upon her an altogether new community, of which she is likely an apprehensive member. As discussed earlier, the hospital itself has a distinctive culture, one that is disorienting and bewildering to those tossed in against their will.

If training "is a matter of intervention and control: a mother decides what behavior to allow, insist on, or ignore, and then tries to shift her child's behavior in the direction she desires" (p. 21), then the hospital thwarts this practice in several ways. First, the hospital environment guarantees that parents are parenting under the "gaze" of others. Ruddick (1989) discusses this reality with regard to general parenting outside the hospital: when under the gaze of others, whether judgmental or not, mothers shift their training practices to accord with expectations, and in "relinquishing authority to others, they lose confidence in their own values and in their perception of their children's needs" (p. 111). It is no surprise, then, that parents of hospitalized children often feel as though they are "parenting in public." No longer do parents have the security and privacy of their home. Their parenting is now the focus of the possibly judgmental attention of hospital staff (Darbyshire, 1995). A sense that one is "parenting in public" is naturally destabilizing to parental confidence. Parental knowledge develops in the private domain of intimate contact, and, in contrast to the professional knowledge developed by hospital staff, it is *by definition* not scientific or objective; it is precisely the closeness of the parent to the child that enables her to be an expert on her child (Callery, 1997). One mother described her experience with nursing staff:

> I can tell sometimes the nurses think that I'm "bugging her," that I should leave her alone. I can tell by their facial expressions and they don't encourage me to touch her. I try to explain to them that I am watching her monitors. . . . I try to make them comfortable with me. But then you know I just have to be able to touch her, do those little things. It makes me feel bad, though, to think that some nurses think I'm being selfish. (Hurst, 2001, p. 72)

Certainly, this quote demonstrates just one family's experience with one set of nurses and may not be the experience of all or most families. However, it does offer us at least one example of how nurse-parent interactions can deeply affect a parent's ability to parent as they desire.

Second, like any family crisis, a childhood illness requiring hospitalization will threaten the biographies of both child and parent. Being thrust into such a rare and unfamiliar environment, parents will often lack a stable and well-informed set of lay beliefs or resources for managing their experiences, expectations, or ability to construct meaningful narratives around that experience.

Young et al. (2002) suggest that one of the primary roles mothers assume after a diagnosis of childhood cancer is "guardians of their child's biography," a role in which mothers seek to protect their sick child's identity, construct narratives about the meaning of the illness, and protect their child's future. In addition, Young and colleagues have discovered that the experience of parenting a child with a chronic illness triggers a "biographical shift" in mothers, requiring them to discover and develop new self-identities, which invite new emphases on certain parenting practices (e.g., protection and responsibility) and new practices altogether (technical caregiving skills).

Why Parental Role Empowerment Matters to Decision-Making

As I transition from a discussion of the ways in which the hospital destabilizes and disempowers the parenting role to a discussion of why this matters to decision-making, I want to be careful and clear about my view of parenting. I do not believe the non-hospitalized world of parenting to be easy or straightforward or without its own fair share of disruptions of central parenting practices. As a parent, myself, making such a claim would be inconsistent with my own parenting experiences. As children grow and situations change, parents will naturally encounter seasons or specific domains where their parental role is disturbed. The point here is not that outside the hospital a parent's role is preserved perfectly and inside the hospital it is thwarted irreparably. The point is, however, that a child's hospitalization presents perhaps one of the most jarring and disorienting experiences for a parent and that we should expect and respond to this reality.

Thus far I have explored three primary parenting practices and how they might be fundamentally thwarted or distorted either by the bare fact of a child's illness, or by the cultural and sociological forces of the hospital environment. My aim here is to clearly depict the possibility that parents not only are practically disoriented or inconvenienced by these forces, but also might be thrown into a state of radical ontological destabilization relative to their self-understanding and their identity as a parent. This state of destabilization and disempowerment, I will argue next, affects parents' ability to make good medical decisions for their children. Further, ethicists, physicians, and nurses have a responsibility to explicitly acknowledge and work to empower and re-stabilize the central practices of parenting, both as an end in itself, but also as a means of promoting better decision-making. Here, I will discuss the epistemic and psychological effects of parental empowerment on decision-making.

Before delving into the details of how parental role empowerment might affect decision-making, we must first explore how we conceptualize the task of medical decision-making. Clinical decision-making is often depicted as a simple and isolated process of reasoning with relevant medical information and weighing risks and benefits to come to a decision. A clinician's responsibility in the decision-making process is framed as a simple matter of disclosing the relevant information in a consumable way. Indeed, this is how many medical ethics textbooks describe the responsibility of the clinician in the informed consent process: it is a simple matter of disclosing the right information, facilitating patient understanding of that information, and ensuring the patient acts in a voluntary manner when communicating a choice (Junkerman & Schiedermayer, 1998). Surely, these are all important components of an informed decision by a patient or surrogate. However, this is not nearly the whole picture of actual decision-making, and this simple conceptual model can easily obscure the complexities and factors involved in real-life decision-making by real-life patients, parents, and surrogates.[2] Further, it can obscure or misrepresent the responsibilities of clinicians and ethicists within that space. As a result, we neglect certain iatrogenic sources of "bad" decision-making, leaving clinicians susceptible to judge or label decisions or decision-makers as "bad" without considering the possibility that the medical enterprise itself has contributed to that decision. For example, high-stakes medical decisions (e.g., whether to perform a tracheostomy for long-term mechanical ventilation) are often presented to parents abruptly, without significant goals of care conversations and after a period where the child's treatment plan was decided without much input from parents. In circumstances like these, where parents have had little time to reorient themselves as parents, to discern and explore their values and goals, or to practice applying those values to medical decisions, it should not surprise us that some parents withdraw from the decision or refuse to entertain any limitations of care. Thus, my contention here is the fact that many parents engage in medical decision-making for their children from a position of disempowerment and instability in their parental role which is ethically significant and requires a response from clinicians and ethicists.

---

[2] One recent example of how bioethicists are expanding their understanding of decision-making to better account for actual decision-making processes looks to the social-psychological framework of mindset theory to help explain why research participants so often display the concerning phenomenon of therapeutic error (Jansen, 2014).

Epistemic Effects of Parental Role Empowerment

As described above, many parents of hospitalized children experience a profound destabilization in their epistemological parenting practices in at least three important ways: first, the content of "relevant" or "important" knowledge has shifted from the intimate knowledge of a parent to the technical knowledge of a medical or nursing professional; thus, second, epistemic authority—or the tendency to let the truth claims of a supposedly authoritative voice "stand in" for one's own attempts to gain knowledge—shifts from the parent to the healthcare team; and finally, that due to these two factors, parents lose "epistemic self-trust" (Zagzebski, 2012) with regard to their parenting. Consider a common scenario: a small child is upset and crying. In a typical environment, a parent would use their knowledge of their child and the situation, knowledge developed over years of parenting experience with that particular child, and make a decision about how best to respond: perhaps a tender hug, or a distraction, or a removal from the environment for a talk, or perhaps something different altogether (think of all the many idiosyncrasies of a particular child). Now, it is important to acknowledge here that not all these attempts will be "correct" or "successful" (as any parent knows, many are not); children are strange and unpredictable and no one has a perfect understanding of their needs and desires. But regardless of whether any individual attempt succeeds or fails, what exists underneath is parental epistemic self-trust: while they might get it wrong sometimes, no one is better positioned to get it right, and they have at their disposal a deep reservoir of relevant knowledge, experience, and confidence from which to draw to get it right. Now consider this same scenario, but in the hospital: perhaps the child is in a hospital bed connected to several monitors, a peripherally inserted central catheter (PICC) line, and other mysterious pieces of technology, and gets upset and starts crying. The parent is faced with same decision as before, but in a radically different epistemic context. There now exist new dimensions of essential knowledge about her child that do not belong to her. Can she climb into bed with her child or will that somehow "hurt" the child or interfere with care? Is she even *allowed* to climb into bed with her child, or must she ask permission from a nurse? Can she offer the distraction of a special food treat, or would the sugar disrupt a delicate nutritional balance?

This example is a small one, and perhaps some parents of hospitalized children would encounter it without much strain. But the point remains that there are plenty of opportunities, both big and small, during the hospitalization of a child for a parent to question his or her knowledge of her child. Consider another common (if not daily) phenomenon in the hospital: parents frequently look outside themselves—specifically to nurses and physicians, or even to monitors and screens—to learn how their child is doing. Or yet another common example: as the medical needs of an ill child become more significant and chronic, parents will often have to be educated by nursing staff about how to provide care for their child. Here I refer to the "technical" tasks of caregiving discussed above: giving medications, managing technologies, suctioning, wound care, giving feeds, and so on. The physical tasks of caregiving shift dramatically, and either a medical professional must educate the parent in detail on how to complete these tasks, or the professional simply takes over these tasks altogether.

As any good pediatric bioethicist knows, medical decision-making for children requires not only the technical medical knowledge of medical professionals, but also the knowledge of an intimate and invested parent of the child and family in question. This is, purportedly, the basis of "shared decision-making." But as demonstrated above, if parents are engaging in the task of decision-making from a position of epistemic disadvantage and self-doubt, then we should not be surprised when the process is difficult, communication is strained, or the decisions, themselves, are questionable.

Psychological Effects of Parental Role Empowerment

The literature suggests that decision-making patterns between parents and professionals change over the time of a child's illness and hospitalization, tracking specifically with changes in parental familiarity, security, and competence in the hospital setting (Dixon, 1996). Parents progress from allowing the healthcare professional to make the decisions during the initial phase of the illness (Jerret, 1994), to desiring participation in decisions (Cohen, 1995), to challenging decisions made by the professionals (Burke et al., 1991; Callery & Luker, 1996), to finally collaborating with healthcare providers on decision-making (Gibson, 1995; Thorne & Robinson, 1988). In bioethics parlance, we might describe this progression as a swinging pendulum, from one extreme of paternalism, to another extreme of exaggerated parental authority, and finally settling in the ideal territory of collaborative, shared decision-making. This progression is consistent with other sources describing parental coping strategies in contexts of unfamiliarity and insecurity. One study suggests that parents deploy three major strategies to re-secure themselves and their children: (1) security through leaving care to staff, (2) security through obtaining control over care, and (3) security through relying on knowing one's child best (Kristensson-Hallstrom & Elander, 1997). This study suggests two important conclusions about parental experience. First, despite efforts toward "family-centered care" and "parental partnership," all parents feel a sense of threat, insecurity, and disempowerment. Second, in the face of these threats, parents engage *different* strategies for re-establishing security at different times, strategies that span from passive disengagement in care (which may appear to some like detachment, laziness, or disinterest) to a strong sense of what should and should not be done by staff (which may be experienced by some as controlling and domineering).

How to Re-Empower Parents in Their Parenting Role

Finally, we turn to the question: If parents are, indeed, experiencing these destabilizing and disempowering forces, and these experiences affect their ability to engage in decision-making, how, then, should we respond? This section outlines several simple, but targeted, strategies for re-empowering parents in their parenting role while their child is ill or hospitalized. Readers can find these strategies summarized in Table 12.1. The aim of re-empowerment is treated both as a means toward the goal of better parental decision-making and as an important end in itself.

First, our response requires awareness—awareness not just that "parenting a child in the hospital is hard," but that parents may be experiencing a myriad of destabilizing forces which could be deeply affecting how they engage the tasks of parenting. Further, our awareness should also extend into an understanding and expectation that parents will engage in various strategies to re-secure themselves and their children, strategies that might look like inappropriate parenting, spanning from passive withdrawal to an aggressive assertion of control and influence.

Second, with this knowledge, the healthcare team should regularly solicit parental thoughts and preferences about day-to-day experiences. For example, nurses and physicians could ask questions like, "What is the hardest thing about being a parent right now?"; "What can we do that would help you feel like a good parent?"; "What would make your time in the hospital easier for you and your child?"; or "What is your preference for how and when we communicate with you?" Preceding these questions with normalizing statements can help to put parents at ease and know their experience is not unusual, for instance: "Parents here often feel off-kilter or disoriented and sometimes it might feel difficult to parent." Soliciting parental experiences and preferences and responding with supportive and reasonable accommodations (where appropriate) should be an ongoing aim of the medical team. For example, if a mother communicates that she gets easily confused by the information presented to her by various medical professionals, it might be appropriate to create a communication plan with her, establishing a primary medical contact who will present "big picture" information, and a few supportive staff members who can help the mother digest that information and write down clarifying questions. The role of the nurse here cannot be underestimated. While the physician is often seen as the primary clinical contact for the *medical* decisions, I believe nurses, as the primary physical

Table 12.1 Suggestions for Clinicians Toward Re-Empowering Parental Roles

Category	Suggestions for Clinicians	Time Frame
Awareness	Be aware that parents are often experiencing powerful forces which are destabilizing and disrupting their ability to understand and enact their parenting role.	Ongoing
Inquiry	Normalize the experience of disorientation, with statements like "Most parents here feel off-kilter at times and sometimes it may feel difficult to be a parent in this environment."	Intermittently
	Regularly solicit parent experiences and preferences, using questions like: "What's the hardest thing about being a parent right now?"; "What would make your and your child's hospital stay easier?"; or "What can we do to help you feel like a good parent?"	Intermittently
Encourage parenting practices: *Epistemic*	Invite parental knowledge before sharing clinical information in clinical encounters. "How is she doing today?"; "What have you noticed in the past 24 hours?"	Regularly, perhaps even daily
	Emphasize how essential parental knowledge is to the care of their child. "While I might know more about her cancer treatment, you know the most about who she is and what she needs."	Regularly, perhaps even daily
Encourage parenting practices: *Biographical*	Ask parents to share their story of the child's illness, "How have you been describing this experience to your friends and family?"	Intermittently
	Ask parents to reflect on their values, beliefs and goals. "What values or beliefs are most important to you right now?"; "What is your biggest fear moving forward?"; and "What are you most hoping for right now?"	Intermittently, ideally before a conversation about a particular treatment decision

(continued)

Table 12.1 Continued

Category	Suggestions for Clinicians	Time Frame
Encourage parenting practices: *Caregiving*	Inquire about parent preferences regarding participation with clinical caregiving tasks. Correct any misinformation, e.g., "I know it's scary to diaper her with a feeding tube, but I'll teach you how to do it without hurting her."	Intermittently
	When desired, invite parents to participate in the clinical caregiving practices required for their child, including things like tracheostomy care, wound care, bathing, and administering feeds.	Regularly, perhaps even daily
	Regardless of parental preference for participation, emphasize and reinforce other non-clinical parent caregiving practices, such as: reading to their child, soothing their child, expressing physical affection. Make suggestions where appropriate.	Regularly, perhaps even daily

caregivers for a hospitalized child, are far more powerful in creating a day-to-day environment that feels secure for parents. Parents often feel more comfortable and at ease talking about these issues with a familiar bedside nurse, rather than the physician who happens to be on service that week.

Finally, the healthcare team should explicitly offer opportunities for parents to engage in practices—epistemic practices, biographical practices, and caregiving practices—that will help re-establish their typical parenting role, held with a sense of openness to the comfort level of any particular parent. First, *epistemic practices* aim to re-establish the parent as the primary knowledge-bearer of their child. This can be achieved, in part, by beginning daily clinical encounters not by sharing clinical information with parents, but instead by asking the parent, "How is your child doing today?"; "Anything you've noticed in the past 24 hours that we should be aware of?"; or "What can we do to help your child today?" At times, these questions will be met with confusion or skepticism: "Why are you asking me? Shouldn't you know?" Certainly, the clinician will know, better than the parent, the results of the chest x-ray or cerebrospinal fluid (CSF) studies, but by waiting to communicate these clinical updates and instead begin by affirming the parent's knowledge first, the clinician communicates a powerful reality: a present and involved parent will almost always know far better than the clinicians how the child *is*. Is she in pain? Has she had a good day? Has she been in good spirits? What's been bugging her? What does she find comfort in today? These are important questions of parental knowledge, not clinician knowledge. Further, an awake and alert child should also be seen as a primary source for this information, but even in this scenario, the parental perspective will be an important supplement.

Second, clinicians can invite parents to participate in *biographical practices*, as well, by offering a parent the opportunity to tell and retell their story, apply their own sense of values and meaning to the situation, and craft meaningful goals for the journey ahead. The aim of these biographical practices is to re-establish the parent's role as primary meaning-makers for their child and family. As opposed to the epistemic practices described above, this will not be a daily practice. Instead, when the child's clinical course reaches a point of transition or stability, this is often a good occasion to have a longer conversation with parents, and ask questions like "How have you been telling this story to yourself, your other children, concerned friends and family?"; "What values or beliefs are most important to you right now?"; "What is your biggest fear moving forward?"; and "What are you most hoping for right now?" Allow parents to contemplate these questions alone or with family if they are hesitant to answer right away. And if possible, try to engage in this conversation apart from conversation about a particular treatment decision. Separating the two takes off the pressure and gives more space for a parent to explore and reflect.

Finally, parents should be invited to participate in *caregiving practices* for their child, including daily tasks of clinical caregiving (e.g., trach care, wound care, bathing), but importantly, including many other caregiving practices, as well. Many pediatric hospitals do this as a matter of standard practice. In fact, completing parent training on these tasks is frequently a condition of discharge to home. In situations where parents must be trained by hospital staff on skills related to clinical caregiving, it may appear that the parents are relearning what it means to be a parent. However, we should heed the earlier warning of MacIntyre here, who cautions against the tendency for the practices of parenting to be reduced to a set of technical skills, dislocated from the parenting context. Parenting as a social practice is far more than a set of technical skills. While learning the technical skills might be an appropriate requirement for discharge home, parents should also be encouraged to continue practicing the many other parental caregiving practices that they are already expert in: comforting and soothing, providing environments of play and learning, providing physical affection, enforcing boundaries and providing discipline, telling stories and reading, connecting children to larger communities of support and meaning, and, of course, the profound act of loving their child.

Conclusion

It is likely unsurprising to learn that parents of ill and hospitalized children are often disoriented and disempowered in their ability to parent. Clearly, parenting a hospitalized child is difficult. However, my contention here has been that it is not merely difficult or disruptive. Instead, we should view the wilderness of the hospital environment as a powerful force that can dramatically impact a parent's ability to engage in the essential practices of parenting, and parents' disempowerment in their parenting role can be the underlying cause of troubling decision-making effects. If a parent feels as though she no longer knows her child, can care for her child, or can protect her child, she will naturally seek out ways to re-stabilize her role, which might include behavior like withdrawing from the hospital context altogether or exerting control and influence in demanding ways. Bioethicists and pediatric clinicians should attend more directly to the effects of hospitalization on the parenting role and attempt to curtail those effects. In particular, pediatric nurses are in a unique position to reorient and re-empower parents in their parenting role, as many of practices previously performed by parents are now performed, in part, by nursing staff. Nurses have significant power in this domain, and by working to reorient and re-empower parents of ill children in their role as parents, they can further equip parents to do the hard work of medical decision-making for their children.

References

Amato, P. R. (1998). More than money? Men's contributions to their children's lives. In A. Booth & A. Crouter (Eds.), *Men in families* (pp. 241–278). Lawrence Erlbaum Press.

Brighouse, H., & Swift, A. (2014). The goods of parenting. In F. Baylis & C. McCloud (Eds.), *Family making* (pp. 11–28). Oxford University Press.

Brotherson, S. E., & White, J. M. (2007). *Why fathers count: The importance of fathers and their involvement with children.* Men's Studies Press.

Burke, S., Kauffmann, E., Costello, E., & Dillon, M. (1991). Hazardous secrets and reluctantly taking charge: Parenting a child with repeated hospitalizations. *Image, 23*(1), 39–46.

Callery, P. (1997). Maternal knowledge and professional knowledge: Cooperation and conflict in the care of sick children. *International Journal of Nursing Studies, 34*(1), 27–34.

Callery, P., & Luker, K. (1996). The use of qualitative methods in the study of parent's experiences of care on a children's surgical ward. *Journal of Advanced Nursing, 23*(2), 338–345.

Cohen, M. (1995). The stages of the pre-diagnostic period in chronic, life-threatening childhood illness: A process analysis. *Research in Nursing and Health, 18*(1), 39–48.

Coyne, I. (1995). Partnership in care: Parents' views of participation in their hospitalized child's care. *Journal of Clinical Nursing, 4,* 71–79.

Darbyshire, P. (1995). Family-centered care within contemporary British pediatric nursing. *British Journal of Nursing, 4*(1)31–33.

Dixon, D. (1996). Unifying concepts in parents' experiences with health care providers. *Journal of Family Nursing, 2*(2), 111–132.

Espezal, H., & Canam, C. (2003). Parent-nurse interactions: Care of hospitalized children. *Journal of Advanced Nursing, 44*(1), 34–41.

Ford, K., & Turner, D. (2001). Stories seldom told: Paediatric nurses' experiences of caring for hospitalized children with special needs and their families. *Journal of Advanced Nursing, 33*(3), 288–295.

Gibson, C. (1995). The process of empowerment in mothers of chronically ill children. *Journal of Advanced Nursing, 21*(6), 1201–1210.

Hallström, I., Runesson, I., & Elander, G. (2002). Observed parental needs during their child's hospitalization. *Journal of Pediatric Nursing, 17*(2), 140–148.

Heerman, J., Wilson, M., & Wilhelm, P. (2005). Mothers in the NICU: From outsider to partner. *Pediatric Nursing, 31*(3), 176–200.

Hurst, I. (2001). Mothers' strategies to meet their needs in the newborn intensive care nursery. *The Journal of Perinatal and Neonatal Nursing, 15*(2), 65–82.

Jansen, L. (2014). Mindsets, informed consent, and research. *Hasting Center Report, 44*(1), 25–32.

Jerret, M. D. (1994). Parents experience of coming to know the care of a chronically ill child. *Journal of Advanced Nursing, 19*(6), 1050–1056.

Jeynes, W. H. (2016). Meta-analysis on the roles of fathers in parenting: Are they unique? *Marriage and Family Review, 52*(7), 665–688.

Junkerman, C., & Schiedermayer, D. (1998). *Practical ethics for students, interns and residents: A short reference manual* (2nd ed.). University Publishing Group.

Kristensson-Hallstrom, I., & Elander, G. (1997). Parents' experience of hospitalization: Different strategies for feeling secure. *Pediatric Nursing, 23*(4), 361–368.

Leonard, V. W. (1996). Mothering as a practice. In S. Gordon, P. Benner, & N. Noddings (Eds.), *Caregiving: Readings in knowledge, practice, ethics and politics* (pp. 124–140). University of Pennsylvania Press.

MacIntyre, A. (1999). *Dependent rational animals: Why human beings need the virtues.* Carus.

MacIntyre, A. (2007). *After virtue* (3rd ed.). University of Notre Dame Press.

Meyer, E. C., Ritholz, M. D., Burns, J. P., & Truog, R. D. (2006). Improving the quality of end-of-life care in the pediatric intensive care unit: Parents' priorities and recommendations. *Pediatrics, 117*(3), 649–657.

Pochard, F., Azoulay. E., Chevret, S., Lemaire, F., Hubert, P., Canoui, P., Grassin, M., Zittoun, R., Le Gall, J. R., Dhainaut, J. F., & Schlemmer, B. (2001). Symptoms of anxiety and depression in family members of intensive care unit patients: Ethical hypothesis regarding decision-making capacity. *Critical Care Medicine, 29*(10), 1893–1897.

Ruddick, S. (1989). *Maternal thinking.* Beacon Press.

Salter, E. K. (2012). Deciding for a child: A comprehensive analysis of the best interest standard. *Theoretical Medicine and Bioethics, 33*(3), 179–198.

Thorne, S., & Robinson, C. (1988). Reciprocal trust in health care relationships. *Journal of Advanced Nursing, 13*(6), 782–789.

Ygge, B. M., & Arnetz, J. E. (2004). A study of parental involvement in pediatric hospital care: Implications for clinical practice. *Journal of Pediatric Nursing, 19*(3), 217–223.

Young, B., Dixon-Woods, M., Findlay, M., & Heney, D. (2002). Parenting in crisis: Conceptualizing mothers of children with cancer. *Social Science and Medicine, 55*(10), 1835–1847.

Zagzebski, L. (2012). *Epistemic authority: A theory of trust, authority and autonomy in belief.* Oxford University Press.

13

Consent and My Chronically Ill Child

Emily A. Largent

When I think about decision-making in pediatric practice, I think about my chronically ill daughter. She was very young when she was diagnosed. As a result, I have had most of my daughter's lifetime to familiarize myself with the facts of her condition. Here are the facts that you should know: my daughter dislikes missing school for doctors' appointments; despises having labs drawn; chafes at the routines of medication, *particularly the injections* (she asked that I emphasize that); resents their side effects. She feels deeply that it is unfair she is sick when other children are not. But she has no choice in the matter.

As it happens, I've had longer than my daughter's lifetime to familiarize myself with the field of bioethics. Working as a bedside nurse in an intensive care unit (ICU), I found deep satisfaction in the labor of caring and advocating for my patients—particularly those lacking decision-making capacity—and their families. Nursing brought me into contact with many ethical challenges. Sometimes, I used my voice successfully to navigate them. Other times, speaking up felt ineffective, and so I remained silent. I feared conflict with other team members or was uncertain how to handle the gradient of authority between nurses and physicians (Okuyama et al., 2014).

Unfortunately, silence of this kind is not uncommon and can have troubling implications for patient care. So, a decade ago, I stepped away from the bedside toward bioethics with a goal of raising my voice and, through scholarship, helping patients in a systematic and enduring way—patients, as it turns out, like my daughter, and families, as it turns out, like my own.

My various perspectives—as a bioethicist in my professional life and as the mother of a chronically ill child in my personal life—have intersected to inform my views about decision-making in pediatric practice. By turns of geography and fate, my daughter has always received her medical care at leading children's hospitals, hospitals with tripartite missions encompassing excellent patient care, innovative research, and the education of future pediatric leaders. Each prong of such missions affects the patient experience. Our family, for instance, routinely confronts decisions not only about my daughter's care, but also about her involvement in research and about the involvement of nursing students, medical students, residents, and other trainees in her care.

I find making decisions about my daughter's medical care to be relatively straightforward. The members of my daughter's extraordinary care team are highly trained specialists expert in medicine, and the members of my family are expert in my daughter's (and our family's) needs and interests. In partnership, we are able to enumerate goals of care and, with those goals to guide us, to make thoughtful decisions about what treatments and interventions we will or will not pursue. More challenging for me are the decisions that must be made about my daughter's involvement in research and training activities. Such decisions are difficult because, whereas my daughter's care is intended solely for her benefit, research and training are intended to benefit future patients—by producing either generalizable knowledge to guide their care or better doctors to treat them. This changes the ethical calculation: the risks and burdens of research and training must be weighed not just against the benefits for my daughter, but against benefits to the broader society.

That my daughter's capacity to make autonomous decisions is still developing adds significant complexity to the decision-making process. I want to foster her emerging capacity for self-determination but realize, too, that while her decision-making capacities develop, she is dependent on me to make decisions that promote and protect her well-being. Thought must therefore be given to when it is appropriate to solicit her opinions and how much weight to give them. In my own experience, these determinations depend on whether we are considering medical care, research, or involvement of trainees, as well as on additional context-specific factors. For example, is the intervention under consideration medically necessary or not? If the former, seeking her input without the possibility that it will meaningfully influence our ultimate choice risks ringing hollow and undermining her trust; if the latter, her input may helpfully guide our decision-making.

In this chapter, I will reflect on what my daughter's care has revealed to me about decision-making in pediatric practice. My purpose here is threefold. First, I will provide a conceptual framework for consent in pediatric practice. Then, I will address consent for research involving children, and finally, a topic that receives relatively less attention, consent for involvement of trainees in the care of children.

Conceptual Framework for Consent in Pediatric Practice

Informed consent has roots in both ethical theory and in law (Beauchamp, 2011; Berg et al., 2001; Faden et al., 1986) The ethical underpinning is respect for autonomy, which is typically understood as independence and self-rule or self-determination. The legal underpinnings can be found in case law addressing

battery (i.e., unconsented touching) and malpractice (i.e., negligent professional conduct) (Faden et al., 1986). Given these roots, we can use "informed
consent" to convey two distinct ideas: first, to describe a process that culminates
in morally transformative authorization; and, second, to describe a process that
culminates in legally transformative authorization. Acting in the absence of informed consent in the first sense is an ethical violation, whereas acting in the absence of informed consent in the second sense is a legal violation.

As it has evolved in theory and in practice, informed consent has four
recognized elements. First, there must be a decision-maker with *decision-
making capacity*. Capacity is the task-specific ability to appreciate a situation and
its consequences, to understand relevant information, to reason about options,
and to communicate a choice (Appelbaum, 2007). Second, there should be
disclosure of relevant information. Such information encompasses the nature
of the illness or condition, as well as the risks, benefits, and alternatives to the
proposed treatment or intervention (including the alternative of doing nothing).
Typically, this information should be disclosed at the level of detail that a reasonable person would want and in language that the decision-maker can understand. Third, the decision-maker should *comprehend* the information disclosed
to them. Finally, the decision-maker should make a *voluntary choice* to accept or
refuse an intervention.

A challenge immediately arises when applying this framework in the pediatric clinical care setting. Children generally lack the ability to act independently, either because they're minors and not considered legally capable of
medical decision-making, or because developmentally, they have limited or no
capacity to engage in medical decision-making. Stated otherwise, they cannot
give informed consent in the sense of *legally* transformative authorization.
(There are exceptions. Emancipated minors can, for instance, give informed
consent for medical care, and some laws allow minors to consent to reproductive healthcare and other sensitive services [Coleman & Rosoff, 2013; Lane &
Kohlenberg, 2012].) Some children may be capable of giving morally transformative consent, and even those who cannot may still be able to evince a preference.
Therefore, in pediatric practice, modifications to the informed consent framework are necessary: a child's parents or guardians provide *informed permission*
for medical intervention, while the child gives *assent*, or affirmative agreement,
if and to the degree it is developmentally appropriate (Bartholome, 1989; Katz
et al., 2016; Kohrman & Clayton, 1995).

Informed permission includes the elements of standard informed consent.
Parents have a legal right to raise their children according to their own values, as
well as a corresponding responsibility to act with the children's best interests in
mind. It has been acknowledged that "best interests" is not an easy standard to
define or apply in healthcare (Kohrman & Clayton, 1995; Ross, 2019). Children

have a variety of interests, including self-regarding and other-regarding interests. Even if people agree on what a child's relevant interests are, they may not agree about the relative weights to assign to them, and thus can reach different conclusions about what is, in fact, best. Moreover, children are situated within families. Decisions about a child's healthcare may result in intrafamilial trade-offs between the interests of the child and the interests of the parents or of siblings, if any. Though there is general agreement that the latter interests are relevant to healthcare decision-making for children, there is controversy over the extent to which they may permissibly influence it. While these ethical challenges must be acknowledged, from a legal standpoint, parents' choices will typically be upheld unless they are neglectful or harmful. The crucial point for our present purposes, then, is that parental informed permission is generally necessary in the clinical care context.

Assent is intended to demonstrate respect for children as individuals by engaging them in an interactive decision-making process and allowing them to express their treatment preferences *when it is reasonable to do so*. It would, for instance, be unreasonable to seek a child's assent if a procedure is necessary to advance the goals of care agreed upon by the clinical team and the family. In such cases, the procedure can and typically will be provided even over the child's objections. To borrow an example from my own life, neither the medical team nor I seek my daughter's assent for her annual flu shot given the shot's clear value for chronically ill children. It would be inappropriate to ask her opinion (likely a "NO!") when we don't seriously intend to weigh her opinion in our decision-making. Instead, we talk with her about why she needs the flu shot and what she can expect when she gets it. Additionally, we allow her to make simple decisions like choosing where to get the shot. This approach allows us to build her trust, recognize her emerging capacity for rationality and autonomy, and to foster her knowledge and understanding of healthcare decision-making.

When it is reasonable to obtain assent, what does the process of seeking a child's agreement look like? The American Academy of Pediatrics asserts that assent should, at the very least, include the following elements:

1. Helping the patient achieve a developmentally appropriate awareness of the nature of his or her condition;
2. Telling the patient what he or she can expect with tests and treatments;
3. Making a clinical assessment of the patient's understanding of the situation and the factors influencing how he or she is responding (including whether there is inappropriate pressure to accept testing or therapy); and
4. Soliciting an expression of the patient's willingness to accept the proposed care (Katz et al., 2016).

The goal is to empower children to the extent of their capacity (Kohrman & Clayton, 1995). When a child is asked to give assent, she must: understand what is being asked, have a notion that her permission is being sought, and make a choice (Emanuel [Ed.], 2003). Children will obviously have more or less ability to do this. Therefore, a developmental approach to assent expects different levels of understanding from children as they age. Around age seven, many children enter a developmental stage characterized by the ability to develop a reasoned decision, though there are questions about if that is the "right age" (Waligora et al., 2014). Additionally, children with more extensive medical experience due to chronic illness often have the ability to engage more effectively in decision-making (Katz et al., 2016).

Particularly for older children, assent serves a number of functions. It helps the child achieve awareness of her situation and calibrate her expectations, which may enhance cooperation with medical care. Assent also creates an opportunity for shared decision-making that can foster the autonomy of young patients and prepare them to assume an ever-greater role in their own healthcare, preparing them to eventually replace their parents as the primary medical decision-makers. Fostering autonomy is particularly important to me as the parent of a child with a chronic illness because I know that years of treatment and countless health-care decisions lay ahead of her. Additionally, I want my daughter to know that her body is her own to control. I am all too aware of the possibility that she may come to believe that her body is controlled by well-intentioned adults who make and execute decisions without her input in the service of making her "better" (Robertson, 2019).

I recently baked a cake for my daughter's seventh birthday. Six of the seven times she's blown out the candles on her birthday cake, we've known that she has a chronic illness. Due to this confluence of age and illness, questions about when and how to seek her assent are particularly salient to me at the moment. This has led me to look increasingly critically at how my daughter's healthcare is delivered, focusing on the consent practices she and I encounter. Her clinical team routinely seeks my permission and her assent as appropriate, closely following the contours of consent for pediatric practice just outlined.

Yet, as a mother, a nurse, and a bioethicist, I see areas for reflection and improvement—particularly when decisions are made around her research participation and around involvement of trainees in her care. As I noted at the outset, these decisions are different than decisions about her clinical care. Whereas my daughter's clinical care is for her benefit, her involvement in research and in training is for the benefit of other, future patients. When we recognize that the goals of research and training are different from the goals of care, it becomes apparent that there are important *moral* differences between these activities as well. And so, I will now turn to decisions about research and training.

Decisions About Research

Much remains unknown about my daughter's chronic condition. As often as not, when I ask a question of my daughter's medical team, the response is a variation on the following: "We don't know." "We're trying to figure that out." Or, "We have some preliminary data suggesting that . . ." Because there are so many open questions, our family has been approached numerous times with opportunities to participate in research to understand biological processes and develop effective treatments. I've been told that we're "a good family for research." I suspect this statement reflects, in part, that we're highly compliant with my daughter's care and attuned to the significant need for research.

At the hospital and in the doctor's office, my professional identity as a bioethicist recedes, allowing my personal identity as a mother to come to the fore. It recedes but does not disappear. Once, during a family meeting, my daughter's medical team floated the idea of having her participate in a clinical trial. Let me assure you, nothing plunges a family meeting into a surprised silence like when an attending asks what you're thinking and you reply:

> "Well . . . actually . . . I've been thinking about the lecture I gave on informed consent yesterday."
>
> "Remind me what you do?"
>
> "Oh, I teach bioethics."

For the decade-plus that I have worked in bioethics, I have focused primarily on ethical and regulatory oversight issues in human subjects research. I am a fierce champion of research. Moreover, I understand that children have long been "therapeutic orphans"—overlooked by investigators and denied the benefits of pharmaceutical research (Stiers & Ward, 2014).

Yet, the prospect of enrolling my own daughter in research can put my role as a mother and my commitment to research in tension. Participating in an observational longitudinal cohort study that uses my daughter's de-identified data? That was fine. There was no prospect of medical benefit for her, but the social value seemed high and the risks very low. But participating in a study that would require tapering her current medications according to a protocol rather than in a bespoke fashion? That felt very different. Despite appreciating the social value, I worried it was not in her best interests to forgo personalized care. I worried despite knowing there was more intuition than evidence informing her team's tapering decisions. My daughter was, as it turned out, ineligible for the tapering study, meaning that the decision about participation was not ultimately mine to make. But even now I feel the tension between wanting to advance the science and wanting to do what is best for her.

Research and care have long been considered distinct activities. Central to the distinction is the idea that the purpose of research—to create generalizable knowledge—is fundamentally different than that of clinical care—to provide personalized care (Largent et al., 2011). Other defining characteristics of research include research methodologies (e.g., randomization, blinding, placebo controls) that sacrifice personalization of care in pursuit of scientific and methodologic rigor and the justification of research-related procedures in light of their social and scientific value, rather than a prospect of direct medical benefit to the patient. Although research can provide care for a child that is good (or even optimal), the fact is that there are often aspects of research that are not in the child's best interest. This helps to explain why research and care are understood to be governed by distinct ethical commitments. Though there is growing pressure on the research-care distinction as efforts to integrate research into clinical care grow (e.g., in learning healthcare systems and embedded pragmatic trials), the distinction continues to have value as we seek to understand key normative commitments governing each (Faden et al., 2013; Largent et al., 2013).

From my mother-bioethicist vantage point, two key ethical issues have arisen around informed consent for research. The first is "dual-role" consent, and the second is the importance of both assent and also a lack of dissent when children are enrolled in research.

Dual-Role Consent

Unsurprisingly—given that my daughter's condition is uncommon, that much about it remains unknown, and that my daughter is fortunate to be cared for by leading experts in the field—members of my daughter's medical team tend also to be the principal investigators (or at least the site investigators) for many relevant studies. Classic statements of research ethics advise against permitting physician-investigators to obtain consent from patients with whom they have a preexisting treatment relationship. I refer to this as "dual-role" consent (Morain et al., 2019).

Reticence about dual-role consent reflects the view, discussed above, that distinct normative commitments govern research and care—and, by extension, clinician-patient and investigator-participant relationships. One implication of this view is that blurring the line between research and care could lead to ethical transgressions. There are three general concerns about dual-role consent. First, it may create role conflict for the physician-investigator who is torn between obligations to the patient and obligations to the research. Second, it can compromise the voluntariness of consent by making the patient or family feel they must consent to research or risk losing their primary treatment relationship. And third, it can promote therapeutic misconceptions—that is, the mistaken confla-tion of research and care (Horng & Grady, 2003).

In my academic work, I have written that although these concerns are valid, they are not dispositive in all cases (Morain et al., 2019). Rather, their force—and thus the ethical acceptability of dual-role consent—varies with study-specific features. As the key features of research participation—particularly the risks, burdens, and anticipated benefits—approach those associated with usual care, it becomes increasingly acceptable for physician-investigators to seek consent from their own patients. In some instances, it will even be preferable. By con-trast, when a trial deviates in important ways from what is typical of clinical care, having a neutral third party lead the consent process is ethically preferable.

Supporting this view, the existing empirical evidence (albeit limited) suggests that at least some patients prefer to discuss research participation with their treating physician (Cho et al., 2015; Kelley et al., 2015; Morain et al., 2023). This makes sense to me as both a bioethicist and a mother of a chronically ill child. Physician-investigators may, in light of the preexisting treatment relationship with a patient and family and their knowledge of the patient's medical and psy-chosocial circumstances, be best positioned to engage in shared decision-making about research participation. Moreover, a physician-investigator's recognition of their fiduciary role could minimize the likelihood that they recommend studies contrary to patients' best interests. This has been my experience.

Ultimately, I believe that the consent processes should typically be the effort of a team—the physician-investigator and a third party—rather than any single individual. This third party is often a research coordinator. One advantage of a team-based approach is that it capitalizes on the benefits of dual-role consent while minimizing the associated ethical concerns. This approach seems par-ticularly important in specialty pediatric care, where treatment often occurs in the context of research, and physician-investigators may be particularly adept at exploring families' goals and values, integrating these insights with their exper-tise, and helping guide decisions about research participation.

Lack of Dissent

Informed consent is generally understood as an ethical requirement in both care and research (Emanuel et al., 2000). Consent for research, however, typically requires higher levels of information-sharing, formality, and oversight than con-sent for care. This is because participation in research is not generally considered obligatory—indeed, it is generally considered supererogatory. Therefore, it is important that prospective participants have the opportunity to determine for themselves through the informed consent process whether enrolling in a particular study is consistent with their preferences, values, and interests. Some ethicists have argued, contrary to the common view and compellingly, that we have a *prima facie* moral duty to participate in research because biomedical knowledge is a public good (Schaefer et al., 2009). They are clear, however, that requirements for informed consent persist, even though participation is morally obligatory. On both accounts, whether participation in research is supererogatory or obligatory, informed consent is important. Yet, as discussed above, children are unable to give informed consent. That is why they are considered a vulnerable population requiring additional protection from research risks.

The federal government has special regulations governing research with children. The Federal Policy for the Protection of Human Subjects or "Common Rule" (45 CFR 46) is "a uniform regulatory floor for human subjects research . . . which generally requires informed consent, independent ethical review, and the minimization of avoidable risks" (Gutmann et al., 2011). The Common Rule requirements apply to children. There is, however, a set of regulations called "Subpart D" that follows the Common Rule and affords *additional* protections to children involved in research. Some of the protections pertain to permissible levels of risk and benefit. Other protections, the ones I will focus on here, are related to consent.

In most cases, the regulations allow children to participate in research only when their parents provide permission. In addition, Subpart D requires "that adequate protections are made for soliciting the [child's] assent" (§46.408). In this context, assent is defined as "a child's affirmative agreement to participate in research" (§46.402). A child's mere failure to object cannot be construed as assent. Subpart D's clear mandate to obtain assent from the child applies unless the child is not capable of providing assent or the research holds out a prospect of direct benefit that is important to the child's well-being and is only available in the context of research. Unfortunately, the federal regulations provide almost no guidance for how the assent requirement should be satisfied and no specific age beyond which assent is required. Many people think that children's assent should be required from age seven onward for developmental reasons discussed above, though this is a matter of debate (Gutmann et al., 2011). As a result of this regulatory ambiguity and lack of practical or ethical consensus about assent, these determinations are left to the discretion of individual institutional review boards (IRBs). This has resulted in problematic variability in practice (Kon, 2006). Clearly, "IRBs need guidance to ensure that the assent requirement is implemented in a way that appropriately respects pediatric research subjects" (Whittle et al., 2004, p. 1751).

Because my daughter only recently turned seven, she and I are just entering the period in which it is practically feasible to seek her assent for research participation. Years ago, when she was far too young to assent, I unhesitatingly gave my permission for my daughter to be enrolled in a longitudinal cohort study of children with her condition. The study employs medical records review, as well as surveys about quality of life and activities of daily living. Though the surveys are completed during routine clinical care appointments, they are for research purposes only. For years, I completed the surveys, meaning that my daughter was not encumbered by any research-related burdens (and only minimal privacy risks) as a result of her participation. At our most recent appointment, however, the research coordinator handed the clipboard with the sheaf of surveys not to me, but to my daughter because she is now old enough to complete the surveys herself. This necessitated that she and I have a sustained discussion about why her participation in research is important. While I told her that completing the surveys was optional, I also emphasized that studying her medical records can provide important insights that might help other kids and that it was consistent with our family values to help others. She ultimately agreed to continue participating and filled out the surveys. Of course, future studies for which my daughter is eligible will carry different risks and burdens and offer different prospects for direct medical benefit. Then, we will have to determine how to navigate the assent process in those circumstances.

A more protective alternative to requiring assent to research participation would be to adopt a lack-of-dissent standard. On this approach, a child's persistent refusal to give assent or sustained dissent (whether verbal or nonverbal) should be given greater ethical weight in the context of research than it does in the context of care. It should generally be determinative of the question of participation, particularly when participation in research offers the child no direct benefit or only a slight prospect of direct benefit (Leikin, 1993). Overriding a child's dissent is disrespectful both because it excludes them from the decision-making process and because it "represents a failure to stop research that may be causing a child distress or pain" (Wendler, 2006, p. 233). Notably, dissent does not require a reason or justification, and a child generally does not have to demonstrate any understanding of a research project in order for her dissent to be respected. This is key. It means that even young children—children who cannot developmentally give assent—can dissent and influence decision-making about their participation in research. Thus, there can be either agency-based or welfare-based reasons for respecting dissent.

Sustained dissent might be repeatedly saying "no," or engaging in prolonged crying or flailing. Of course, there will be times when—if it is a matter of safety or direct medical benefit—sustained dissent cannot be determinative. For example, if a child is enrolled in an ongoing study of a novel drug, it may be necessary to proceed with a scheduled lab draw to monitor for drug-induced liver injury over the child's vociferous dissent. Even in instances where sustained dissent should be respected, it is reasonable to try to address the child's concerns before abandoning research participation altogether.

A potential challenge is that, as I've already noted, my daughter is tired of medical encounters and treatment, but further research to understand and to treat—possibly even to cure—her chronic condition is essential. If, as I think it is reasonable to assume, my daughter's experience mirrors that of other chronically ill children in these ways, allowing for sustained dissent to protect these children could have the perverse consequence of resulting in less research overall being done that could improve their care and their lives. I don't believe this is a devastating objection to the sustained dissent view. Rather, it is indicative that more work is needed to identify the right balance of protections.

Decisions About Training

A primary goal of our medical education system is to produce clinicians qualified to promote health, prevent and treat disease, and relieve suffering. Though many aspects of the practice of medicine or of nursing can be learned in classrooms, from textbooks, or with simulators, others can only be learned through the direct provision of patient care (Largent et al., 2020). Nursing school, medical school, and graduate medical education programs offer trainees supervised educational experiences that support their acquisition of knowledge, skills, and professional judgment.

Trainees have been part of my daughter's medical care from the very beginning because she receives much of her care in teaching hospitals partnered with medical and nursing schools. I have routinely accepted trainees' presence at my daughter's bedside for a variety of reasons (Largent, 2020). Some reasons are highly specific to me. As a student nurse, I completed my pediatrics clinical in the very same children's hospital where my daughter presently receives her care. My nursing education depended on the willingness of families to let me learn at their children's bedsides. I feel like this is a favor I should repay. As a medical school faculty member, I'm committed to the education of excellent doctors. I believe my obligation to the students goes beyond the lecture halls to the hospital floors. Other reasons reflect the particular nature of my daughter's illness. Given the relative rarity of my daughter's condition, her case will likely be one of just a handful that trainees see. A closely related argument is that, in the absence of specific tests for her condition, experience with the physical exam is extremely important. I know this to be true because of my background in nursing. Neither preceptors nor trainees have ever taken the time to explain the importance of my daughter's involvement in training activities to her or to me. This is a missed opportunity.

Beyond these quite personal reasons, I think there is a moral obligation to say "yes" to trainees. Above, I noted that some ethicists feel that biomedical knowledge is a public good and, therefore, that there is a moral obligation to participate in research. Similarly, I would argue that biomedical knowledge as embodied by clinicians is a public good. All of us take advantage of this public good, and therefore, I would argue that we all have a *prima facie* obligation to contribute to training unless we have a good reason not to contribute (Largent, 2020).Yet, changing the default such that pediatric patients and their families appreciate that they should contribute to training unless it is too burdensome will require education that fosters and cultural change that appeals to a sense of duty.

Trainees need to hone their skills on patients to become better healthcare providers; society ultimately benefits from well-trained doctors and nurses. Though patients may benefit from trainees' time and focused attention, they don't necessarily benefit. They may be burdened or even harmed when trainees participate in their care, for example, by performing procedures that would otherwise be performed more efficiently or more effectively by a more experienced member of the team. These incremental risks and burdens are justified not by any prospect of direct medical benefit to the patient, but by the social value that results. This echoes the logic of research, not of care (Jagsi & Lehmann, 2004).

Because consent is an ethical centerpiece of research and because training is highly (though not perfectly) analogous to research, it is striking to me that it has been an exception rather than the norm that I am asked for my permission or that my daughter is asked for her assent to have trainees involved in her care. Our experience is consistent with research suggesting that there are gaps between ethical norms and actual practice regarding patient consent to participation in training activities for doctors and nurses more broadly (Torrance et al., 2012; Ubel et al., 2003). When I look to the literature on pediatric decision-making, I find that consent to involvement of trainees receives scant attention compared to consent for either care or research. The 2016 American Academy of Pediatrics policy on informed consent in pediatric practice doesn't, for example, address consent to trainee involvement at all (Katz et al., 2016).

Of course, I acknowledge that trainees will be included in my daughter's care when I sign the Bill of Patient and Family Rights and Responsibilities when we check her in for appointments. Blanket consent is, however, insufficient—"proximity of consent to individual procedures is crucial" (Jagsi & Lehmann, 2004, p. 332). Some may argue that context matters. I knowingly seek care for my daughter at a teaching hospital, and during visits, each person's place on the medical hierarchy is meticulously detailed for me. There are introductions, badges, and shorter or longer white coats. Therefore, the argument goes, my permission is implied. I have three responses to this argument.

First, medical education is opaque to many people. In one survey of emergency room patients, only half of respondents knew what "medical student" meant, and only a third knew what "intern" and "resident" meant (Pallin et al., 2008). We cannot assume that parents understand the import of meticulous introductions, read badges, or intuit the meaning of the length of a doctor's white coat or the color of a nursing student's uniform. Disclosure of trainee involvement in the absence of parental comprehension does not—indeed, cannot—constitute informed consent. Therefore, the process of obtaining parental permission should include a discussion of the trainee's role, as well as of what steps are taken to promote patient safety when trainees are involved in care, such as assuring appropriate faculty supervision.

Second, even if parents understand the roles and responsibilities of the various team members, if they do not know—or do not feel—they can make a voluntary choice about trainee involvement, a mere lack of objection cannot be equated to morally transformative agreement to having trainees involved a child's care. Given my background in nursing and bioethics (and as a lawyer who has actually read the Bill of Patient and Family Rights), I know that I can say "no" without adverse consequences for my daughter's care. But we cannot assume that all parents know they have the right to say "no." Though this is purely anecdotal, my husband only recently came to appreciate that he could say "no" despite years of attentive involvement in our daughter's care. As an aside, information asymmetries around who trainees are and whether they must be involved may help to explain why physicians' children are less likely to be seen by trainees than are other children (Diekema et al., 1996). The process of obtaining parental permission should make it clear that families can opt out while also appealing to their sense of moral duty.

My third reply is that any argument that relies on parental permission for trainee involvement in pediatric care problematically overlooks the centrality of the pediatric patient. If, for the reasons just outlined, we cannot argue that a parent's permission for trainee involvement is implied, we certainly cannot argue that a child's assent is implied. Children should typically be asked for their assent to trainee involvement in their care because their bodies are the site of learning. For my young daughter, I would often be satisfied with the attending simply saying: "This is Alison. She goes to school like you do, but at her school, she is learning to be a doctor. Is it okay with you if Alison helps me with your exam today?" At shift change, the beside nurse might explain that she is working with a nursing student and ask if the student can take vital signs or help with the day's medication administrtaion and ambulation. The detail and complexity of the assent process may change with the child's developmental stage as well as the trainee's role in care (e.g., observational vs. interventional). Above, I noted that in pediatric research there is a regulatory requirement to obtain the child's assent. I argued that there is also an ethical requirement to respect a child's sustained dissent in most cases, which allows even younger children to have a say in their research participation. I would argue that the same lack-of-dissent standard could be extended to involvement of trainees in a child's care.

For any child, there is potentially added discomfort and inconvenience in submitting to examinations or procedures performed by trainees. When a child is chronically ill, the cumulative burden can feel overwhelming. For instance, every few months, my daughter is seen in clinic. There is an essential albeit uncomfortable component of the exam for which she must sit absolutely still. Given her age and temperament, stillness is elusive. In the hands of an experienced clinician, this component of the exam can be completed in under a minute. In the hands of a trainee, it can take significantly longer—and then the exam must be repeated by a more experienced clinician to verify the trainee's assessment. My daughter's patience rapidly decays when she finds herself undergoing this exam at the hands of a trainee. She grows increasingly frustrated. In cases like this, I would hope she would say "yes" if asked to let a trainee examine her, but also that she would have the chance to draw a line, to say "enough" if the exam wears on too long. Children may find value in knowing that they have the option to say "no" even if they never exercise it.

Admittedly, there may be some times when it is easier to respect a child's sustained dissent than others. For example, in an emergency, a resident may be the only clinician immediately available to perform a medically necessary intervention (Largent et al., 2020). Moreover, there may be instances where it is impossible to parse whether a child is objecting to a medical intervention per se (where their dissent may not carry weight) versus objecting to the trainee's involvement (where it should carry weight). It may be fruitful in such circumstances to decide when or under what conditions a trainee will hand care over to a more experienced provider. For instance, a student nurse might be allowed two opportunities to insert an IV before the preceptor steps in.

A final point in closing is that communication and professionalism are taught at the bedside—not just clinical skills. When a trainee is involved in my daughter's care without my explicit permission and without her assent or lack of dissent, both the trainee and my daughter learn ethically troubling lessons. The trainee's sense of the importance of consent erodes (Ubel et al., 2003). And my daughter intuits a lack of autonomy from what is said and unsaid (Robertson, 2019). By contrast, asking for my permission and her assent demonstrates respect for my daughter as a person, rather than treating her as a convenient teaching tool.

Conclusion

As a nurse, a bioethicist, and a mother, I know that getting consent right, particularly in pediatric practice, is challenging. In this chapter, I have considered three major types of decisions that must be made—decisions about care, about research, and about training—and have identified the unique considerations when decisions are being made for and with a child. Fortunately, being mindful of our ethical obligations to patients—and patients' obligations to the health-care system—can make decision-making easier for pediatric patients and their families—patients, as it turns out, like my daughter, and families, as it turns out, like mine. Moreover, ethical reflection can show us where we still have room to improve.

Acknowledgment

I would like to thank my daughter for her assent to publishing this chapter.

References

Appelbaum, P. S. (2007). Assessment of patients' competence to consent to treatment. *New England Journal of Medicine*, *357*(18), 1834–1840.

Bartholome, W. G. (1989). A new understanding of consent in pediatric practice: Consent parental permission, and child assent. *Pediatric Annals*, *18*(4), 262–265.

Beauchamp, T. L. (2011). Informed consent: Its history, meaning, and present challenges. *Cambridge Quarterly of Healthcare Ethics*, *20*(4), 515–523.

Berg, J. W., Appelbaum, P. S., Lidz, C. W., & Parker, L. S. (2001). *Informed consent: Legal theory and clinical practice*. Oxford University Press.

Cho, M. K., Magnus, D., Constantine, M., Lee, S. S. J., Kelley, M., Alessi, S., Korngiebel, D., James, C., Kuwana, E., Gallagher, T. H., Diekema, D., Capron, A. M., Joffee, S., & Wilfond, B. S. (2015). Attitudes toward risk and informed consent for research on medical practices: A cross-sectional survey. *Annals of Internal Medicine*, *162*(10), 690–696.

Coleman, D. L., & Rosoff, P. M. (2013). The legal authority of mature minors to consent to general medical treatment. *Pediatrics*, *131*(4), 786–793.

Diekema, D. S., Cummings, P., & Quan, L. (1996). Physicians' children are treated differently in the emergency department. *The American Journal of Emergency Medicine*, *14*(1), 6–9.

Emanuel, E. J. (Ed.) (2003). *Ethical and regulatory aspects of clinical research: Readings and commentary*. Johns Hopkins University Press

Emanuel, E. J., Wendler, D., & Grady, C. (2000). What makes clinical research ethical? *JAMA*, *283*(20), 2701–2711.

Faden, R. R., Beauchamp, T. L., & King, N. M. P. (1986). *A history and theory of informed consent*. Oxford University Press.

Faden, R. R., Kass, N. E., Goodman, S. N., Pronovost, P., Tunis, S., & Beauchamp, T. L. (2013). An ethics framework for a learning health care system: A departure from traditional research ethics and clinical ethics. *The Hastings Center Report*, *43*(s1), S16–S27.

Gutmann, A., Wagner, J., Allen, A. L., Hauser, S. L., Arras, J. D., Kucherlapati, R. S., Atkinson, B. F., Michael, N. L., Farahany, N. A., Sulmasy, D. P. & Grady, C. (2011). Moral science: Protecting participants in human subjects research. *Presidential Commission for the Study of Bioethical Issues.* Washington, DC.

Horng, S., & Grady, C. (2003). Misunderstanding in clinical research: Distinguishing therapeutic misconception, therapeutic misestimation, & therapeutic optimism. *IRB: Ethics and Human Research, 25*(1), 11–16.

Kohrman, A., & Clayton, E. W. (1995) Informed consent, parental permission, and assent in pediatric practice. *Pediatrics, 95*(2), 314–317.

Jagsi, R., & Lehmann, L. S. (2004). The ethics of medical education. *British Medical Journal, 329*(7461), 332–334.

Katz, A. L., Webb, S. A., Macauley, R. C., Mercurio, M. R., Moon, M. R., Okun, A. L., Opel, D. J., Statter, M. B., & Committee on Bioethics. (2016). Informed consent in decision-making in pediatric practice. *Pediatrics, 138*(2), e20161485.

Kelley, M., James, C., Alessi Kraft, S., Korngiebel, D., Wijangco, I., Rosenthal, E., Joffe, S., Cho, M. K., Wilfond, B., & Lee, S. S. J. (2015). Patient perspectives on the learning health system: The importance of trust and shared decision making. *The American Journal of Bioethics, 15*(9), 4–17.

Kon, A. A. (2006). Assent in pediatric research. *Pediatrics, 117*(5), 1806–1810.

Lane, S. H., & Kohlenberg, E. (2012). Emancipated minors: Health policy and implications for nursing. *Journal of Pediatric Nursing, 27*(5), 533–548.

Largent, E. A. (2020). Consent to trainee involvement in pediatric care. *New England Journal of Medicine, 383*(12), 1097–1099.

Largent, E. A., Joffe, S., & Miller, F. G. (2011). Can research and care be ethically integrated? *Hastings Center Report, 41*(4), 37–46.

Largent, E. A., Miller, F. G., & Joffe, S. (2013). A prescription for ethical learning. *Hastings Center Report, 43*(s1), S28–S29.

Largent, E. A., Newman, R., Gaw, C. E., & Lantos, J. D. (2020). When a family seeks to exclude residents from their child's care. *Pediatrics, 146*(6), e2020011007.

Leikin, S. (1993). Minors' assent, consent, or dissent to medical research. IRB: Ethics and Human Research, 15(2), 1.

Morain, S. R., Barlevy, D., Joffe, S., & Largent, E. A. (2023). Physician-Investigator, research coordinator, and patient perspectives on dual-role consent in oncology: A qualitative study. *JAMA Network Open, 6*(7), e2325477.

Morain, S. R., Joffe, S., & Largent, E. A. (2019). When is it ethical for physician-investigators to seek consent from their own patients? *The American Journal of Bioethics, 19*(4), 11–18.

Okuyama, A., Wagner, C., & Bijnen, B. (2014). Speaking up for patient safety by hospital-based health care professionals: a literature review. *BMC Health Services Research, 14*(1), 61.

Pallin, D. J., Harris, R., Johnson, C. I., & Giraldez, E. (2008). Is consent "informed" when patients receive care from medical trainees? *Academic Emergency Medicine, 15*(12), 1304–1308.

Robertson, A. D. (2019). What I learned from my childhood as a patient: Internalized messages about bodies. *JAMA Pediatrics, 173*(8), 719.

Ross, L. F. (2019). Better than best (interest standard) in pediatric decision making. *Journal of Clinical Ethics, 30*(3), 183–195.

Schaefer, G. O., Emanuel, E. J., & Wertheimer, A. (2009). The obligation to participate in biomedical research. *JAMA, 302*(1), 67–72.

Stiers, J. L., & Ward, R. M. (2014). Newborns, one of the last therapeutic orphans to be adopted. *JAMA Pediatrics, 168*(2), 106.

Torrance, C., Mansell, I., & Wilson, C. (2012). Learning objects? Nurse educators' views on using patients for student learning: Ethics and consent. *Education for Health, 25*(2), 92–97.

Ubel, P. A., Jepson, C., & Silver-Isenstadt, A. (2003). Don't ask, don't tell: A change in medical student attitudes after obstetrics/gynecology clerkships toward seeking consent for pelvic examinations on an anesthetized patient. *American Journal of Obstetrics and Gynecology, 188*(2), 575–579.

Waligora, M., Dranseika, V., & Piasecki, J. (2014). Child's assent in research: Age threshold or personalisation? *BMC Medical Ethics, 15*(1), 44.

Wendler, D. S. (2006). Assent in paediatric research: Theoretical and practical considerations. *Journal of Medical Ethics, 32*(4), 229–234.

Whittle, A., Shah, S., Wilfond, B., Gensler, G., & Wendler, D. (2004). Institutional review board practices regarding assent in pediatric research. *Pediatrics, 113*(6), 1747–1752.

14

How Confucian Values Shape the Moral Boundaries of Family Caregiving

*Helen Yue-lai Chan, Richard Kim, Doris Yin-ping Leung, Ho-yu Cheng,
Connie Yuen-yu Chong, and Wai-tong Chien*

Confucian ethics have been fundamental to many East Asian cultures in structuring social and moral norms and ethical duties, thereby promoting social solidarity. Of the five cardinal relationships (*wu lun* 五倫) identified in Confucianism, three are within the family: father–son, elder brother–younger brother, and husband–wife (the other two are ruler–subject and friend–friend). This suggests that family, on the Confucian view, is the basis of a society. The concept of self-identity is often intertwined with social identity in the interpersonal relationships within the Confucian tradition, and thus the family shares in happiness, manages challenges, and endures suffering together, as a part of a single unit (Chang & Basnyat, 2017; Sun & Fan, 2019). Family continues to play a fundamental role in caregiving in both East Asian and Chinese communities in Western countries. In Confucian-based familism, maintaining family continuity is essential not only for the good of the family, but also for ensuring that one is able to receive adequate care in late adulthood. Family remains the locus of care for many, and its role of providing holistic support to aged relatives is particularly clear in an aging society (Bedford & Yeh, 2019; Xie & Fan, 2020).

The aim of this chapter is to analyze the ethical duties commonly observed in family caregivers in Confucian culture. In this chapter, we first review the fundamental values in Confucian ethics and then identify the ethical issues emerging in family caregiving through cases drawn from our recent research. This is followed by discussion of family caregiving in the context of Confucian values and its impacts. We explore transcultural commonalities and examine the discrepancies in traditional teachings and contemporary understanding of Confucian values. We also offer suggestions to enhance cultural competence in the practice of nursing.

The Moral Significance of Confucian Values

Confucian values emerged from the teachings of Confucius, or Kongzi (孔子) (trad. 551–479 BCE), one of the most influential thinkers in the history of Eastern culture and society. Confucius claimed that *ren* (仁, often translated as "humaneness," "goodness," or "benevolence") is the underpinning value defining the ethical norms of attitudes, beliefs, and conduct in interpersonal relationships. As stated in the *Doctrine of the Mean* (*Zhong Yong* 中庸), one of the Four Books in the Confucian traditions, "benevolence is the characteristic element of humanity, and the great exercise of it is in loving relatives" (20:5). Family members are expected to provide good care for, and meet the needs of, their loved ones despite limited support during the caregiving process. In the *Book of Rites* (*Liji* 禮記), one of the Five Classics in the Confucian traditions, the following values are listed:

> Kindness on the part of the father, and filial duty on that of the son; gentleness on the part of the elder brother, and obedience on that of the younger; righteousness on the part of the husband, and submission on that of the wife; kindness on the part of the elders and deference on that of juniors; with benevolence on the part of the ruler, and loyalty on that of the minister. (Li Yun 9:19)[1]

These ten normative values shape the expectations and obligations for the five Confucian interpersonal relationships in a society, including those within a family. Although modernization and Westernization have generally identified "family" as the nuclear family and have, according to some sociologists, lessened both the interdependence of family members and the influence of filial beliefs (Bedford & Yeh, 2019; Xia & Xu, 2017), family remains the primary source of caregiving in Confucian societies (Fan, 2006).

It is worth noting that there are a number of Confucian values and norms that those who live in contemporary, Western societies may find challenging, with perhaps the subordination of wives being the most challenging.[2] Moreover, in passages throughout the classical Confucian texts, the duties of family appear to be both far less contingent on context and much more demanding than those commonly found in the West. For example, some Western scholars have argued that whether or not adult children have a duty to obey their parents and take care of them in their old age depends on the extent to which parents

---

[1]   Translation from Legge, Legge, Chai, & Chai (1967, pp. 379–380).
[2]   Discussions of gender relations in Confucianism have been an important topic of scholarly exploration in recent years. What has emerged from discussions on gender relations is that, while there are patriarchal elements in classical Confucian texts that would trouble many contemporary readers, there is considerable room for debate concerning whether Confucianism is intrinsically connected to these patriarchal values. See Li (1994) and Raphals (1998).

fulfill their parental responsibilities.[3] Indeed, there are some deep and fundamental differences in ethical worldviews between Confucian and contemporary
Western societies. There is, of course, much more to say here, and we return to
this topic when discussing transcultural values.

Regarding the basic account of filial duty in Confucianism, "filial piety" (*xiao*
孝) is a well-known and fundamental Confucian value requiring grown children
to express indebtedness and reverence. Filial piety is a cornerstone of Confucian
ethics and is also known as fraternal submission. As Master You said:

> A young person who is filial and respectful of his elders rarely becomes the kind
> of person who is inclined to defy his superiors, and there has never been a case
> of one who is disinclined to defy his superiors stirring up rebellion. The gent-
> leman applied himself to the roots. "Once the roots are firmly established, the
> Way will grow." Might we not say that filial piety and respect for elders consti-
> tute the root of Goodness? (Analects 1:2)[4]

Hence, being a filial son or daughter is the foundation of moral development
(Nie, 2020; Slingerland, 2003). This explicates a traditional saying, "Filiality
is prioritized as the first among a hundred kinds of behaviors," that inculcates
moral values into our daily lives. The Chinese character for filiality (*xiao* 孝) is
the combination of two characters, with "old" (*lao* 老) placed just above "son"
(*zi* 子), suggesting a son carrying an older person on his shoulders. In modern
language, this character is usually used in the term *xiao shun*, (孝順) meaning
that filial children are required to be obedient to parents. The focus of the term is
squarely on adult children's duty to take care of their parents, a value that remains
deeply entrenched in East Asian cultures and societies. From this standpoint,
families provide the initial environment for not only physical but also moral development: it is through our parents that we gain our moral sensibilities, which
in turn shape our moral identity.

In recent decades, there has been significant scholarly treatment of
Confucianism as a form of virtue ethics, a normative theory that takes virtues—
excellent dispositions of character or mind—as central to the ethical life
(Ivanhoe, 2007).[5] By developing virtues, one becomes properly disposed to feel,
think, and act well in a variety of situations. Virtue ethics also tends to focus
on the kind of person one should become and on what constitutes a flourishing
human life. Debates about whether Confucianism is a form of virtue ethics not-
withstanding, it is clear that early Confucian thinkers paid much attention to the

---

[3] This view is argued by English (1979).
[4] Translation from Slingerland (2003, p. 1).
[5] The scholarly literature on virtue ethics is vast and continues to grow (see Tiwald, 2010).

kind of moral character one ought to develop in the course of one's life and to the reshaping of one's motivations, emotions, thoughts, and behaviors through constant self-examination, ritual practice, and conscientious social intercourse. As a number of scholars have argued, filial piety is a cornerstone virtue, playing a pivotal role in the Confucian tradition (Ivanhoe, 2007; Kim, 2020; Sarkissian, 2010). Following the account of virtue offered by Nussbaum (1988), as connected to distinct "spheres of human experience," we might locate the virtue of filial piety as the excellence that allows one to act properly with regard to one's relationship to parents. In fact, the Confucian tradition is on solid ground when it comes to the view that the child-parent relationship is a key experience in the lives of most humans. Filial piety, then, is the virtue that allows us to act well in this important, complex, and intimate part of human lives.

In the next section we explore the complexities of familial relationships and how the virtue of filial piety can be exemplified in concrete human experiences.

Understanding Family Caregiving in the Context of Confucian Values

In this section, we present four cases involving Chinese family caregivers managing chronic disease, including the perspectives of parents and adult children drawn from recent studies, to illustrate how they grapple with complex moral situations involving familial care. We hope to show that care for dependents often involves challenging, morally complex features. Nevertheless, we find in these cases the manifestation of the Confucian ethical outlook regarding the responsibilities that family members have toward the sick and dependent.

Case 1: Care for Child with Developmental Disorder

Ms. M cares for her eight-year-old son with Asperger's syndrome. Her son often cries, screams, and threatens Ms. M by saying, "If you do not follow my requests, I am going to starve myself to death!" On one occasion, Ms. M insisted on declining his request for an expensive toy. To validate his threat, her son refused to eat for a whole day. Eventually, Ms. M bought the toy for him. Ms. M's son has continued to use this strategy, leading to a pattern wherein Ms. M often feels that she has no choice but to give in to her son's demands. This situation has been escalating since Ms. M found that her son would threaten to engage in self-harm, such as attempting to jump from a great height, if his demand is not obeyed. Ms. M shared, "Every time when my son blames me ruining his experience at school [...], and says that he has suffered enough, although I know what he says is wrong, I still find myself anxious with doubts, 'Am I wrong? Am I not good enough?' If I do not satisfy his requests, I worry so much that he will really hurt himself.'"

Case 2: Care for Child With Mental Disorder

A father recalls, "My son has recently become more agitated and emotional over the past few months. One day, he told me that he would like to escape from the family because he thought it was over-controlling. He said to me that I am so stringent and demanding. He said he did not want to continue living in such a family and would commit suicide. [...] I felt very disappointed and I am fearful that I may lose my son, whom I love very much. From that time, I have been very afraid of upsetting him and making our relationship worse. [...] From the bottom of my heart, I am very fearful of never seeing him again in my life if he runs away from home. My son showed courtesy and filialness before the illness, but now he has become so emotional and uncooperative. Whenever I asked him to do trivial things, he would become very defensive and argue with me. [...] He has also threatened to attack me if I treat him badly, although I think he would not hurt me, as I am his only significant person in the world."

Case 3: Care for Aged Parent

Ms. X is a single middle-aged woman living with her mother, who suffered from a massive hemispheric stroke in a public housing estate. To prevent her mother from moving to a residential care facility, Ms. X quit her job to be her primary caregiver. Ms. X did not seek emotional and financial support from her younger brother, as she believed he had to manage his own family issues and that it was the obligation of an elder daughter to take care of her mother. She tried to send her mother to respite care, but her mother refused to eat without her companionship. Hence, despite muscle pain and other physical distress related to the caregiving tasks, Ms. X insisted on her mother staying at home, perceiving this as her responsibility as a daughter.

Case 4: Care for Parent with a Life-limiting Condition

Mr. B's father, who was diagnosed with advanced dementia, was admitted to the hospital due to fever. Given his unstable condition, the healthcare team asked Mr. B and his younger sister to decide whether life-sustaining treatments should be used should their father's condition deteriorate. Years ago, Mr. B was offended by the healthcare providers when they raised issues about end-of-life care. He even did not allow his father, who was still mentally competent at that time, to participate. The father preferred comfort care at the end of life, but avoided bringing up the conversation with Mr. B for fear of upsetting his son. When the disease progressed, Mr. B opted for a feeding tube for his father because he regarded forgoing life-sustaining treatments as giving up on his father's life. During this current situation, Mr. B again argued adamantly that they should preserve their father's life at all costs. Mr. B's sister knew their father's wish for end-of-life care but she would not dare to speak up given Mr. B's hard stance.

The preceding examples reveal a range of attitudes, beliefs, and behaviors of Chinese family caregivers which in different ways have been influenced by Confucian sociocultural values. As noted above, many scholars have interpreted Confucian ethics as a form of virtue ethics that, like Aristotelianism, takes the life of virtue as enjoyable for the virtuous agent. However, in the aforementioned cases, the moral commitments rooted in Confucian ethics seem to result in the feeling of entrapment among family caregivers. In the following paragraphs, we analyze the dynamics between caregivers and care recipients.

Cultural expectations place enormous pressure on those who are expected to take care of sick family members (usually adult children) in Confucian societies. Family members with ill health are generally regarded as vulnerable and are expected to be protected from further physical and emotional harms. As we observed in the above cases, caregivers often try to please their loved ones to prevent them from experiencing negative emotions or feelings of abandonment, sometimes to the extent of overindulgence, and in doing so they may even reinforce the caregiver's subservient role, as well as keep the recipient of care locked into their own position (Chien et al., 2001; Kasl & Cobb, 1966; Williams, 2005). In Cases 1 and 2, the caregiving parents are pressured by intimidation tactics to comply with their children's demands. The parents demonstrated fear that the children would cause self-harm or even commit suicide. The two cases involving the adult children of aging parents are more complicated, as these caregivers may be expected to conform to the sociocultural expectations of filial piety. For example, Ms. X internalized the role expectations of family caregiving, prioritizing her mother's welfare over her personal life (Ng et al., 2016).[6] Mr. B also seemed to internalize a duty to provide unconditional support for one's parents. He appeared to be afraid of violating the duties arising from filial piety by insisting on life-sustaining treatment as a moral obligation. His intention to prolong his father's life as much as possible may be explicated by his perception of the death of his father as personal failure (Chow, 2017).

It is worth clarifying that we are not endorsing these values or the way the participants in the cases handled their situation. Rather, we are trying to show how the moral psychology at work in these cases is anchored in certain Confucian values that have become deeply embedded within many non-Western cultures and societies. While determining whether these values are worth reflective endorsement would require a separate, normative inquiry, it seems increasingly accepted by moral philosophers that morality arises within specific cultures and societies, and so normative reflection must also address the norms and values that shape a particular society. This does not mean that we cannot engage critically and offer reasons for revising or even discarding certain values, but that such work needs to be done carefully, by first doing the hard work of understanding *why* some values gained a foothold in certain communities.

The overprotective acts of family caregivers can create tension and conflict in relationships, resulting in the caregivers' feelings of guilt (Chong et al., 2018; Han et al., 2019; Ng et al., 2016). The reflective questions asked by Ms. M concerning her actions may be an indication of her sense that she was failing in her role as a caregiver (Johncock, 2018). The fear of her mother harming herself drove Ms. X to insist on having her mother live with her at the cost of her own psychological and physical health. Mr. B, who refused to discuss end-of-life care issues with his father, had a similar aim to protect him, in this case from emotionally draining conversations and anxiety (Pang, 1999). The topic of death remains a cultural taboo; thus, discussing issues such as end-of-life care with sick relatives can feel intrusive and impolite and may be perceived (whether rightly or wrongly) as abdicating caregiving responsibility. The feeling of obligation to care for and protect the old and sick prompted Mr. B to act paternalistically by not allowing his father to make treatment decisions (Luichies et al., 2019). His decision to disregard his father's wishes may also have been made out of a sense of failure to live up to expectations of him as a caregiver. These expectations are linked to the sense of self-worth in Chinese culture. We elaborate upon this concept in the following section.

---

[6] It is worth noting that when it comes to intimate relationships, there is not a sharp boundary between one's own "personal well-being" and the well-being of those one deeply cares about.

Transcultural Commonalities and Differences in Family Caregiving

Some of the behaviors in the above examples may seem irrational, particularly through the lens of modern liberalism that focuses on the values of rights and autonomy. To a certain extent, we agree and would argue that these undesirable psychological sequelae observed in the caregiving practices of the case studies result from a distorted understanding of Confucian values. Clearly, the nature of family caregiving is highly influenced by cultural context. Below, we will attempt to understand the differences in sentiment and behavior of family caregivers in both the East and West (Nie & Fitzgerald, 2016). We will also draw upon the four models of family interests to discuss different perspectives on balancing the interests between the sick individuals and their family members (Groll, 2014). The following section seeks to compare caregiving practices inherent in these specific cultural perspectives to reveal their possible commonalities and differences. Our intention is not born out of rivalry; we believe that the ethical values underlying family caregiving practices in different cultures are not absolutely dichotomous or contradictory.

Family Interests Versus Individual Autonomy

Inevitably, dedication to fulfilling a caregiving obligation can conflict with individual interests and goals (Johncock, 2018; Luichies et al., 2019). Seidlein et al. (2019), who explored caregiving burden in the long-term care setting, noted that caregiving responsibilities can be differentiated into the obligatory or supererogatory. To offer a brief explanation of distinction: the obligatory pertains to actions that are morally required. A failure to perform these actions would imply that one is morally blameworthy. Supererogatory actions are good to perform, but not morally required. A failure to perform such actions would not make a person morally blameworthy. For example, intimate social and emotional support are morally obligatory for family caregivers (Xu, 2021). According to the Special Goods Theory (Keller, 2006), such kind of care is special goods, irreplaceable by outsiders. On the other hand, responsibilities are considered supererogatory if they infringe on the caregiver's health or personal life (Seidlein et al., 2019). In the direct model of family interests, family members are encouraged to openly discuss and weigh their competing interests in the caregiving process. Family caregiving may draw upon each other's strengths and conserve resources through collaboration (Bamm & Rosenbaum, 2008; Coyne et al., 2017). It might also be justifiable to outsource some support to paid caregivers in the private market. This distinction, if it exists at all, is far less clear in the context of East

Asian cultures (Xu, 2021). What would often be considered a supererogatory ac-tion in the West may be understood as obligatory in East Asian societies (Keller, 2006). This difference helps explain why the family remains the backbone of care-giving in Confucian societies: a failure to give proper care to a family member would imply moral culpability and a downgrading of one's moral status as a filial child or concerned parent (Cheng et al., 2018; Leung et al., 2020). Here we may also notice a different conception of morality at work. Because Confucianism takes morality as tightly connected to the fulfillment of fundamental roles, failing to live up to one's role will be taken as failing from a moral point of view.

Apart from protecting their loved ones from harm, an overarching aim of caregivers in Confucian societies is that they work to preserve family harmony. Within such a cultural setting, when disagreements arise, direct confrontation is generally avoided, and it goes against the norm to "speak one's mind" (Bedford &Yeh, 2019). In Case 4, both Mr. B's father and his sister were afraid of upsetting him by contradicting his views on end-of-life treatment. Such avoidance of di-rect confrontation may be due to a traditional belief in retaining family and social harmony (Bond, 1996; Kwan, 2000). Although the father figure is tradi-tionally an authoritative position in the family, they can became submissive once they became care dependent (Bowman & Hui, 2000; Bowman & Singer, 2001). The interests of the whole family are prioritized over individual interests, per-sonal values, and wishes in a collectivistic society. This can be explained by the family interests model in which one may sacrifice for the sake of family members (Groll, 2014). Hence, if preserving face is considered important from a familial perspective, the father would follow the family's decision to prevent family members from feeling ashamed of themselves. A common result of these norms is that honest conversations are often missing within families. People tend to use an indirect approach in communication, which can make interpretation difficult and can cause misunderstandings (Fang & Faure, 2011). Messages in such com-munication are implicit and must be interpreted within their context, taking in-tonation and nonverbal expression into account. This communication style can avoid conflict and maintain harmonious relationships, but it requires listeners to read between the lines and offers little opportunity to ascertain whether their understanding is correct. For example, although Mr. B's father had his own care preferences, he may have avoided explicitly sharing his views by using indirect or subtle language, such as indicating that he preferred to "follow fate," stating that the future is "too hard to predict," and expressing his belief that his son would be able to make the most appropriate decision for him. The superficial meaning of his responses might simply be misinterpreted as indecisiveness or avoidance; his responses give little cue to the family regarding substitute decision-making for him concerning his care. These interpretations are in line with a qualitative study finding that emotional distance is a cultural barrier for reconciliation between parents and adult children at the final phase of life (Chan et al., 2012).

Moral Obligation Versus Reciprocity

The care of sick relatives and aged parents by family members exists across cultures and communities, albeit with subtle differences between the motivations and roles of Eastern and Western caregivers (Han et al., 2019; Johncock, 2018; Luichies et al., 2019; Prunty & Foli, 2019; Teng et al., 2020). The motivation of caregivers to promote the well-being of their sick or frail relatives in the examples provided aligns with the principle of beneficence in Western bioethics, although the Confucian perspective imposes a much more demanding form of care. Luichies et al. (2019) noted that the primary determining factor in the care-giving experience of adult children for their aged parents in Western culture is the quality of the child–parent relationship (Luichies et al., 2019). Western adult children tend to take up caregiving roles because they love their parents and have built good relationships with them. The concepts of "repaying the debt" and caregiving out of moral obligation or cultural norms are more likely to be rejected in Western cultures than in Eastern cultures (Luichies et al., 2019). It is more common in Western cultures that family caregivers consider themselves advocators for and supporters of relatives in need (Han et al., 2019).

In contrast, in Eastern cultures, adult children perceive taking care of those who are sick, weak, or in need as a moral obligation that often holds independent of the emotional quality of the relationship (Chang & Basnyat, 2017; Holroyd, 2001; Liu & Bern-Klug, 2016; Luichies et al., 2019). Ivanhoe (2007) contends that filial piety is more than a sense of gratitude for parental love; adult children owe their parents care because it is believed that parental sacrifices can never be fully repaid. Family caregiving, which is not limited to the child–parent relationship, is an inherited moral responsibility that persists even at a cost to one's own time and personal well-being. As discussed above, sick or aged relatives are generally deemed weak and vulnerable, and family caregivers bear a responsibility to ensure that the care recipients are free from all kinds of physical and psychological burdens. Examples of caregiving include performing even the most minute task for the recipient (Han et al., 2019) and preventing them from learning of or discussing any potentially emotionally sensitive issues (Pang, 1999). However, as illustrated in the aforementioned examples, overprotective acts can result in psychological and interpersonal injury. The intense nature of this type of caregiving role and the excessive authority, together with scrupulous concern, can have negative consequences for both parties.

Given these facts, it is important that nurses be cautious in assessing family dynamics and interactions when providing care to a family for which caregiving responsibilities are potentially motivated by social expectation stemming from filial piety or Confucian values. Rather than simply relying on family caregivers' perspectives, nurses should also listen to the care recipients' views and preferences for their care, as their voices may have been ignored in the caregiving process, as seen in the example of Mr. B's father (Chan & Pang, 2010). Nurses play a vital role in restoring equity in unbalanced relationships between caregiver and care recipient, and thus safeguard the patient's right to autonomy and informed choices.

Guilt Versus Shame

Both shame and guilt, usually manifested as depression and self-blame, are self-conscious, moral emotions. They are often used interchangeably, but they are considered distinct emotions in the literature (Bedford & Hwang, 2003; Cherry et al., 2017; Shen, 2018; Tangney et al., 2013; Teroni & Denna, 2008). Guilt results from a feeling of responsibility for wrongdoing, whereas shame results from an eroded self-image due to wrongdoing or failure to meet social expectations (Bedford & Hwang, 2003; Deem & Ramsey, 2016).

Contemporary scholarship suggests that family caregivers are vulnerable to self-stigmatized feelings, including shame, guilt, and embarrassment (Han et al., 2019; Yang, 2015). Guilty feelings among family caregivers have been divided into various categories. A study of guilt in Chinese bereaved adult children found that caregivers' guilt may stem from a broad range of issues, including bearing responsibility for the death (even absent any action of theirs leading to the death), survivor guilt, and indebtedness guilt (Chow, 2017). These negative emotions can be interpreted on the basis of the Confucian tradition wherein bereaved family members are expected to mourn for years (three years according to ancient practice) and are not entitled to any joyful experiences for a period of time (Chow, 2017). Prolonged expression of grief is still respected in modern Eastern culture, where family members withdraw for months from all kinds of festive events, including weddings, celebrations, and social gatherings. These examples echo Bedford and Hwang's (2003) argument that the sense of guilt may be present despite the obligation being beyond the capacity of the caregiver.

Nevertheless, empirical studies have shown that family caregivers are generally confused by these negative emotions. They commonly report a sense of guilt when they perceive themselves to be incompetent in caregiving responsibilities, even in the absence of a transgression (Holroyd, 2001; Nuyen, 2004). The guilt arises when caregivers perceive their own inadequacy in meeting the role expectations (positive duties) of caregivers (Johncock, 2018; Luichies et al., 2019; Prunty & Foli, 2019). In Case 3, Ms. X is afraid that she would fail in her role as a dutiful daughter if her mother is placed in a care facility, which is often regarded in Confucian society as escaping caregiving responsibility. This also helps to explain why Mr. B, in Case 4, insisted on employing every means nec-essary to preserve his father's life, regardless of the consequences; decisions to withhold or withdraw life-sustaining treatment from family members are seen as a failure to fulfill filial obligations (Teng et al., 2020). Liu and Bern-Klug (2016) maintain that worry about performance is a secondary stressor of caregiving burden among Chinese adult children.

Clearly, some of the guilty feelings reported by family caregivers may be shame. Confucian culture has been known as a shame-oriented culture in which shame (or "losing face") plays a key role in promoting self-regulated conduct and behavior (Geaney, 2004; Shen, 2018). "Face"—interpreted as the situated self-identity in Western social psychology—broadly refers to one's self-respect and dignity in Confucian society and has been well recognized in the litera-ture (Bedford & Hwang, 2003; Han, 2016). Hwang and Han (2010) divide the concept of face into social face (*mianzi*) and moral face (*lian*), the latter being based on the social evaluation of the integrity of an individual's moral character. Studies report that moral face is related to one's concern about cultural norms, such as filial piety, and an evaluation regarding to what extent one can act in so-cially accepted ways (Han, 2016; Yang, 2015). Preserving the good as well as the face of the family is an overarching duty of each family member (Fan, 2006; Han et al., 2019). Family caregivers exhibiting greater concern about protecting their moral face tend to internalize pressure from social norms or others' evaluation and thus feel shame and worthlessness if they fail to fulfill the expected moral obligations (Geaney, 2004).

Negative self-appraisal of the caregiving performance has been widely documented and is not limited to caregivers in Confucian society (Han et al., 2019; Johncock, 2018; Luichies et al., 2019; Prunty & Foli, 2019; Teng et al., 2020). This has important implications for nurses, who must be able to distin-guish shame from guilt. Although both emotions are primarily "social" emotions arising from a sense of duty imposed by cultural values and social expectations (Tangney et al., 2013), the strategies for managing the two emotions differ vastly. Unlike the feelings of guilt that motivate people toward reparative action, people with feelings of shame tend to exhibit maladaptive behaviors, such as denial or hiding from the situation, and externalize the emotion in the form of anger and blame put on others to reclaim a sense of control (Deem & Ramsey, 2016; Tangney et al., 2013). Shame drives family caregivers to be defensive or to deny wrongdoing (Cherry et al., 2017; Shen, 2018). There is substantial evidence of a significant positive association between families' level of expressed emotion, which is marked by high levels of criticism, emotional over-involvement, and/ or hostility, and patients' relapse rates in mental health problems (Cherry et al., 2017).

The overprotective and paternalistic acts taken by the family caregivers in the provided case studies may be partly due to an intention to avoid feeling shame as a caregiver. Hence, nurses should be sensitive to identifying shame through verbal or behavioral cues and risk factors. Being female, co-residing with the ailing family member, and having a close emotional relationship with the care recipient are associated with secondary anxiety, which can exacerbate feelings of shame (Liu & Bern-Klug, 2016). Nurses may find themselves scapegoats, drawing the irrational, hostile behavior or disproportionate expressions of anger associated with shame experienced by family caregivers, as they have the most frequent contact with patients and their families. In facing these situations, nurses should tactfully empower family caregivers to address the self-stigmatized feelings to strengthen their emotional capacity for caregiving. Nurses may discuss with the caregiver to explore the reasons for their guilt and shame. Given that shame is a social emotion stemming from perceived norms, it requires a multidisciplinary approach that includes peer support and public education to cultivate a compassionate culture that supports family caregivers in transcending the negative evaluative stance of self-disapproval and self-directed rumination and instilling conciliatory behaviors, such as appreciation of one's own efforts in the caregiver role within the practical constraints of medicine. Through constructive self-exploration, the caregiver can achieve greater self-understanding and become more open to healthy ways of dealing with the complex challenges that arise out of responsible caregiving. This does not mean the caregiver needs to abandon their fundamental Confucian values or moral outlook, for discarding one's deeply held cultural values is often neither practical nor helpful. Rather, the goal is to help the caregiver come to a deeper appreciation of her own motivations and goals, and the strong emotions attached to the situation. Through subtle, intelligent guidance, an effective nurse can help nudge the caregiver toward deeper self-understanding, leading to better long-term decisions for both the caregiver and the family.

Reflection on Confucian Ethics in Family Caregiving

The cited cases reveal that family caregiving guided by Confucian values may lead to fear and guilt due to perceived moral obligations. However, in classical Confucian ethics, we find not only a hierarchical authority embedded in social interactions to maintain social order in relationships (Bond, 1996), but also the need for the affectionate care of the elderly, who are among the most vulnerable people in society. When Ziyou asked Confucius the meaning of filial piety, the Master said, Nowadays, 'filial' means simply being able to provide one's parents with nourishment. But even dogs and horses are provided with nourishment. If you are not respectful, wherein lies the difference?[7]

The concept of reverence highlighted in this statement suggests that filial piety means more than merely providing parents with material and financial support; rather, it is rooted in care and respect. Rather than perceiving obligation as the driving force of caregiving, families should regard caregiving as a duty of compassion intended to express gratitude (Xu, 2021). To achieve this, nurses can act as facilitators for open communication that enables family members' frank expression of emotion, fosters connection, and promotes the interests of family caregivers when they are in conflict with those of the care recipients (Chan et al., 2012).

Returning to the discussion of the earlier case studies, we might worry that some of the behaviors of both caregivers and their recipients appeared detrimental to the participants. While we can observe that the behaviors were partially driven by a sense of responsibility connected to Confucian filial piety, it is apparent that certain negative emotions such as guilt, shame, or fear were also playing a substantial role in their decisions. In our view, it is important to take seriously the foundational Confucian values such as filial piety, but it is also important to critically evaluate whether a certain action is, in fact, advancing the good of the family and its members. For while it may appear that Mr. B was simply acting out of filiality in insisting on every type of life-saving procedure for his father, he may have been driven more by fear and guilt than considerations of what is best for his father. In fact, aside from what Mr. B should have done in this particular case, genuine expression of the virtue of filial piety would require acting in the best interest of one's parents. There is a world of difference between genuine virtue and mere simulacrum of virtue. This is a key point found in early Confucianism. Mencius, one of the most important Confucian thinkers, attributes to Confucius the following thought:

> I hate that which seems but is not. I hate weeds out of fear that they will be confused with grain sprouts. I hate cleverness out of fear that it will be confused with righteousness. I hate glibness out of fear that it will be confused with faithfulness. I hate the tunes of the state of Zheng out of fear that it will be confused with vermillion. I hate the village worthies out of fear that they will be confused with those who have Virtue.[8]

---

[7] *Analects* 2:7. From Slingerland (2003).
[8] *Mengzi* 7B37. From Van Norden (2008).

The village worthy is someone who is respected by the people in the village but isn't actually virtuous. To outsiders, the village worthy's behavior appears virtuous. But, as Mencius cautions, there is a large gap between the truly virtuous and one who is merely apparently virtuous. Often our behaviors, even when appearing to be decent, do not spring from the right motives. We act kindly toward a superior because we really want that promotion; we give to the beggar to feel better about ourselves. This is a crucial element of Confucianism that needs to be highlighted because even those who take themselves to be acting out of filial piety may in fact be acting for self-serving purposes. In noting this we do not mean to condemn Mr. B or other caregivers and care recipients in the case studies. Given the emotionally fraught and extremely challenging nature of the situation, acting well in such contexts is a truly heroic feat.

Confucianism is taken as a form of virtue ethics by many scholars, focusing on a set of Confucian virtues such as filial piety (*xiao*), reverence (*jing*), loyalty (*zhong*), and benevolence (*ren*) that are constitutive of well-being and human flourishing (Kim, 2020). We can now more clearly see how understanding these virtues may be important for the practice of nursing, particularly within a Confucian social context. Without an adequate understanding of the significance of these values in shaping the moral conception of the duties and responsibilities of caregivers and care recipients, nurses will not be able to attend to the needs of caregivers and their recipients with the sensitivity necessary for navigating complex situations. Virtue ethicists tend to eschew focusing on moral principles, and focus, rather, on cultivating proper feelings and thoughts, and the development of practical wisdom. But as we've observed through our case studies, family caregiving, due to its emotionally charged nature, will often involve a variety of challenging feelings connected to one's moral identity. So, for those nurses working within Confucian social and cultural contexts, the sort of guidance, intervention, and help they offer will need to consider those Confucian values that are shaping the participants' understanding of their moral responsibilities as both caregivers and care recipients.

Conclusion

This chapter has discussed family caregiving in the context of Confucian values, but the underlying goals and impacts of caregiving are universal across cultures. Because Confucianism highlights many of the moral features of care ethics, we might view Confucianism as taking up a more specific, culturally embodied form of care ethics that also focuses on the centrality of care, empathy, and human relationships, while also incorporating such values as loyalty, filial piety, and deference to elders—values that do not play as significant a role in the ethics of care literature. In the way that care ethicists have challenged the impartial, justice-based perspective of the concept as inadequate to capture the moral experience, Confucianism (along with other non-Western moral traditions) can provide a challenge to the Western system of moral values by showing that there are certain moral values, such as shame, deference, loyalty, and commitment, that ought to be given serious attention from an ethical point of view. However, there is a dearth of discussion in the literature about how to address ethical issues in relation to Confucian values, particularly in the context of family caregiving. We have attempted to provide some insights on nursing care in this chapter to spark more in-depth discussion to address this gap.

Acknowledgement

Some of the quotes in this chapter are fictitious and were developed based on the authors' clinical encounters. Other quotes are based on data gathered during a research study "Effects of a Motivational-Interviewing-Tailored Programme for Promoting Advance Care Planning Behaviours on Patients with Palliative Care Needs: A Randomised Controlled Trial" funded by General Research Fund (ref. no.: 14168417), Research Grants Council, The Hong Kong SAR Government. The funder had no influence on data collection, data analysis, or data interpretation. Ethical approval for the study was granted by the Joint Chinese University of Hong Kong—New Territories East Cluster Clinical Research Ethics Committee (ref. no.: 2017.414-T). The authors would like to express thanks to the participants for their support to our study.

References

Bamm, E. L., & Rosenbaum, P. (2008). Family-centered theory: Origins, development, barriers, and supports to implementation in rehabilitation medicine. *Archives of Physical Medicine and Rehabilitation, 89*(8), 1618–1624.

Bedford, O., & Hwang, K. K. (2003). Guilt and shame in Chinese culture: A cross-cultural framework from the perspective of morality and identity. *Journal for the Theory of Social Behaviour, 33*(2), 127–144.

Bedford, O., & Yeh, K. H. (2019). The history and the future of the psychology of filial piety: Chinese norms to contextualized personality construct. *Frontiers in Psychology, 10*, 1–11.

Bond, M. H. (1996). *The handbook of Chinese psychology.* Oxford University Press.

Bowman, K. W., & Hui, E. C. (2000). Bioethics for clinicians: 20. Chinese bioethics. *Canadian Medical Association Journal, 163*(11), 1481–1485.

Bowman, K. W., & Singer, P. A. (2001). Chinese seniors' perspectives on end-of-life decisions. *Social Science and Medicine, 53*(4), 455–464.

Chan, C. L. W., Ho, A. H. Y., Leung, P. P. Y., Chochinov, H. M., Neimeyer, R. A., Pang, S. M. C., & Tse, D. M. W. (2012). The blessings and the curses of filial piety on dignity at the end of life: Lived experience of Hong Kong Chinese adult children caregivers. *Journal of Ethnic and Cultural Diversity in Social Work, 21*(4), 277–296.

Chan, H. Y. L., & Pang, S. M. (2010). Let me talk: An advance care planning programme for frail nursing home residents. *Journal of Clinical Nursing, 19*(21–22), 3073–3084.

Chang, L., & Basnyat, I. (2017). Exploring family support for older Chinese Singaporean women in a Confucian society. *Health Communication, 32*(5), 603–611.

Cheng, H. Y., Chair, S. Y., & Chau, J. P. C. (2018). Effectiveness of a strength-oriented psychoeducation on caregiving competence, problem-solving abilities, psychosocial outcomes and physical health among family caregiver of stroke survivors: A randomised controlled trial. *International Journal of Nursing Studies, 87*, 84–93.

Cherry, M. G., Taylor, P. J., Brown, S. L., Rigby, J. W., & Sellwood, W. (2017). Guilt, shame and expressed emotion in carers of people with long-term mental health difficulties: A systematic review. *Psychiatry Research, 249*, 139–151.

Chien, W. T., Kam, C. W., & Lee, I. F. K. (2001). An assessment of the patients' needs in mental health education. *Journal of Advanced Nursing, 34*(3), 304–311.

Chong, Y. Y., Leung, D., & Mak, Y. W. (2018). When control exacerbates distress: A qualitative study exploring the experiences of Hong Kong Chinese parents in caring for a child with asthma. *International Journal of Environmental Research and Public Health, 15*(7), 1372. doi:10.3390/ijerph15071372

Chow, A. Y. (2017). Death in the family: Bereavement and mourning in contemporary China. In X. Zhang & L. Zhao (Eds.), *Handbook on the family and marriage in China* (pp. 373–391). Edward Elgar.

Coyne, E., Dieperink, K. B., Østergaard, B., & Creedy, D. K. (2017). Strengths and resources used by Australian and Danish adult patients and their family caregivers during treatment for cancer. *European Journal of Oncology Nursing, 29*, 53–59.

Deem, M. J., & Ramsey, G. (2016). Guilt by association? *Philosophical Psychology, 29*(4), 570–585.

Fan, R. (2006). Confucian filial piety and long term care for aged parents. *HEC Forum, 18*(1), 1–17.

Fang, T., & Faure, G. O. (2011). Chinese communication characteristics: A Yin Yang perspective. *International Journal of Intercultural Relations, 35*(3), 320–333.

Geaney, J. (2004). Guarding moral boundaries: Shame in early Confucianism. *Philosophy East and West, 54*(2), 113–142.

Groll, D. (2014). Four models of family interests. *Pediatrics, 134*(Suppl 2), S81–S86.

Han, K. H. (2016). The feeling of "face" in Confucian society: From a perspective of psychosocial equilibrium. *Frontiers in Psychology, 7*, 1055. doi:10.3389/fpsyg.2016.01055.

Han, M., Diwan, S., & Sun, K. (2019). Exploring caregiving-related experiences among Chinese American and European American family caregivers of persons with mental illness. *Transcultural Psychiatry, 56*(3), 491–509.

Holroyd, E. (2001). Hong Kong Chinese daughters' intergenerational caregiving obligations: A cultural model approach. *Social Science and Medicine, 53*(9), 1125–1134.

Hwang, K. K., & Han K. H. (2010). Face and morality in Confucian society. In E. H. Bond (Ed.), *Oxford handbook of Chinese psychology* (pp. 479–498). Oxford University Press.

Ivanhoe, P. (2007). Filial piety as a virtue. In P. J. Ivanhoe & R. L. Walker (Eds.), *Working virtue: Virtue ethics and contemporary moral problems* (pp. 297–312). Oxford University Press.

Johncock, W. (2018). How much care is enough? Carer's guilt and Bergsonian time. *Health Care Analysis, 26*(1), 94–107.

Kasl, S. V., & Cobb, S. (1966). Health behavior, illness behavior and sick role behavior: I. Health and illness behavior. *Archives of Environmental Health: An International Journal*, 12(2), 246–266.

Keller, S. (2006). Four theories of filial duty. *Philosophical Quarterly*, 56(223), 254–274.

Kim, R. (2020). *Confucianism and the philosophy of well-being*. Routledge.

Kwan, K.-L. K. (2000). Counseling Chinese peoples: Perspectives of filial piety. *Asian Journal of Counselling*, 7(1), 23–41.

Leung, D. Y. P., Chan, H. Y. L., Chiu, P. K. C., Lo, R. S. K., & Lee, L. L. Y. (2020). Source of social support and caregiving self-efficacy on caregiver burden and patient's quality of life: A path analysis on patients with palliative care needs and their caregivers. *International Journal of Environmental Research and Public Health*, 17(15), 5427. doi:10.3390/ijerph17155457.

Li, C. (1994). The Confucian concept of Jen and the Feminist ethics of care: A comparative study. *Hypatia*, 9(1), 70–89.

Liu, J., & Bern-Klug, M. (2016). "I should be doing more for my parent": Chinese adult children's worry about performance in providing care for their oldest-old parents. *International Psychogeriatrics*, 28(2), 303–315.

Luichies, I., Goossensen, A., & van der Meide, H. (2019). Caregiving for ageing parents: A literature review on the experience of adult children. *Nursing Ethics*, 28(6), 1–20.

Ng, H. Y., Griva, K., Lim, H. A., Tan, J. Y. S., & Mahendran, R. (2016). The burden of filial piety: A qualitative study on caregiving motivations amongst family caregivers of patients with cancer in Singapore. *Psychology and Health*, 31(11), 1293–1310.

Nie, J. (2020). The summit of a moral pilgrimage: Confucianism on healthy ageing and social eldercare. *Nursing Ethics*, 28(3), 316–326.

Nie, J., & Fitzgerald, R. (2016). Connecting the East and the West, the local and the universal: The methodological elements of a transcultural approach to bioethics. *Kennedy Institute of Ethics Journal*, 26(3), 219–247.

Nussbaum, M. (1988). Narrative emotions: Beckett's genealogy of love. *Ethics*, 98(2), 225–254.

Nuyen, A. T. (2004). Filial piety as respect for tradition. In A. Chan & S. Tan (Eds.), *Filial piety in Chinese thought and history* (pp. 212–223). Routledge.

Pang, S. M. C. (1999). Protective truthfulness: The Chinese way of safeguarding patients in informed treatment decisions. *Journal of Medical Ethics*, 25(3), 247–253.

Prunty, M. M., & Foli, K. J. (2019). Guilt experienced by caregivers to individuals with dementia: A concept analysis. *International Journal of Older People Nursing*, 14(2), 1–13.

Raphals, L. (1998). *Sharing the light: Representations of women and virtue in early China*. State University of New York Press.

Sarkissian, H. (2010). Recent approaches to Confucian filial morality. *Philosophy Compass*, 5(9), 725–734.

Seidlein, A. H., Buchholz, I., Buchholz, M., & Salloch, S. (2019). Relationships and burden: An empirical-ethical investigation of lived experience in home nursing arrangements. *Bioethics*, 33(4), 448–456.

Shen, L. (2018). The evolution of shame and guilt. *PLoS ONE*, 13(7), 1–11.

Slingerland, E. (Ed.). (2003). *Confucius Analects: With selections from traditional commentaries*. Hackett.

Sun, S., & Fan, R. (2019). To relieve or to terminate? A Confucian ethical reflection on the use of morphine for late-stage cancer patients in China. *Developing World Bioethics*, 20(3), 130–138.

Tangney, J. P., Stuewig, J., Malouf, E. T., & Youman, K. (2013). Communicative functions of shame and guilt. In K. Sterelny, R. Joyce, B. Calcott, & B. Fraser (Eds.), *Cooperation and its evolution* (pp. 485–502). MIT Press.

Teng, C., Sellars, M., Pond, D., Latt, M. D., Waite, L. M., Sinka, V., Logeman, C., & Tong, A. (2020). Making decisions about long-term institutional care placement among people with dementia and their caregivers: Systematic review of qualitative studies. *Gerontologist*, 60(4), e329–e346.

Teroni, F., & Deonna, J. A. (2008). Differentiating shame from guilt. *Consciousness and Cognition, 17*(3), 725–740.

Tiwald, J. (2010). Confucianism and virtue ethics: Still a fledgling in Chinese and comparative philosophy. *Comparative Philosophy, 1*(2), 55–63.

Van Norden, B. W. (2008). *Mengzi: With selections from traditional commentaries.* Indianapolis: Hackett Pub. Co.

Williams, S. J. (2005). Parsons revisited: From the sick role to . . . ? *Health, 9*(2), 123–144.

Xia, Y. R., & Xu, A. (2017). Changes in Chinese urban family structure. In X. Zang & L. X. Zhao (Eds.), *Handbook on the family and marriage in China* (pp. 42–52). Edward Elgar.

Xie, W., & Fan, R. (2020). Towards ethically and medically sustainable care for the elderly: The case of China. *HEC Forum, 32*(1), 1–12.

Xu, H. (2021). What should adult children do for their parents? *Nursing Ethics, 28*(3), 346–357.

Yang, X. (2015). No matter how I think, it already hurts: Self-stigmatized feelings and face concern of Chinese caregivers of people with intellectual disabilities. *Journal of Intellectual Disabilities, 19*(4), 367–380.

15

Constructing Avenues for Agency

A Role for Nurses in Caring for Persons With Disabilities

Laura K. Guidry-Grimes

Disability is a complex phenomenon. People with the exact same diagnosis can have vastly different experiences of disability depending on a host of factors. Those without a disability, including clinicians, tend to undervalue quality of life with disability when compared to first-person reports (Agaronnik et al., 2019; Iezzoni et al., 2021; Shakespeare et al., 2009; Skotko et al., 2011; VanPuymbrouck et al., 2020; Wilson & Scior, 2014). In a review of representations of disability in nursing and healthcare literature, the researchers conclude:

> Nurses should advocate cooperatively with those living with disability in an attempt to educate and transform negative labelling and stigmatization against those viewed as helpless, dependent, and as less able to contribute to society. Before this can be achieved, nurses must further the understanding of disability and recognize their own values, beliefs, views, prejudices and thoughts about disability. (Boyles et al., 2008, p. 434)

Nursing curricula have a number of gaps when it comes to addressing the needs, interests, and diversity of disabled people (Colbert & Kronk, 2020; Smeltzer et al., 2005). A 2010 review found that "textbooks widely used in undergraduate nursing education contribute to the lack of attention to the health, health care needs, and nursing of PWDs [persons with disabilities]" (Smeltzer et al., 2010, p. 152). An audit of nursing curricula found that the majority of programs did not require content focused on intellectual disability (ID), and a majority of nursing students "are emerging from their pre-registration studies with little to no knowledge of the needs of people with ID," which "is likely to contribute to the poor practices in hospitals that people with ID often experience" (Trollor et al., 2016, p. 76). According to a 2012 study, nurse educators exhibited a strong preference for able-bodied persons; their implicit bias scores against persons with disabilities[1] were even worse than scores from the general

---

[1] There is ongoing discussion among activists and scholars about whether "disabled persons" or "persons with disabilities" is the better term. I alternate between these terms out of respect for

public (Aaberg, 2012). Taken altogether, these data indicate that the nursing profession has opportunities for improvement in this area of patient[2] care and advocacy.

Disabled people are at risk of having their needs, interests, and values misunderstood or neglected in many spheres of life. The disability rights movement's slogan, "nothing about us without us," emphasizes this point: their inclusion and first-person experiences and self-identified needs should be prioritized, especially when others' decisions will affect them. In healthcare environments, these concerns can become especially acute. Prevalent misconceptions about disability, such as those about poor quality of life and the inability to participate in decisions, can quickly lead to harming or wronging the patient and endangering therapeutic trust.[3] When a person with a disability stays in the hospital, nursing home, or other healthcare facility, nurses (and often nursing assistants) become enmeshed in their daily life. Nurses are privy to sensitive details of what makes their patient's day go better or worse, and they take responsibility for some of the most intimate aspects of caregiving. Nurses should be ethically attuned to how a range of decisions, from the implementation of policies to bedside interactions, can support the patient as a person. In order to do this careful work well, nurses need to understand how sociopolitical and institutional structures affect experiences of disability.

The aim of this chapter is to show how disabled people can be rendered vulnerable in clinical contexts, which has implications for how nurses should identify and address different types of barriers for patients' agency. This chapter begins by distinguishing standard biomedical interpretations and social interpretations of disability. This discussion includes physical, intellectual, and psychiatric disabilities. Conceptions of disability differ in how they frame vulnerability and how they suggest vulnerabilities should be ameliorated. This chapter focuses on how institutional environments, such as hospitals and nursing homes, can limit opportunities for agency. Discussions of agency in bioethics tend to focus exclusively on autonomy, but there are a host of moral interests at stake with agency that ought to be protected. I then make this theoretical analysis more concrete by applying it to a specific area of agential interests—medication decisions. This chapter concludes with reflection on how healthcare facilities should proactively mitigate vulnerabilities for patients with disabilities.

this debate. It is important for nurses (and others) to use the self-identified language of people with disabilities, and norms and expectations can vary (see Ladau, 2021).

[2] For the sake of avoiding cumbersome sentences, I use the word "patient," but my analysis and recommendations also apply to those who live in healthcare facilities as residents.

[3] To learn more about the relationship between disability studies and bioethics, including discussion of quality-of-life judgments, reproductive justice, chronic illness, and end-of-life issues (among others), see Reynolds and Wieseler (2022).

Ways of Understanding Disability

The dominant medical narrative portrays disabilities as limitations that hinder worthwhile life pursuits and disrupt agency, as something wrong within the body of the individual. Nursing textbooks mostly focus on this interpretation of disability (Iklhani et al., 2016; Smeltzer et al., 2010). According to biomedical models,[4] deficiencies in quality of life are a direct and inevitable result of physiological facts of the impairment (e.g., the paralysis, genetic abnormality, neurological difference). Biomedical models can acknowledge the importance of discrimination, stigma, and other sociocultural and political factors that impact the lives of disabled people. However, according to this interpretation, impairment *always* threatens quality of life and the ability to function well in society, regardless of how accommodating the environment is. Biomedical models are also sometimes referred to as individual models, since the "disability is regarded as a problem at the individual (body-mind) level" (Barnes & Mercer, 2011, p. 2).

Biomedical models frame disability as personal tragedy. On this view, the root problem of impairment needs to be addressed through medical intervention. A just healthcare system would be aimed toward improving the quality and accessibility of treatment and prevention. Although proponents of biomedical modeling often claim that it is value-free and objective, "they also tend to regard normal functions as presumptively desirable and many, though not all, impairments as disadvantageous in causing various limitations and in denying or restricting valuable experiences or opportunities" (Wasserman, 2001, p. 221). As a result, anyone who does not try to minimize or prevent impairment (such as by seeking medical interventions or taking proactive steps through reproductive choices) would be making an irrational decision at best, a morally irresponsible decision at worst. To recover, the "disabled person is expected to make the best of their diminished circumstances and focus on individual adjustment and coping strategies with appropriate professional direction" (Oliver & Barnes, 2012, p. 19). As far as what counts as high quality of life, standards are based on ableist norms. Ableism refers to societal attitudes and practices that discriminate against and devalue people who have or are perceived to have disabilities: "This form of systemic oppression leads to people and society determining who is valuable or worthy based on people's appearance and/or their ability to satisfactorily produce, excel and 'behave'" (Lewis, 2019, n.p.). An ableist norm, then, suggests that only nondisabled functioning, behavior, or appearance is valuable. Daily reliance on a ventilator at home, caregiving support, or assistive technology, for

---

[4] Disability studies and disability bioethics have extensive discussion of these models, and I do not have space in this chapter to delve into the numerous nuances and debates on this topic. The basic distinction between biomedical and social models of disability has been hugely influential in scholarship and activism.

example, would be viewed as a necessarily diminished quality of life according to ableist norms.

Disability activism and disability studies challenge this narrative. This shift in perspective makes a difference for identifying the causes of disability, what it could mean to any given person, and how disabilities should be addressed. Despite the emphasis on biomedical models in nursing textbooks, social models (see Table 15.1) warrant more attention in nursing curricula (Colbert & Kronk, 2020; Iklhani et al., 2016). One benefit is that "if nurses are to be prepared to provide care that is empowering. [. . .] use of [social] models may encourage students to become advocates for the removal of barriers to health care and to examine how society and health professionals contribute to discrimination by constructing disability as an abnormal state" (Smeltzer et al., 2005, p. 215). According to this alternative interpretation, "impairment" designates a biological condition, whereas "disability" signifies a sociopolitical condition.[5] The extent to which someone is disabled will be a function of their specific context:

> the disability in a given situation is often created by the inability or unwillingness of others to adapt themselves or the environment to the physical or psychological reality of the person designated as "disabled"; and people with disabilities often regard the accommodations they make to their physical conditions as ordinary living arrangements and their lives as ordinary lives, despite their medicalization by professionals and most people's insistence that they are unusually helpless or dependent. (Wendell, 1996, p. 30)

While a condition may justifiably receive a medical diagnosis, that condition is not necessarily *disabling* on this view of disability. Disability bias, discrimination, stigma, lack of accommodation, and limited access can pose the exclusive or primary threat to the person's agency and flourishing potential—rather than one's impairment or embodied diversity. One implication is that disabled people have an epistemic privilege (a distinctive and superior source of knowledge and understanding) into their condition, which includes insights into which limitations are significant and from whence disadvantage arises (Asch, 2001).

A central claim of social models of disability is that a positive self-identity— an identity that opens doors for novel modes of being, new communities, and empowerment—can be available for persons with impairments and embodied difference (Shakespeare, 2010). Even if proponents of biomedical models insist

---

[5] Tom Shakespeare, Anita Silvers, Jenny Morris, Sally French, Julie Mulvany, Liz Crow, and others have all raised concerns about social models that rely on a sharp contrast between impairment and disability, since biological and environmental features interact in important ways. It is also important to recognize that some people who identify as Deaf or as neurodivergent reject impairment/disability language altogether.

Table 15.1 Contrasting Key Aspects of Medical and Social Models of Disability

	Medical Model	Social Model
Core values	Non-impaired functioning, behavior, appearance; independence, self-sufficiency, control	Expanding notions of valuable and normal human diversity; interdependence and relationality; nothing about us without us; disability justice (Invalid, 2017), equity
Central cause(s) of disability—what is often most *disabling*	Impaired or defective body, brain, genetics; significant biological losses or abnormalities	Environmental factors (social, legal, economic, architectural), lack of accommodation/access, stigma, discrimination, ableist norms
Quality of life with impairment	Necessarily diminished, less than what it would be without impairment	Not necessarily diminished; potential for positive self-identity, community, flourishing, meaningful living, agency
Appropriate interventions	Medically treating, removing, or preventing the impairment; coping strategies	Equitable restructuring of the sociopolitical environment; appropriate inclusion of persons with disabilities in decision-making; comprehensive accommodations and access
Just healthcare system	Would improve quality and accessibility of treatment or prevention of impairment	Would address environmental factors that contribute to disabling experiences, eliminate disability bias and discrimination from healthcare interpersonally and structurally, remove access barriers
Presumed expert perspective on disability	Medical professionals	Persons with disabilities

that they can recognize the empowerment of the disability community, they would nonetheless have to add a "but" in their assessment: They are capable of being empowered as a community, *but* each individual will inevitably struggle against the limitations posed by impairment and would be better off without it. Based on the social model, a just healthcare system would address *environmental* factors that contribute to disabling experiences for diverse patient groups.

Accommodating disability would have to include overhauling the structures of society that are built around ableist norms.

Of course, there is no monolithic experience of disability, and some impairments can cause pain and limitations. However, "[t]he claim that certain impairments preclude valuable experiences does not mean that they thereby make life any less rich or valuable overall; it may rather support the conclusion that there is an indefinite variety of ways in which human lives can flourish" (Wasserman, 2001, p. 222). Many in the disability community emphasize that their conditions can be associated with gifts, community, and enriched experiences; thus, it is not the case that all rational and responsible people, other things being equal, would (and should) take a "magic pill" to rid themselves of their impairment (Goering, 2008). Disability can be a form of human difference that is not "bad-difference" but instead "mere-difference," so that we "needn't deny that disabled people miss out on some intrinsically good abilities or experiences—it's just that they have access to other, different good things" (Barnes, 2019, p. 58).

Social model proponents emphasize that many perceived features of disability that are deemed to be undesirable—such as losses to independence, self-sufficiency, and control over one's life—are actually common facets of human existence or do not necessarily pose problematic limitations to individuals with disabilities as is commonly believed (Asch, 2001). Multiple studies have shown that healthcare professionals tend to assume, mistakenly, that disabled people have a lower quality of life due to their medical condition (Agaronnik et al., 2019; Iezzoni et al., 2021; Shakespeare et al., 2009; VanPuymbrouck et al., 2020). Many quality-of-life judgments are based in ableist norms or tacit subjective judgments from a nondisabled person about their own fears of having a certain impairment or disability. Given these issues, in addition to the vast diversity of disabled people, first-person reports are more reliable for quality-of-life assessments than outsider judgments.

Many disability activists and scholars contend that biomedical models err by misconstruing and overemphasizing the value of independence and control. As Adrienne Asch puts it:

> self-direction, self-determination, and participation in decision making about one's life are more genuine and authentic measures of independence or, better, interdependence. It is no more demeaning to obtain help in dressing or washing from a personal assistant than it is to get services from an auto mechanic, a plumber, or a computer technician. (2001, p. 313)

In the same vein, Carolyn Ells (2001) argues that any lack of control that is associated with impairment if often due to lack of accommodation and inaccessibility. To promote agential opportunities and support flourishing potential, barriers need to be reduced, and opportunities need to be created. This requires careful perceptiveness and creative problem-solving, along with ongoing partnership with people who have a range of disabilities. Unfortunately, none of this may be commonplace in facilities that are run by persons without disabilities.

Layers of Vulnerability With Disability

The human condition is one of frailty[6] and interdependence; we are always at risk of suffering harms, of losing what is important to us, of having some part of our support system lost. Humans are finite creatures in every sense—when it comes to our life span, our rationality, our abilities. We rely on innumerable features of our environment and our relationships to get through the day. This is evident in everything from our upbringing and education to the food we eat to our transportation to the basic means of recreation. Complex networks make our lives possible. If a person imagines themselves to be truly independent, that is likely a function of privilege: "the privileged have their dependency needs met almost invisibly—meals appear, beds are made, bills paid, suits are pressed—and in socially acceptable ways that honor norms of independence" (Holstein et al., 2010, p. 115).[7]

It is therefore a bizarre and tragic myth that disabled people are deeply dependent, while nondisabled people are completely independent. What makes this myth tragic is that cultural presumptions in favor of independence lead to denigrating assumptions about persons with disabilities. This is not to deny that certain disabilities may require more assistance with activities of daily living, such as washing, dressing, or toileting. But we are all interdependent, and features of our relationship and environment can further undermine *or* facilitate what we want to do in any given day. Jackie Leach Scully describes "permitted

---

[6] Some authors use the term "vulnerability" to cover the ontological condition of humanity in this way. Barry Hoffmaster, e.g., describes vulnerability as a universal feature of humanity that binds us together: "Vulnerability means that one is controlled by, rather than in control of, the world" (2006, p. 43). Christine Straehle argues that "[b]ackground conditions of vulnerability are a fact of human life" (2016, p. 35). Mackenzie, Rogers, and Dodds describe *inherent* vulnerability as the "capacity to suffer that is inherent in human embodiment" (2013, p. 4). For the sake of protecting "vulnerability" as a helpful term in bioethics, I use "frailty" to make the ontological point about humanity and "vulnerability" more narrowly (see Guidry-Grimes & Victor, 2012).

[7] This also highlights the invisibility of care work and other forms of labor that norms of independence gloss over. Caregiving, in domestic and professional spaces, is disproportionately done by women. Low-paid labor that makes the basic functioning of society possible is frequently done by racial minorities. Norms of independence, then, reflect complex histories and discriminatory patterns of ableism, classism, sexism, and racism (among other forms of bias and discrimination).

dependency" as those dependencies that are commonly shared and have been made invisible in industrialized society for those with a certain level of privilege. Scully (2014) makes the point that these permitted dependencies do not "show up as exceptional vulnerability" (p. 217). The dependencies associated with disability are not all inevitable consequences of impairment but are instead "established and maintained through implicit decisions made by the people, usually not disabled, who have the power to do so" (Scully, 2014, p. 217). Even if some impairments or different forms of functioning involve dependencies, those dependencies lie on a spectrum of human diversity, and they only cause distinctive *problems in living* if the environment or social system does not accommodate or support them (Scully, 2014, pp. 210–220).

There are many conceptions of vulnerability in bioethics, but I will use the term to refer to the disadvantaged placement of an individual within the context of certain practices (e.g., economic, social, healthcare), which results in threats to some aspect of their agency or well-being (Guidry-Grimes & Victor, 2012). This view of vulnerability is heavily influenced by the work of Florencia Luna, who emphasizes that situations *render* someone vulnerable. She uses the metaphor of layers to describe how one person can have different vulnerabilities that are highly contextual and may overlap (Luna, 2019). Luna's account has some similarities to Mackenzie, Rogers, and Dodds's (2014) concept of *situational* vulnerability, which is context-dependent and changing. This view of vulnerability is useful for understanding how environments can be disabling for persons with impairments, neurologic differences, or other forms of diversity that fall outside of medical norms of health. It is simplistic and unhelpful to just label a school-age child with cerebral palsy as vulnerable, for instance; such a child can acquire layers of vulnerability due to their parents' insurance status, lack of access to regular physical therapy, school buildings without proper accommodations, ostracization from peers, and teachers' biases or discomfort that lead to distanced interactions and subpar instruction. By identifying these layers, we avoid viewing the child's vulnerabilities as inevitable, singular, and rigid.

Further, it is useful to analyze how vulnerabilities relate to systems of power. When systemic or institutional conditions intersect to create additional barriers to a person's ability to exercise their agency or achieve well-being, those vulnerabilities have been compounded (Guidry-Grimes & Victor, 2012). If teachers and administration wrongly misinterpret the child with cerebral palsy as necessarily being cognitively impaired, they might move the child into poorly funded, segregated, and stigmatized special education classes with inadequately trained teachers. This would make it even more difficult for the child to learn, gain self-confidence, and engage in recreational play with peers. In this situation, the child's multilayered vulnerabilities have been further compounded. We can similarly identify *pathogenic* vulnerabilities, which arise when something "intended to ameliorate vulnerability has the paradoxical effect of exacerbating existing vulnerabilities or generating new ones" (Mackenzie et al., 2014, p. 9).

Agential Vulnerability

For the rest of this chapter, I will focus on *agential vulnerability*—when someone has been rendered vulnerable in a way that thwarts or distorts their agency. The philosophical literature on agency is vast, but very simply, I use the term to refer to the exercise of the capacity to act or choose (Schlosser, 2019).[8] Again, agency does not presume or rely on independence; our agency is socially embedded, relational, and interdependent. When we enable someone's agency, we are respecting that the person might not merely want others to provide benefits; they should instead be engaged as active participants. This is part of what it means to respect someone as a person,[9] as a distinct individual with values and a sense of self.

Successful agency has two parts: the *capacity to set ends* and the *opportunity to achieve ends*, where *end* is used here as basically synonymous with *goal*. Each of these parts needs to be deconstructed a bit further, since agential vulnerability can relate to either or both of these parts.

In ethics, when we are concerned about enabling agency,[10] it is because we associate agency with the ability to identify for oneself what matters, what the person is invested in, or what is authentic. But, of course, an agent might not act or choose in ways that reflect any of those values, even from the agent's own perspective. In order to be well-positioned to set ends that the agent thinks are actually *worth* setting for themselves, the agent needs a certain amount of self-knowledge (enough to understand what matters to them), self-trust and self-respect (to feel sufficiently invested in their own ends), a sense of ongoing-ness into the future (so it is worthwhile to plan for the future), and a sense of

---

[8] I added the caveat to act *or to choose* because efficacious action might not be possible (for reasons described in this chapter). Schlosser acknowledges: "Further, it seems that genuine agency can be exhibited by beings that are not capable of intentional action, and it has been argued that agency can and should be explained without reference to causally efficacious mental states and events" (2019, p. 1). The capacity *to choose* involves intentionality, which is a philosophically complex topic outside the scope of this chapter.

[9] The criteria for personhood are outside the scope of this paper, but Eva Feder Kittay and others have challenged ableist criteria for personhood.

[10] This chapter is not about the ethics of intention or action. The focus is instead on the ethics of enabling agency, regardless of whether that agency is used for laudable ends, neutral ends, or even problematic ends. This is closely parallel to the classic focus in bioethics on enabling autonomy, even while recognizing that respecting autonomy means that certain immoral intentions and actions may result.

self-efficacy (so trying to set ends has a point from their perspective).[11] This might seem like a tall order, but these are not cognitively complex prerequisites with high thresholds. Even significant doubt or insecurity does not necessarily prevent someone from having enough self-trust (and other capacities) to plan for the future.

Disabled people often encounter mistaken assumptions about their agential capabilities. Consider the common phenomenon called "Does He Take Sugar?" syndrome, where a nearby able-bodied person (such as the person pushing a wheelchair) is asked questions instead of the person receiving the drink (the person in the wheelchair) (Scully, 2014). Multiple studies and surveys indicate that healthcare professionals often avoid sharing in decisions with patients with psychiatric disabilities, even though a process of sharing expertise and partnering can be feasible and productive in psychiatric treatment (Guidry-Grimes, 2020; Hamann et al., 2009; Langer et al., 2015; Slade, 2017; Song et al., 2019). Disability advocacy groups have long emphasized that persons with intellectual, developmental, and psychiatric disabilities are often wrongfully excluded from decision-making—a concern which ultimately made its way into the 2006 Convention on the Rights of Persons with Disabilities (CRPD) (United Nations Department of Economic and Social Affairs, 2006). Disability activists discourage courts (and, by extension, healthcare institutions that would petition the court system) to assign guardians for decision-making, since this process can mistakenly minimize the agential capabilities of the would-be ward. Based on the CRPD, *supported* decision-making is the preferred mechanism for enabling the agency of disabled people who would otherwise have that power given to a guardian. The exact meaning and parameters of supported decision-making are outside the scope of what can be covered here, but it may include designation of support person(s) who can help facilitate conversations, relay details of accommodation or modification needs, provide a safe and respectful environment for decision-making, and, importantly, underscore the personhood and rights of the person with a disability (Davidson et al., 2015; National Resource Center for Supported Decision-Making, n.d.; Peterson et al., 2021; Shogren et al., 2017).

A person can have a robust capacity for setting ends in all the ways described, but if they do not have adequate *opportunities* to exercise that agency, then their agency will be impeded. Opportunities for achieving ends are mediated by a host of factors, many of which are outside the control of any one agent. Most basically,

---

[11] Paul Benson (2000) emphasizes self-trust and self-respect. McLeod and Sherwin (2000) emphasize self-trust as well, which they describe as the ability to trust the "capacity to make appropriate choices, given her beliefs, desires, and values [. . .] her ability to act on her decisions; and also that she trusts the judgments she makes that underlie those decisions" (pp. 262–263). Jodi Halpern (2001) describes the importance of having a sense of ongoingness into the future and a sense of self-efficacy. These philosophers are discussing *autonomous* agency, but I believe that they apply to (efficacious) agency as well. I explain my understanding of this distinction later in the chapter.

there have to be choices available. In some contexts, giving someone a choice, even a trivial one, can be a sign of respecting their agency. Through coercion or other undue pressures, one person can (even unintentionally) restrict viable choices for another, which disrespects their agency. Ethically, providing choice for the sake of choice is of limited value. What is far more important is providing choices that actually matter to the agent. A jailer might offer me a choice between a wooden spoon or a plastic spoon, but this could indicate the jailer was mocking my agency, not respecting it. Which opportunities *matter* will depend on numerous personal factors, such as family traditions, culture, religion, and idiosyncratic preferences. As long as a person has the potential for agential growth, it is also important to offer opportunities to learn and experiment—which also means opportunities to fail and take risks. This last point is worth emphasizing, given that people with psychiatric disabilities often have these opportunities substantially limited for them as a protective measure, which might not be justified in the circumstances. Patricia Deegan comments: "But now that you have been labeled with mental illness, the dignity of risk and the right to failure have been taken from you" (Deegan, 2000, p. 361).

Attending to capacities and opportunities for agency is a complicated matter. The ethical importance of enabling agency may seem less than obvious at times for nurses and other healthcare professionals, such as when patients make seemingly irrational decisions. Paternalism reigned in medical practice for hundreds of years; healthcare professionals (especially physicians) took on the responsibility of making decisions on behalf of their patients in the name of beneficence. Even today, in the age of informed consent, healthcare professionals may try to minimize burdens of decision-making for certain patients. Nurses and other caregivers may not act paternalistically in a traditional sense and yet still fall into patterns of choosing *for* patients, which is often infantilizing and disrespectful. This is another example of pathogenic vulnerability—well-intentioned actions meant to address vulnerability that actually worsen vulnerability. Whenever healthcare professionals fail to enable a patient's agency, there is a moral risk of wronging the patient and missing what actually matters from the patient's perspective.

Regarding Capacity Evaluations

Questions about agency in clinical contexts tend to revolve around a particular type of evaluation: capacity assessments.[12] There is substantial literature on

---

[12] Capacity is importantly distinct from competence. Competence is a legal presumption of all legal adults, whereas capacity is a clinical determination that can override that presumption if there is concern that a patient cannot provide legally and ethically legitimate informed consent or refusal.

capacity assessments from medical, legal, and ethical perspectives, but I want to emphasize how these assessments can be mistaken when a patient has a disability. Additionally, the *entirety* of a patient's agential potential can be erroneously viewed through the lens of a capacity assessment, even though an incapacitated patient can still have preferences and values that should be incorporated in healthcare decisions.

In order to be authorized as their own decision-maker in clinical settings, patients need to show four elements of capacity—the ability to sufficiently understand, reason through, appreciate, and communicate a choice (Appelbaum, 2007). Whether someone has capacity is supposed to be judged according to a particular decision, since someone could have adequate capacity for some decisions and not others, and capacity may change over time. Capacity is a threshold concept that admits of degrees, and a patient needs to demonstrate robust capacity for high-stakes or complex decisions (e.g., leaving against medical advice when in danger of acute deterioration) (Buchanan & Brock, 1990). Capacity status can also wax and wane, so it should be regularly reassessed. An accurate and precise capacity evaluation is necessary for protecting patients' autonomy interests and well-being. Nurses may or may not have the legal or clinical responsibility for assessing capacity,[13] but regardless, through the course of their work, nurses can gain detailed evidence about the extent of a patient's decisional capacity. In addition, nurses can learn when patients are at their "decisional best" and help communicate that to the rest of the team in order to maximize the chances the patient can meaningfully contribute to decisions.[14]

Capacity assessments are prone to a multitude of errors, however, especially when healthcare professionals are not sufficiently trained to adjust for various forms of disability. Misperceptions about certain diagnoses or symptoms can contribute to errors, such as when healthcare professionals overgeneralize psychiatric and intellectual disabilities and wrongly assume that patients with any of these conditions should not be their own decision-makers. Many people with psychiatric disabilities have capacity for all or most decisions (Okai et al., 2007). Persons with intellectual disabilities can have sufficient capacity for decisions, especially when given the benefit of a support person or assistive technologies (Devi, 2013). Most adults with mild dementia retain capacity, and even moderate dementia does not necessarily eliminate the possibility for capacitated

---

[13] Licensed physicians may be the only members of the healthcare team who are allowed to make formal capacity evaluations, but that is not universal; e.g., the 2017 Adult Capacity and Decision-Making Act of Nova Scotia extended this authority to nurses (NPs and RNs) who have completed necessary training (Nova Scotia College of Nursing, 2018).

[14] For more on capacity assessments, including how a multidisciplinary team can gather evidence regarding capacity, see Ganzini et al. (2004).

decision-making (Moye et al., 2004). Communication barriers can also lead to mistaken capacity evaluations. For example, a patient could have a motor or neurological disorder that makes speaking difficult, and the healthcare team may misunderstand the patient's baseline cognitive status (especially if the patient does not have family or other caregivers present to correct the team).

Clinicians can miss important nuances to what the patient does and does not understand. The patient's capacity status could also fluctuate, but if the healthcare team does not notice those fluctuations or what precipitates dips in capacity, then the patient might not be empowered as a decision-maker when they are most capable. Vulnerabilities related to capacity assessments are exacerbated when clinicians are inadequately trained, when time is too constrained for an in-depth interview over time, and when the patient's medical needs are acute. Moreover, in residential settings like nursing homes, standard capacity assessments are not built for non-medical decisions in daily living, such as those related to sexual activity (Victor & Guidry-Grimes, 2019).

Even if a patient lacks capacity, perhaps to such an extent that someone else should have decision-making *authority*, that does not mean that the person thereby lacks any perspective on who they are or what makes their life go well. It would be a significant mistake to assume that an incapacitated patient must lack *all* awareness or self-knowledge (Guidry-Grimes, 2018). The presumption, in fact, should be that patients with diminished cognitive faculties "will be capable of participating in collaborative decision-making with a surrogate and medical professional and should have the opportunities to do so, as they are willing and able"; even patients who have no apparent understanding of the medical situation "may be able to express wishes and preferences concerning their lives, or these preferences may be evident to caregivers" (Berlinger et al., 2013, p. 141). The healthcare team's moral work, then, includes being able to suss out the details of a patient's preferences (which may be communicated through nonverbal means) and then understanding how those preferences factor into the patient's valuing system. Especially in situations where nurses have extended contact with a person who is deeply reliant on them for their activities of daily living, such as in long-term care facilities, nurses have a crucial role in identifying enduring preferences and contextualizing decisions. In fact, for long-term patients/residents who are otherwise isolated or alone, a certified nursing assistant or nurse may have more of an impact than anyone else in that person's life. A better understanding of the patient's behavioral patterns, likes and dislikes, regular activities, and personality should all inform decision-making, so decisions are individualized to the person *as a person*. Below I describe forms of valuing that carry moral weight, which go beyond what is captured by a capacity assessment.

Forms of Valuing

Questions of *agency* are tightly linked to questions of *valuing* in bioethics; given all of the macro- and micro-level decisions that have to be made in a clinical setting, the involved parties need to know whether the patient has the ability to form and act on relevant values. There are many ways in which someone can value something; the relevant capacities can be relatively simple or cognitively complex. How we conceive of the ability to value makes a significant difference for how we should treat persons in our care. If valuing is construed as the sort of thing that is only available to sophisticated reasoners who reflectively endorse their preferences based on their understanding of their life as a whole, then it would become a rarefied issue. In healthcare settings, misunderstanding *who* can have capacities for valuing and *why* this matters can result in not soliciting patients' views, overriding preferences, or failing to provide supports and opportunities that patients need to live out what they value for themselves. Often patients will be able to express what kind of care or support they need, but nurses' moral work can also involve paying attention to what a patient values and what is integral to their sense of self, even when not stated or documented explicitly.

Autonomy is the form of valuing discussed most in the bioethics literature. Etymologically, "autonomy" means self-legislation or self-governance. There are numerous conceptions of autonomy, but fundamentally it refers to the ability to reflect critically on motivations or values without being unduly influenced, so the resulting decision is "owned" by the person making decisions (Dworkin, 1988, pp. 15–16). Many persons with disabilities (physical, intellectual, and psychiatric) are capable of autonomous decision-making. In clinical settings, capacity assessments (described above) serve as an *approximate* check for whether a decision is autonomous. A decision can meet the bar for capacity and still raise red flags for being autonomous, however; undue influence and inauthenticity would not be captured by a standard capacity assessment. This means that a person could give ethically valid informed consent/refusal for a procedure and yet feel that this decision was driven by internal or external forces that were not *owned* by the decision-maker.[15] Jodi Halpern, a psychiatrist and bioethicist, gives the example of Ms. G, a woman who declines life-saving treatment as a result of sudden and profound grief that overwhelms her after her husband cruelly leaves her in the hospital. Ms. G's decision met the bar for capacity, but Halpern (2001) shows how this decision likely did *not* meet the bar for autonomy because of how her husband's actions and her grief "took over" the decision-making process and resulted in a decision that the patient would not have reflectively endorsed if able to think more like herself. This example shows a danger of giving too much

---

[15] I am grateful to Jamie Carlin Watson for helping me develop this argument.

weight to capacity assessments; simply letting Ms. G die is not necessarily respecting her autonomy. The bar for autonomous decision-making is a also relatively high one; many of our everyday decisions probably fail to be autonomous because we do not expend the mental resources to critically deliberate or ensure authenticity. A problem with focusing exclusively on autonomy in evaluating agential interests, then, is that doing so neglects less cognitively intensive decision-making. And as a result, people with diminished autonomy—such as those with advanced dementia, significant intellectual disabilities, or profound psychiatric disabilities—can have meaningful aspects of their agency neglected.

Agnieszka Jaworska (1999) shows how the capacity to value is more fundamental than the capacity for autonomy. She describes what it means to value something: the individual believes that what they want is worth wanting; achieving what they want is connected to their sense of self-worth; and they believe it has importance even if it does not currently give them pleasure or satisfaction. Jaworska conceives of valuing as having a relatively "stable set of purposes and preferences" (1999, p. 128). On her view, valuing is not equivalent to high-order reflection; that is, something can have personal value even if it has not been endorsed in a process of critical deliberation. This means that valuing is possible for individuals who fit in a broad range of cognitive abilities; valuing is not limited to persons who are intellectually engaged at the highest levels with their choices. Jaworska argues that someone could be capable of valuing even if unable to "devise and carry out the means and plans" for following their values, due to (e.g.) perpetual confusion or memory lapses (1999, pp. 127–129). Moreover, she argues that valuing is possible even if it "becomes uncoupled from the person's grasp of the narrative of her whole life" (1999, p. 117). In other words, someone could retain the capacity to value even when not completely alert or oriented or cognizant of details of their life as a whole. Jaworska makes this point by examining cases of patients with dementia, who are still able to value certain things even if they no longer know their precise age, date, or location (1999). Similarly, most individuals with intellectual and psychiatric disabilities will be able to reach the cognitive threshold needed for some form of valuing.

Valuing is contrasted with merely desiring. Mere desires are fungible and fleeting, so their being obstructed does not pose significant harms to the agent as an agent.[16] Jaworska describes mere desires as distinctive in that "a person could contemplate being free of a mere desire with a sense of relief" (1999, p. 114).[17] It is constitutive of mere desires that they do not occupy a place of importance to the person, that they could have those desires go unsatisfied without feeling much in the way of regret or indignation.

---

[16] This is not to deny that repeatedly obstructing someone's mere desires can have a cumulative effect that end up being significant, maybe especially for individuals who have diminished moral interests.

[17] According to Jaworska, persons can "distinguish between desires and attitudes that merely occur within him and those that are truly his own" (2007, p. 538).

Caring is an important form of valuing.[18] Jaworska provides the following account of caring:

> [I]t is best understood as a structured compound of various less complex emotions, emotional predispositions, and also desires, unfolding reliably over time in response to relevant circumstances. Typical components of caring include: joy and satisfaction when the object of one's care is flourishing and frustration over its misfortunes; anger at agents who heedlessly cause such misfortunes. (Jaworska, 2007, p. 560)

Caring is a special kind of emotional investment that directs the person's actions, intentions, emotional responses, and end-setting. As a structured compound, carings "forge a vast network of rational and referential connections that support the agent's identity over time" (Jaworska, 2007, p. 561). In other words, what someone cares about will relate to and build on other things they care about over time. When someone cares about something, they "structure [their] plans and intentions to promote it" (Jaworska, 2007, p. 563, n. 97). As a result, carings support the individual's sense of self and their own agential perspective—which is what makes them authoritative in "speaking for" who the agent is.[19]

Jaworska suggests that children and many people with Alzheimer's are capable of both the cognitive and affective dimensions of caring. Cognitive limitations will not always preclude the possibility of caring. Caring involves capacities that are complex but not overly demanding. Jaworska argues that caring provides the most basic structure of human agency, and she distinguishes it from the highly intellectualized capacities for second-order volition or autonomy (Jaworska, 1999, 2007). These more sophisticated capacities are more complex forms of valuing (see Figure 15.1). Jaworska's point is that these sophisticated capacities are not necessary for an agent to be capable of valuing; the emotional attunements involved in caring are sufficient for an agent to have a differentiated sense of self with agential projects they can consider their own. Given that a person can still care about the same things over time while experiencing memory losses or failures in means-end reasoning, even significant intellectual or psychiatric disabilities will often not eliminate the possibility of this form of valuing.

---

[18] Whether caring is a type of valuing on Jaworska's account is open to interpretation. I offer a plausible reading, since caring would not fall into the category of merely desiring. Further, Jaworska's analysis of valuing among individuals with dementia has striking parallels to her analysis of caring among these individuals. Valuing is not a highly intellectualized notion on her account, so the emotional capacities involved in caring could constitute a form of valuing.

[19] Jaworska explains: "any attitude, reflexive or not, has the right kind of authority to speak for the agent, so long as it is part of its function to support the psychological continuities and connections that constitute the agent's identity and cohesion over time" (2007, p. 552).

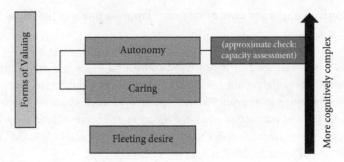

Figure 15.1 Forms of valuing in terms of cognitive complexity.

We thus have a broad sense of what it means to value something. Persons with a wide range of cognitive and affective abilities can experience agential vulnerability in healthcare settings, which can significantly impact capacities and opportunities for valuing. Ethical tensions that can arise should not be reduced to threats to autonomy alone. Incapacitated patients can still be capable of valuing and having their agency undermined, and there should be more explicit discussion and guidance around this point. In the next section, I describe applications of this theoretical framework in enabling agency for disabled people.

In Application: Agential Vulnerability in Healthcare Environments

Agential vulnerability is evident in healthcare environments. When sick or ill or in pain, a person's end-setting capacity can be diminished. Hospitals, nursing homes, and other facilities are built for particular purposes and have myriad constraints on opportunities for achieving individually chosen ends. So, some degree of agential vulnerability will be inevitable for many patients and long-term residents of healthcare facilities.[20] The specifics of a patient's agential needs can get lost in the hustle and bustle of healthcare due to time pressures, patient loads, emergent and urgent issues that arise, and general burnout. The result can be fights for control.

Because of their dedicated time at the bedside and the intimacy of their care work, nurses and nursing assistants have an essential role in understanding the nuances of a patient's agency. Their attunement to agential vulnerability can

---

[20] There are notable instances where someone's agential vulnerability is actually worse outside the hospital or facility; by having regular meals, medications, a restful place to sleep, and people to safely interact with, some people will be more agentially supported inside the healthcare environment than they would be in their homes or on the streets.

make all the difference for whether a patient's perspective is understood and cen-tered in decision-making. This can also impact trust and the therapeutic alliance, especially for patients who tend to have multilayered vulnerability to begin with and are at high risk for having those vulnerabilities compounded—such as those with new or preexisting disabilities. I will now make these points more concrete by discussing an area of agential vulnerability in healthcare environments for disabled persons: medications. This is not the only area of agential vulnerability, but it highlights ethically complicated issues related to medical decision-making as well as everyday living.

Agency With Medications

Adult patients are presumed to have capacity for medication decisions unless healthcare professionals have reasons for doubting their capacity status. Capacity assessments can be sources of agential vulnerability for reasons described pre-viously, so healthcare professionals should approach their evaluation with care and attention to detail. If a guardian, healthcare power of attorney (POA), or surrogate is instead authorized as the decision-maker, it may not seem neces-sary to include the patient in these discussions. The medical team may initiate these discussions outside the patient's room and leave it to the guardian/POA/surrogate to decide what they tell the patient afterward. In such a situation, the medical team's interactions with the patient could then be focused on eliciting the patient's assent or acquiescence. Nurses and nurse assistants are often heavily engaged with the patient in these scenarios, though the engagement may be more in terms of coaxing and getting the patient to trust what the nurse is telling them to do. This kind of engagement can end up being infantilizing, with elements of pressuring or even manipulation, such as when patients are told they can have a desired food item only if they swallow whatever the med-ication is. Even decisionally incapacitated patients should be included in these decisions to the greatest extent possible, however. For one, the patient may gain a greater degree of understanding and appreciation if regularly engaged in their care. Additionally, as described above, incapacitated patients can still be capable of valuing, and their perspective should remain central in decision-making. Along the same lines, decisionally incapacitated patients should not be treated as objects to be managed, but instead should have their status as persons con-firmed and reaffirmed in their daily interactions with caregivers. If members of the healthcare team worry that these discussions could be confusing or upsetting for the patient, they should broach this concern explicitly with specialists (such as speech pathologists or psychiatrists) and those who are closest to the patient, so they can give guidance for creating a comfortable and safe space for including the patient in an appropriate manner.

Although I do not have the space here to give the topic justice,[21] I want to briefly analyze the practice of covert administration of medication. This occurs when caregivers give medication without the patient's knowledge, using some form of deliberate deception in the act of disguising or concealing the medication (Munden, 2017). The purpose is to treat incapacitated patients who would otherwise refuse the medication. This practice is relatively common, yet there is a dearth of legal and professional guidance for this form of deception (Guidry-Grimes et al., 2021; Munden, 2017). Covert medication administration may arise if it seems the only alternatives are either to permit dangerous decompensation or to force medication in some way. Deception can take many forms in these situations, from overt lying (e.g., "this IV bag only contains liquid for hydration") to subtler concealment (e.g., "this medication is just to help you sleep" when it is primarily being given as a mood stabilizer).

There are substantial moral risks to covert medication, though. Caregivers could find themselves in a deception loop without a clear end when the patient chronically experiences diminished capacity as a result of dementia or psychiatric impairment, for example. If the patient's symptoms or medical condition improves as a result of the medication, the patient would be unable to associate the improvement with the medication. From the patient's perspective, it may seem the medical recommendations were incorrect after all, since the patient improved on their own![22] The patient could then continue to refuse the medication, even though caregivers are *more* convinced that the medications are beneficial. They may decide never to disclose the truth to the patient if the patient is not expected to regain capacity. As long as the patient retains the ability to participate in discussions but remains in the dark about receiving medications, they are ignorant of important health information that could impact their preferences and decision-making. They also might not be able to report side effects accurately as a result of the deception. This is a concern for patients who are below the threshold for decisional capacity but who still have the ability to discuss their preferences and values. At any point that caregivers do choose to reveal the truth, they risk losing the patient's trust and the patient declining the medication anyway. If the patient discovers the truth on their own, then they may reject support offered by caregivers or family (especially if family either consented to or participated in the practice), which opens up the patient to additional vulnerabilities in terms of their relationships and potentially their housing and finances as well. Practices and rituals around eating and feeding are cared about by people of all cognitive

---

[21] In this subsection, I draw from Guidry-Grimes et al. (2021).
[22] This concern is based on actual clinical experiences.

levels, so it is no small risk for food to become a potential source of betrayal and distrust. Covert administration of medication, therefore, carries significant risk of compounding a range of vulnerabilities.

Given these concerns, healthcare facilities (whether acute care, long-term care, or other) should have clear guidelines for this practice.[23] Diligent attempts at shared decision-making should be exhausted before this option is considered. The potential benefits for the patient in the short *and* long term should be sig-nificant enough to outweigh the many risks and harms at stake. Any decision to attempt covert medication administration should first be discussed with all relevant caregivers, including any nurses who are asked to participate and those who know the patient best (such as family, a group home manager, or long-term psychiatrist). Guidelines should include a continual re-evaluation process with explicit benchmarks and expected endpoints. In any given situation, it could turn out that providing medication in a transparently involuntary manner will have more ethical benefits than costs (Guidry-Grimes et al., 2020). This example shows how one area of healthcare decision-making can carry high stakes for patients who have preferences and values that conflict with the medical plan. Especially given the relational nature of agency, patients may wish to build relationships with nurses and nurse assistants that make it more likely that those preferences will be respected. Medications are an important area of agency for any patient, and the ethical challenges with enabling agency become complex when a simple capacity assessment does not settle the issues.

The Need to Address Institutional Barriers

This chapter has provided a framework for understanding disability in rela-tion to the policy decisions and built and social environment. Environmental features can render a person vulnerable in ways that are not inherent to their impairment or medical condition; moreover, healthcare institutions can com-pound a range of vulnerabilities, even when caregivers are well-intentioned. Nurses and nurse assistants, along with other members of the healthcare team, have *critically important*—and *sensitive*—moral work in enabling the agency of patients. This work can make a significant difference for whether the patient is able to live out their values within the constraints of a healthcare environment. Nurses often have the most extended contact time with patients in acute care settings, and in the context of long-term care, nurse assistants can have an enor-mous impact on residents' capacities and opportunities for everyday agency. The healthcare system and institutional structures can make this moral work even

---

[23] To see an example of such a policy, see NHS Northamptonshire Healthcare (2017).

more complicated and difficult. As was shown in the example of taking medication, policies and guidance from leadership are necessary if nurses and other caregivers are to provide person-centered care for their patients.

The COVID-19 pandemic has further emphasized how healthcare environments can worsen preexisting vulnerabilities. Disabled people, especially those in congregate care facilities like nursing homes, have experienced exceptionally high rates of mortality and other harms. Despite the herculean efforts of clinical leadership, nurses, and other staff during this public health crisis, many healthcare environments produced pathogenic vulnerabilities for patients with disabilities. Disability activists have been calling for drastic overhaul of these facilities for years. In hospital settings with visitor restrictions, disabled people have not always had their regular caregivers or support persons present, which can make a difference for the quality and safety of their care, as well as their ability to communicate more effectively with strained healthcare teams (Guidry-Grimes et al., 2020).

Institutions should be making it as easy as possible for nurses to provide attentive care for patients with diverse needs. Those in leadership positions should be constantly assessing barriers that caregivers experience in trying to do the right thing for their patients. Enabling capacities and opportunities for patients' agency is a momentous and ongoing task. Mitigating vulnerabilities and identifying potential sources of pathogenic vulnerabilities should be prioritized by those with the most power in the healthcare system. It should not be left to nurses to constantly struggle to find solutions in a broken system.

References

Aaberg, V. A. (2012). A path to greater inclusivity through understanding implicit attitudes toward disability. *Journal of Nursing Education, 51*(9), 505–510.

Agaronnik, N., Campbell, E. G., Ressalam, J., & Lezzoni, L. I. (2019) Exploring issues relating to disability cultural competence among practicing physicians. *Disability and Health Journal, 12*(3), 403–410.

Appelbaum, P. S. (2007). Clinical practice: Assessment of patients' competence to consent to treatment. *New England Journal of Medicine, 357*(18), 1834–1840.

Asch, A. (2001). Disability, bioethics, and human rights. In G. L. Albrecht & K. D. Seelman (Eds.), *Handbook of disability studies* (pp. 297–326). Sage Publications.

Barnes, C., & Mercer, G. (2011). *Disability*. Polity Press.

Barnes, E. (2019). *The minority body: A theory of disability*. Oxford University Press.

Benson, P. (2000). Feeling crazy: Self-worth and the social character of responsibility. In C. Mackenzie & N. Stoljar (Eds.), *Relational autonomy: Feminist perspectives on autonomy, agency, and the social self* (pp. 72–93). Oxford University Press.

Berlinger, N., Jennings, B., & Wolf, S. M. (2013). *The Hastings Center guidelines for decisions on life-sustaining treatment and care near the end of life* (2nd ed.). Oxford University Press.

Boyles, C. M., Bailey, P. H., & Mossey, S. (2008). Representations of disability in nursing and health literature: An integrative review. *Journal of Advanced Nursing, 62*(4), 428–437.

Buchanan, A. E., & Brock, D. W. (1990). *Deciding for others: The ethics of surrogate decision making.* Cambridge University Press.

Colbert, A., & Kronk, R. (2020). Equity access: Online nursing education on care for people with disabilities. *Journal of Nursing Education, 59*(6), 349–351.

Davidson, G., Kelly, B., Macdonald, G., Rizzo, M., Lombard, L., Abogunrin, O., Clift-Matthews, V., & Martin, A. (2015). Supported decision making: A review of the international literature. *International Journal of Law and Psychiatry, 38*, 61–67.

Deegan, P. E. (2000). Recovering our sense of value after being labeled mentally ill. In M. Adams, W. J. Blumenfeld, R. Castañeda, H. W. Hackman, M. L. Peters, & X. Zúñiga (Eds.), *Readings for diversity and social justice: An anthology on racism, antisemitism, sexism, heterosexism, ableism, and classism* (pp. 359–363). Routledge.

Devi, N. (2013). Supported decision-making and personal autonomy for persons with intellectual disabilities: Article 12 of the UN Convention on the Rights of Persons with Disabilities. *Journal of Law, Medicine & Ethics, 41*(4), 1073–1105.

Dworkin, G. (1988). *The theory and practice of autonomy.* Cambridge University Press.

Ells, C. (2001). Lessons about autonomy from the experience of disability. *Social Theory and Practice, 27*(4), 599–615.

Ganzini, L., Volicer, L., Nelson, W. A., Fox, E., & Derse, A. R. (2004). Ten myths about decision-making capacity. *Journal of the American Medical Directors Association, 5*(4), 263–267.

Goering, S. (2008). "You say you're happy, but . . .": Contested quality of life judgments in bioethics and disability studies. *Bioethical Inquiry, 5*, 125–135.

Guidry-Grimes, L. (2018). In the balance: Weighing preferences of decisionally incapacitated patients. *Hastings Center Report, 48*(3), 41–42.

Guidry-Grimes, L. (2020). Overcoming obstacles to shared mental health decision making. *AMA Journal of Ethics, 22*(5), E446–451.

Guidry-Grimes, L., Dean, M., & Victor, E. K. (2021). Covert administration of medication in food: A worthwhile moral gamble? *Journal of Medical Ethics, 47*, 389–393.

Guidry-Grimes, L., Savin, K., Stramondo, J. A., Reynolds, J. M., Tsaplina, M., Burke, T. B., Ballantyne, A., Kittay, E. F., Stahl, D., Scully, J. L., Garland-Thomson, R., & Fins, J. J. (2020). Disability rights as a necessary framework for crisis standards of care and the future of health care. *Hastings Center Report, 50*(3), 28–32.

Guidry-Grimes, L., & Victor, E. (2012). Vulnerabilities compounded by social institutions. *International Journal of Feminist Approaches to Bioethics, 5*(2), 126–146.

Halpern, J. (2001). *From detached concern to empathy: Humanizing medical practice.* Oxford University Press.

Hamann, J., Mendel, R., Cohen, R., Heres, S., Ziegler, M., Bühner, M., & Kissling, W. (2009). Psychiatrists' use of shared decision making in the treatment of schizophrenia: Patient characteristics and decision topics. *Psychiatric Services, 60*(8), 1107–1112.

Hoffmaster, B. (2006). What does vulnerability mean? *Hastings Center Report, 36*(2), 38–45.

Holstein, M., Waymack, M. H., & Park, J. (2010). *Ethics, aging and society: The critical turn.* Springer.

Iezzoni, L. I., Rao, S. R., Ressalam, J., Bolcic-Jankovic, D., Agaronnik, N. D., Donelan, K., Lagu, T., & Campbell, E. G. (2021). Physicians' perceptions of people with disability and their health care. *Health Affairs, 40*(2), 297–306.

Ilkhani, M., Glasper, A., & Jarrett, N. (2016). Nursing care related to care for disabled children: Literature review. *International Nursing Review, 63*(1), 78–83.

Invalid, S. (2017). Skin, tooth, and bone: The basis of movement is our people: A disability justice primer. *Reproductive Health Matters, 25*(50), 149–150.

Jaworska, A. (1999). Respecting the margins of agency: Alzheimer's patients and the capacity to value. *Philosophy & Public Affairs, 28*(2), 105–138.

Jaworska, A. (2007). Caring and internality. *Philosophy and Phenomenological Research, 74*(3), 529–568.

Ladau, E. (2021). *Demystifying disability: What to know, what to say, and how to be an ally.* Ten Speed Press.

Langer, D. A., Mooney, T. K., & Wills, C. E. (2015). *Shared decision-making for treatment planning in mental health care: Theory, evidence, and tools.* Oxford University Press.

Lewis, T. A. (2019, March 5). *Longmore lecture: Context, clarity, & grounding.* Talia A. Lewis: Blog. https://www.talilalewis.com/blog/longmore-lecture-context-clarity-grounding.

Luna, F. (2019). Identifying and evaluating layers of vulnerability: A new way forward. *Developing World Bioethics, 19,* 86–95.

Mackenzie, C., Rogers, W., & Dodds, S. (2014). Introduction: What is vulnerability and why does it matter for moral theory? In C. Mackenzie, W. Rogers, & S. Dodds (Eds.), *Vulnerability: New essays in ethics and feminist philosophy* (pp. 1–32). Oxford University Press.

McLeod, C., & Sherwin, S. (2000). Relational autonomy, self-trust, and health care for patients who are oppressed. *Philosophy Publications, 345,* 259–279.

Moye, J., Karel, M. J., Azar, A. R., & Gurrera, R. J. (2004). Capacity to consent to treatment: Empirical comparison of three instruments in older adults with and without dementia. *The Gerontologist, 44*(2), 166–175.

Munden, L. M. (2017). The covert administration of medications: Legal and ethical complexities for health care professionals. *Journal of Law, Medicine & Ethics, 45,* 182–192.

National Resource Center for Supported Decision Making. (n.d.). *National Resource Center for Supported Decision Making.* http://www.supporteddecisionmaking.org/.

NHS Northamptonshire Healthcare. (2017). *MMP015 Covert administration of medicines policy and guidelines.* https://www.nhft.nhs.uk/download.cfm?ver=19296.

Nova Scotia College of Nursing. (2018). *Assessing capacity: A guideline for nurses.* https://cdn1.nscn.ca/sites/default/files/documents/resources/AssessingCapacity.pdf.

Okai, D., Owen, G., McGuire, H., Singh, S., Churchill, R., & Hotopf, M. (2007). Mental capacity in psychiatric patients: Systematic review. *The British Journal of Psychiatry, 191*(4), 291–297.

Oliver, M., & Barnes, C. (2012). *The new politics of disablement* (2nd ed.). Palgrave Macmillan.

Peterson, A., Karlawish, J., & Largent, E. (2021). Supported decision making with people at the margins of autonomy. *The American Journal of Bioethics, 21*(11), 4–18.

Reynolds, J. M., & Wieseler C. (Eds.) (2022). *The Disability Bioethics Reader.* Routledge.

Schlosser, M. (2019, Winter). Agency. In E. N. Zalta (Ed.), *The Stanford encyclopedia of philosophy.* https://plato.stanford.edu/archives/win2019/entries/agency.

Scully, J. L. (2014). Disability and vulnerability: On bodies, dependence, and power. In C. Mackenzie, W. Rogers, & S. Dodds (Eds.), *Vulnerability: New essays in ethics and feminist philosophy* (pp. 204–221). Oxford University Press.

Shakespeare, T. (2010). The social model of disability. In L. J. Davis (Ed.), *The disability studies reader* (3rd ed., pp. 266–273). Routledge.

Shakespeare, T., Lezzoni, L., & Groce, N. (2009). Disability and the training of healthcare professionals. *The Lancet, 374,* 1815–1816.

Shogren, K. A., Wehmeyer, M. L., Lassmann, H., & Forber-Pratt, A. J. (2017). Supported decision making: A synthesis of the literature across intellectual disability, mental health, and aging. *Education and Training in Autism and Developmental Disabilities, 52*(2), 144–157.

Skotko, B. G., Levine, S. P., & Goldstein, R. (2011). Self-perceptions from people with down syndrome. *American Journal of Medical Genetics Part A, 155*(10), 2360–2369.

Slade, M. (2017). Implementing shared decision making in routine mental health care. *World Psychiatry, 16*(2), 146–153.

Smeltzer, S. C., Dolen, M. A., Robinson-Smith, G., & Zimmerman, V. (2005). Integration of disability-related content in nursing curricula. *Nursing Education Perspectives, 26*(4), 210–216.

Smeltzer, S. C., Robinson-Smith, G., Dolen, M. A., Duffin, J. M., & Al-Maqbali, M. (2010). Disability-related content in nursing textbooks. *Nursing Education Research, 31*(3), 148–155.

Song, J., Borlido, C., De Luca, V., Burton, L., & Remington, G. (2019). Patient versus rater evaluation of symptom severity in treatment resistant schizophrenia receiving clozapine. *Psychiatry Research, 274,* 409–413.

Straehle, C. (2016). Vulnerability, health agency and capability to health. *Bioethics, 30*(1), 34–40.

Trollor, J. N., Eagleson, C., Turner, B., Salomon, C., Cashin, A., Iacono, T., Goddard, L., & Lennox, N. (2016). Intellectual disability health content within nursing curriculum: An audit of what our future nurses are taught. *Nurse Education Today, 45,* 72–79.

United Nations Department of Economic and Social Affairs. (2006). *Convention on the rights of persons with disabilities (CRPD).* https://social.desa.un.org/issues/disability/crpd/con vention-on-the-rights-of-persons-with-disabilities-crpd#:~:text=The%20Convention%20 is%20intended%20as%20a%20human%20rights,must%20enjoy%20all%20human%20rig hts%20and%20fundamental%20freedoms..org

VanPuymbrouck, L., Friedman, C., & Feldner, H. (2020). Explicit and implicit disability attitudes of healthcare providers. *Rehabilitation Psychology, 65*(2), 101–112.

Victor, E., & Guidry-Grimes, L. (2019). Relational autonomy in action: Rethinking dementia and sexuality in care facilities. *Nursing Ethics, 26*(6), 1654–1664.

Wasserman, D. (2001). Philosophical issues in the definition and social response to disability. In G. L. Albrecht & K. D. Seelman (Eds.), *Handbook of disability studies* (pp. 219–251). Sage Publications.

Wendell, S. (1996). *The rejected body: Feminist philosophical reflections on disability.* Routledge.

Wilson, M. C., & Scior, K. (2014). Attitudes toward individuals with disabilities as measured by the Implicit Association Test: A literature review. *Research in Developmental Disabilities, 35,* 294–321.

16

Emerging Ethical Issues in Dementia Care

Jennifer H. Lingler and Jalayne J. Arias

Recent advances in Alzheimer's disease (AD) research have led to a new era in which the pathological hallmarks of the disease can be detected in the brains of living individuals. With these developments comes increasing prognostic and diagnostic certainty for a devastating neurodegenerative disorder that was once definitely diagnosed only upon examination of post mortem brain tissue. The advent of biomarker testing for AD has also led to a surge of renewed interest in dementia ethics as clinicians, researchers, and ethicists grapple with the implications of providing older adults with the option of learning their AD biomarker status years before advanced cognitive decline manifests. This chapter begins with an overview of the dementia ethics literature, focusing on the work of two of the field's most prominent contributors, Ronald Dworkin and Rebecca Dresser, and outlining efforts to identify ethical approaches to medical decision-making for the decisionally incapacitated. We then discuss the field's transition to an era of biologically defined AD, arguing that a focus on dilemmas concerning medical decision-making in states of advanced cognitive decline has left the field relatively ill-equipped to comprehensively counsel patients who may be contemplating or reacting to tests of their AD biomarker status. We assert that, going forward, nurses will play a key role in offering pretest counseling and post-test support for AD biomarker test candidates. Nurses will play a corresponding key role in identifying and responding to emerging ethical challenges arising during the provision of such services. We outline, in particular, how nurses will have a unique opportunity to reject hypercognitive biases that have limited the field's attention to ethical issues of specific relevance to nursing care. Finally, we describe how nurses are ideally positioned to guide patients, families, and other clinicians toward giving increased consideration to the interpersonal and behavioral (e.g., noncognitve) implications of AD and work to proactively identify plans for promoting dignity throughout the disease course.

Overview of Classic Arguments in the Dementia
Ethics Literature

Ethical issues are pervasive in dementia care. Clinicians face them throughout the trajectory of dementia diagnosis and management, beginning during the earliest of clinical encounters with patients and their families, and continuing through end-of-life decision-making. A common example, arising in the early stages of dementia, involves a family member expressing the desire to exclude their loved one from discussions regarding the changes in thinking and/or behavior that are being observed. For some, this inclination to keep potentially embarrassing, upsetting, or conflict-provoking information from the patient extends to requesting or even pleading with providers to withhold disclosure of the diagnosis from the affected individual. Conversely, clinicians may be confronted with situations where a mildly impaired individual with a new dementia diagnosis requests that their condition be kept confidential despite posing potential risks to others in the community (e.g., by continuing to drive) or in the employment setting (e.g., if one works in an industry like transportation, childcare, or holds position with decision-making responsibilities that impact the lives of others). Yet, despite the wide array of ethical challenges that arise in the care of persons with dementia, one issue has most consistently and disproportionately captured the interest of bioethicists: that is, how should clinicians and families make health-related decisions with, or on behalf of, those who lose the capacity to direct their own care?

While references to the special moral case of mentally incompetent adults in the ethics literature predates both the modern bioethics movement and the growing public health crisis of AD and related dementias (see, e.g., Kant, 2007), recent decades have witnessed a surge in publications featuring analyses focused on the problem of medical decision-making for persons with dementia-imposed decisional incapacity. This section will summarize key concepts and arguments that are frequently articulated in the dementia ethics literature.

Many of these analyses are framed around the question of how to balance competing obligations to promote autonomy and beneficence (generally understood to involve promoting best interests) among individuals with dementia. Prominent ethicists have offered contrasting approaches to the dilemmas associated with dementia-imposed decisional incapacity. In particular, the approaches originally put forth by Ronald Dworkin and Rebecca Dresser represent two conceptual extremes that have dominated the subfield of dementia ethics for nearly 40 years. Dworkin's (1994) view prioritizes autonomous, prospective decision-making through a conceptual tool of precedent autonomy, wherein Dresser (1995) articulates the limits of such an approach and advances a competing concept of the revised best interests standard. The following sections, respectively, summarize these approaches and identify a disproportionate focus on the cognitive symptoms of dementia. This focus on dementia's cognitive symptoms, we argue, is a shortcoming common to both approaches, pointing to the need for caution as the field of dementia care evolves and considers the ethical dilemmas posed by new developments in the science of AD.

Precedent Autonomy

The core assumption underlying Dworkin's (1994) classic analysis of autonomy is that autonomous persons have the right to determine the course of their own lives, including the course of their medical treatment or nontreatment. Dworkin's treatment of dementia ethics is most concerned with issues pertaining to the withholding of invasive medical treatment for persons with advanced dementia who, in their pre-dementia days, expressed the view that life with dementia would be undesirable and undignified. Cognitive symptoms associated with dementia may compromise autonomy by impeding competency to deliberate about courses of action for medical treatment. In this circumstance, Dworkin proposes a means of continuing to respect such persons' autonomy through what he refers to as an "integrity view of autonomy."

His signature concept of precedent autonomy maintains that treatment determinations for persons with dementia ought to regard as binding the views that such persons expressed in their pre-dementia states. Dworkin asserts that this practice of honoring precedent (pre-dementia) expressions of autonomy serves to sustain and promote the integrity of the individual's autonomy. This position is defended on the basis that individual autonomy functions, in large part, to protect one's critical interests.

Critical interests are most clearly understood when contrasted with what Dworkin calls "experiential" interests. Simply put, experiential interests are the pursuits in which one engages because the experience of doing so is enjoyable. Examples of experiential interests can include watching sports, working hard, or listening to music. In contrast, critical interests are those pursued throughout the life course which, taken together, form convictions (whether recognized or unrecognized by the individual) about what's really important in one's life. Dworkin argues that while experiential interests may provide rich and even meaningful experiences, it is the pursuit of critical interests, such as fostering close relationships with family, that truly add value to life and, therefore, warrant protection (by others).

In the context of advanced dementia, Dworkin claims that, embedded within critical interests, are deeply personal preferences and values that emerge out of specific life circumstances and come to command the conviction and

investment of their holders. He ties this notion to both autonomy and competence, suggesting that autonomy promotes the capacity to live out of a "distinctive sense of character" and that competence requires the ability to act out of
such a sense of self (1994, pp. 224–225). Thus, the autonomy of the pre-dementia
self and, therefore, the character of the person, on the whole, may remain intact (even after onset of dementia), since Dworkin thinks it best to honor the
preferences of the "precedent self" rather than heed the potentially random and/
or inconsistent, and experientially driven, wishes of the demented self. He argues
for adhering to such pre-dementia preferences irrespective of the degree of enjoyment derived from experiential interests in the demented state. For Dworkin,
part of the justification for elevating critical interests above the level of experientially tied interests is that critical interests tend to be long-standing, both developing and being sustained over one's lifetime. Experiential interests, in contrast,
are temporally tied to the moments in which they are pursued. Their fleeting
nature is integral to that which renders them noncritical.

Dworkin frames his argument, in part, around a hypothetical example
involving a woman with AD who had, prior to the onset of her dementia, executed a directive that, should she become demented, no life-threatening
conditions that she develops should be treated. This directive, Dworkin claims,
ought to be respected as it represents a statement, born of critical interests, about
the overall kind of life that this woman wishes to live. In theory, this approach
prevents autonomy and beneficence from conflicting, as Dworkin goes on to say
that it is in the best interests of the person on the whole to preserve the autonomy
of the pre-dementia self.

Despite many criticisms of both the practicality (e.g., De Sabbata,
2020) and philosophical soundness (e.g., Byers, 2020; Cowley, 2018; Groves,
2006; Jaworska, 1999) of Dworkin's argument over the years, the essential
threads of this view are prevalent in mainstream approaches to dementia care.
For example, the Alzheimer's Association, a leading international organization
for AD advocacy, education, and support, actively promotes advance directives
in early stage dementia (Alzheimer's Association, 2016), as do the dementia care
guidelines of numerous professional organizations and legislative initiatives,
such as the implementation of a billing code for advanced care planning.
Collectively, these efforts serve to codify and promote as normative this worldview that one's autonomy can and should be preserved in the face of dementia.

An Alternative View: Revised Best Interests

Dresser has been one of the strongest critics of Dworkin's approach over the
years. Importantly, her work extends beyond the task of criticizing Dworkin's

view of precedent autonomy to develop an original paradigm for dementia ethics. Dresser critically analyzes Dworkin's *Life's Dominion*, emphasizing the moral relevance of current interests among persons with dementia and suggesting that such interests be given priority in instances where they conflict with pre-dementia critical interests, even if such preferences are explicitly outlined in an advance directive (Dresser, 1995). Among pragmatic considerations related to Dworkin's claim, Dresser explains the inapplicability of the precedent autonomy argument for the vast majority of dementia sufferers whose pre-dementia preferences, even if grounded in critical interests, are unknown as they never executed advance directives. She also delineates various policy-related problems with respect to designing and implementing the approach, even among those who wish to plan their care in advance. For example, she challenges the feasibility of advance planners to collect all of the experiential information that might be material in cultivating an understanding of what it may be like to live with dementia in the future. She maintains that it is counterproductive, in terms of autonomy maximization, to "give effect to choices that originate in insufficient or mistaken information" (1995, p. 35).

Similarly, Dresser faults advance directives for their inability to incorporate up-to-date prognostic and therapeutic information into treatment preference selections (Dresser, 1986). Citing Buchanan and Brock (1989), she further notes that decisions rooted in advance directives lack the benefit of ongoing discussions with loved ones and healthcare providers that typically facilitate the incorporation of personal values into medical care choices among competent persons.

Dresser's alternative, a revised best interests standard, is grounded in the notion that neither the concerns of an uninformed former self, nor those of a hypothetically derived competent self, should necessarily override the current interests of persons with dementia. However, she maintains that the traditionally invoked best interest standard relies, to a dangerous extent, on the value-laden and socially constructed perspective of a "reasonable person" (Dresser, 1986). For Dresser, a tension arises in viewing the interests of a person with dementia as akin to those of a reasonable person. She argues for revising the best interest standard to attend to the particularities germane to the life of a person with dementia by prioritizing the current experiential interests of the individual (Dresser, 1995).

Dresser notes that Dworkin's argument for the elevation of critical interests beyond experiential ones rests upon an assumption that people want their lives to have narrative coherence. Questioning this claim, she asserts that his argument would not hold should it turn out that a more common life theme is "to accept and adjust to the changing natural and social circumstances that characterize a person's life" (1995, p. 36).

It bears emphasis that the arguments for prioritizing pre-dementia critical interests at one extreme, and immediate, experiential interests at the other, both rely heavily on what would be clinically characterized as moderate- to late-stage AD as the prototypical target for discussions of dementia ethics. Both Dworkin and Dresser frame portions of their discussions around the case of "Margo," a 55-year-old Alzheimer's patient who was the subject of a case report that appeared in the *Journal of the American Medical Association* in the early 1990s (Firlik, 1991). Margo, a woman with what, based on the details of her functional status as provided in the case report, appears to be moderate-stage AD, typifies the kind of person about whom dementia ethicists have been writing. Persons in the moderate stages of AD typically have impairment across multiple cognitive domains, which commonly manifests in the inability to form new or retrieve well-formed memories, consistently identify the correct words when speaking, or find one's way around, even when in a familiar space. As one may suspect, this level of impairment precludes independent decision-making, as key functions like learning new information, engaging in meaningful deliberation about potential courses of action, and communication of a clear choice are all impacted. In advanced dementia, an affected individual may also have minimal capacity for verbal communication and require extensive assistance with self-care.

While the loss of such key abilities for independently living raises important ethical questions, including that of how medical care decisions should be made under such circumstances, the dementia ethics literature to date has been biased by an overt emphasis on advanced AD cases. Unfortunately, this tendency for dementia ethics discussions to be predicated on the portrayal of persons with moderate to severely advanced AD, and prioritizing the ethical issues presented by the late-stage cognitive symptoms of dementia, does not readily square with the clinical experience of, or future directions in, dementia care. In the following section, we present the current professional guidelines that classify the clinical syndrome of Alzheimer's dementia as distinct from biologically defined AD, noting that the latter does not initially entail the cognitive and functional impairment that so strongly influences traditional analyses of ethical issues in dementia care. We then argue that *hypercognitivism*, a form of bias that assigns heightened value to rational thought as a core feature of selfhood, has hindered both the existing and emerging discourse on dementia ethics.

Emerging Paradigm of Alzheimer's Disease as Biological Diagnosis

Alzheimer's Disease as a Spectrum

In 2011, the National Institute on Aging and the Alzheimer's Association published diagnostic criteria that reframed the definition of AD (McKhann et al., 2011). These were the first diagnostic criteria published since the hallmark and prevailing 1984 McKhann Criteria (McKhann et al., 1984). The new criteria represented a significant shift. Since 1984, AD has been defined according to clinical symptoms and primarily at the advanced dementia stage. Additionally, prior to 2011, a definitive diagnosis of AD was only available at autopsy. In vivo individuals were diagnosed with either *probable* or *possible* AD according to their functional capacity and clinical symptoms (e.g., memory loss). In 2011, the new criteria added two new stages of the disease: mild cognitive impairment and preclinical AD. Importantly, they also introduced the use of biological markers (amyloid and tau, as measured by neuroimaging, cerebrospinal fluid, or in plasma) as part of the diagnosis. Most recently, Jack and colleagues (2018) published a new framework for diagnosing AD in the research context. The 2018 framework defines AD first by biological criteria and then according to stages of the disease (preclinical, mild cognitive impairment, dementia) according to the progression of symptoms. Under this model, the clinical syndrome of dementia due to AD represents a later stage of the multi-decade biological process, which begins with a preclinical or "asymptomatic" stage.

Ethical Concerns About AD Biomarker Testing

The shifting from a clinical to biological definition of AD opens a new category of ethical challenges for current and, in particular, future clinicians. Many of these ethical issues harken back to questions raised in the 1990s regarding the disclosure of a diagnosis. However, the questions have evolved to focus on the use of biomarkers to identify asymptomatic individuals with an increased risk for AD based on positive biomarkers. Proponents of testing and disclosing biomarkers to individuals who are asymptomatic or exhibiting minimal cognitive changes reference the value these results could have for advance care planning and the ability to improve lifestyle to reduce risk factors. Additionally, some argue that the doctrine of "right to know" literature applies here, drawing from a history in genetics literature to argue that individuals have an established right to know their own medical information. Comparatively, others have argued that the information provided by biomarkers for asymptomatic individuals would not alter clinical care (without a disease-modifying therapy) and could expose the individual to stigma and potential discrimination (Stites et al., 2018). Still, the prevailing literature has yet to fully address the ethical tensions that will likely face clinicians who could find themselves deciding whether to pursue biomarker information for individuals who are either asymptomatic or presenting with subtle cognitive changes.

Schermer and Richard (2019) examine the ethical acceptability of what has become known as "preclinical AD" (biomarker positivity in the absence of symptoms), and make an explicit case against this terminology and categorization. They argue against the reconceptualization of AD as a biological entity, in the absence of a preventive intervention, arguing that such labeling could do more harm than good. The harms cited by Schermer and Richard are primarily psychological in nature, including anxiety and uncertainty, and these authors bolster their argument by reminding their readers that some of the asymptomatic individuals who test positive for AD biomarkers will never actually develop a dementia syndrome.

Concerns about adverse psychological responses to positive AD biomarker tests are valid, especially given survey data suggesting that AD is the most feared disease of late life (Tang et al., 2017). Indeed, concerns about inducing psychological harm echo those raised by the aforementioned commentators on the ethical implications of AD biomarker testing. However, unlike others who have called for caution in disclosing AD biomarker status to at-risk individuals, Schermer and Richard argue for refraining altogether from the use of labels that link positive results of tests for Alzheimer's pathology to a clinical diagnosis. While these authors' position might be viewed as an extreme restriction of information concerning how clinical interpretations of AD biomarker testing should be communicated to patients, this example highlights an overall pattern that can be observed in the published discourse on implications of AD biomarker testing; that is, a tendency to treat information about the brain as carrying particularly high stakes for affected patients.

Before discussing the potential biases that might incline clinicians, ethicists, and other commentators to treat information about brain health as special and indeed potentially dangerous, it seems prudent to review the literature for empirical evidence that harm can result from disclosing such information. Understanding the nature and extent of such risks, which were originally put forth as theoretical in nature, seems critical to determining how much weight to given them in deliberations about best practices for engaging patients in discussions around such testing.

Empirical Studies of the Impact of AD Biomarker Testing

To the extent that empirical studies can inform normative ethics, it bears emphasis that there is little evidence of psychological harm resulting from AD biomarker testing. A recent review of studies examining psychological outcomes following the receipt of amyloid positron emission tomography (PET) scan results concluded that there is no evidence of elevated depression, anxiety, or suicidal ideation levels following learning the result of this AD biomarker test (Kim & Lingler, 2019). Even the single study that has documented a phenom-enon of post-disclosure emotional upset found that such upset does not translate to clinically actionable depression or anxiety and that participants are over-whelmingly satisfied with their results and do not regret the testing (Lingler et al., 2020). In addition, there are reports, including from our own studies, of qualitative data suggesting that individuals undergoing AD biomarker testing are capable of appreciating the nuanced nature of the test results and their status as being "at heightened risk" for the subsequent development of clinical dementia (Lingler et al., 2016).

In the face of such evidence, one must question the full range of potential factors underlying opposition to biomarker-informed classification of AD risk status. We assert that the same forces of hypercognitivism that bias approaches to dementia ethics and influence the current medical decision-making literature are at play.

Hypercognitivist Bias in the Dementia Ethics Literature

Hypercognitivism

Hypercognitivism is a term coined by bioethicist Stephen Post to describe how a disproportionate focus on the cognitive losses associated with dementia lead to a devaluing and, ultimately, dehumanization of affected individuals (Post, 1995). Post argues that rationality is too strict a requirement for moral standing, arguing that instead it is *who we are*, not how we decide, that makes us human. Drawing on the work of sociologist (Kitwood & Bredin, 1992), Post reminds us of the essential humanness of the capacity for such endeavors as creativity, spir-ituality, and love, and goes on to articulate 12 noncognitive characteristics of the enduring self in the context of dementia.

A hypercognitivist disproportionate focus on the implications of diminishing potential for rational thought is starkly evident in the aforementioned litera-ture on medical decision-making in dementia. Even Dresser's argument for focus on the experiential interests of the current self is grounded in the logic that exploring one's current best interests is an approach to be reserved for when the rational self is inaccessible or absent.

We contend that addressing concerns around the processes for medical decision-making in the context of advanced dementia are not so much inappro-priate as they are *incomplete*. The disproportionate focus on such issues, which emanate from the cognitive symptoms of dementia, has led to general neglect of the everyday ethical issues encountered in dementia care. By everyday ethical issues, we mean those that are often faced by nurses and nursing care assistants who spearhead the day-to-day care of such individuals. Many of these everyday ethical issues reflect not the cognitive symptoms of dementia (like impaired recall and language processing), but the behavioral symptoms of dementia and, oftentimes, their social implications. Examples of such everyday ethical challenges include the moral permissibility (or impermissibility) of lying to patients (or, "therapeutic fibbing") to avoid confrontation in the provision of nursing care (e.g., "No, Ms. S. your bus isn't due for a few hours, so we have plenty of time to go ahead and help you shower"), considerations in managing abusive behaviors by persons with dementia toward vulnerable staff in long-term care relationships (including racist and sexist language and actions), and more recently, use of monitoring technologies to promote the safety of persons who may require more oversight than is feasible based on their living situation. Issues such as these are unlikely to be adequately raised and addressed by clinicians following current protocols for counseling candidates for AD biomarker testing. Although such issues may not have life-or-death stakes, or involve decision-making for medical care, they are pervasive in the day-to-day nursing care of individuals with dementia and have significant implications for the maintenance of quality of life and preservation of dignity within this population.

In effect, the practices of focusing on ethical issues related to loss of the capacity to make medical decisions, and inadequately attending to ethical issues concerning the nursing care of persons with dementia, have positioned the field to approach emerging developments in dementia ethics, specifically questions around the ethics of AD biomarker testing, from a skewed perspective. Stated simply, the prevailing view seems to be that while it might be psychologically devastating to learn of one's AD biomarker status, at least one would have the opportunity to direct one's future medical care. Below, we explain why this hypercognitivist portrayal of this issue is incomplete and how nurses can play a key role in informing and supporting candidates for AD biomarker testing while at the same time identifying and beginning to address a broader range of ethical issues that may be associated with such opportunities.

Revisiting the Exclusive Focus on Cognitive Impairment in Dementia Ethics

There is broad consensus that a major advantage of undergoing AD biomarker testing is to inform one's planning for the future, with the implication being that any ethical concerns about the risks associated with AD biomarker testing (e.g., discrimination and stigma) are outweighed by the value of being able to plan for one's medical care under a future scenario of advanced cognitive impairment.

While the value of executing advance medical directives with a better understanding of one's risk of AD is clear to dementia researchers and care providers, there is growing empirical evidence that candidates for AD biomarker testing rarely, if ever, describe their planning activities as focused on, let alone limited to, medical decision-making in the context of advanced cognitive impairment.

Indeed, several qualitative studies have explored older adults' perceptions regarding the pursuit of biomarker testing for AD. To be sure, these reports document participants to report that they have found AD biomarker testing to be valuable for planning purposes. Scrutiny of such reports suggests that the type of planning valued by patients is neither spontaneously nor exclusively described in terms of future medical decision-making. This is notable because much of the literature on ethical concerns in dementia care focus on medical decision-making in advanced dementia as the primary ethical concern. An example of the wide-ranging, non-medical planning that seems to be of interest to patients is found in Vanderschaeghe and colleagues' (2017) analysis of interviews with patients with mild cognitive impairment following the receipt of amyloid PET scan results. Patients in this study characterized the value of such information as useful for making "practical" arrangements and "enjoying life more." Our own team's interviews with patients following amyloid PET revealed similar findings with practical arrangements, including downsizing of homes and making changes to retirement plans. We also found evidence of a desire to "enjoy life more," often couched in terms of the pursuit of leisure activities and "bucket list" items. The social implications of positive AD biomarker tests were also emphasized. For example, some individuals described plans to mend strained familial relationships. Others explained that having family members better understand the source of their cognitive symptoms would lead to reduced frustration and more social support. One individual voiced a fear of eventually failing to recognize family members, underscoring the significance of concerns about the implications of progressive dementia for deeply valued social relationships.

Overall, findings from both our team's and Vanderschaeghe's interviews with symptomatic patients following biomarker disclosure reveal an interest in using information about one's AD biomarker status to plan for a broad range of activities and to take effect in the near future; that is, planning for the way one wishes to live before reaching a state of advanced cognitive impairment. Findings from our team's 2018 analysis of qualitative interviews with amyloid PET scan candidates following pre-test counseling but prior to disclosure were consistent with these results in that no participants spontaneously spoke of a desire to control medical decisions in the distant future; rather, planning was referenced in more general terms, as exemplified by the quote, "it's going to help me determine what I'm going to do with my life in the future." Even when participants spoke directly of the potential for a positive biomarker result to convey a future with advanced dementia, participants described implications for quality of life and the dehumanizing impact of neurodegeneration, (e.g., "I'm going to wind up like . . . a vegetable"), not decisional incapacity per se (Lingler et al., 2018). Similarly, when the Vanderschaeghe team invited patients to describe their motivations for sharing their results with other people in their life, none mentioned preparing their loved ones to act as proxy medical decision-makers. Rather, responses focused on helping other people in their lives to understand what is happening with them in the present as they experience initial cognitive changes and, relatedly, to enhance their capacity for social support.

While these examples provide evidence that the value of AD biomarker testing has implications for how one wishes to live during the period of time leading up to advanced cognitive decline, it is important to note that analyses of first-person accounts of living with dementia or caring for an affected family member reveal the same overall pattern of prioritizing quality of life and extend to the maintenance of dignity. Within this literature there is also a clear emphasis on the interpersonal and behavioral, rather than the cognitive, implications of dementia. For example, our team's meta-synthesis of qualitative investigations of the lived experience of dementia found that the experience, or fear, of social isolation is one of the most prominent and consistently reported features of late-life cognitive decline, from the perspective of those affected (Lingler & Hu, 2016). Our 2016 review also found preliminary support for the notion that positive interpersonal experiences can ameliorate the existential threats that are often experienced or feared by persons with dementia, including both the threat of loss of self and the threat of loss of self as a valued being living in relationship with others. More recently, Anderson and colleagues' (2021) analysis of 2,345 blog entries of persons impacted by dementia revealed the following priorities for care: perceived value from others, self in relation to others, behavioral respect, and self-value.

This body of literature suggests that the opportunities afforded by AD biomarker testing extend far beyond planning for future decisional incapacity during acute medical crises or at the end of life. This has significant implications for nurses, who can play a key role in educating and supporting individuals who are contemplating or who have recently received AD biomarker test results.

The Role of Nurse in Helping Patients to Navigate AD Biomarker Testing

Given the current state of limited medical treatment options for individuals who test positive for AD biomarker testing, the decision to pursue such information is a classic example of what decision scientists call "preference sensitive"; that is, the decision of whether or not to be tested depends on the potential value, from the testee's personal perspective, of the information to be gleaned. During both pre-test counseling or post-disclosure support, nurses can guide patients to explore their values and preferences in considering the range of implications of a future with a neurodegenerative decline. In addition to basic information about the cognitive changes associated with AD, nurses have expertise in the day-to-day care needs of affected individuals, as well as the interpersonal and behavioral changes that are likely to occur over time among individuals who are biomarker positive. Rather than framing knowledge of AD biomarker status as an opportunity to pre-plan one's future medical decisions, nurses can, more broadly, discuss how one's results might impact plans for how one wishes to live as changes ensue and ways of ensuring that one's dignity is maintained throughout the course of illness; that is, pre-test counseling and post-disclosure support should include planning for the near and distant future. Regarding the latter, nurses, as frontline care providers, are especially well positioned to guide discussions toward the maintenance of dignity over time.

Prioritizing threats to dignity as the starting point for considering the ethical implications of dementia has two key implications for the notion of advance planning. First, rather than focusing on the potential, and theoretical, possibility that the wishes of a pre-dementia self could conflict with those of a self with dementia, the focus shifts to discussing the future of an individual whose humanity will persist and will be worthy of dignity. Second, rather than narrowly focusing on (distinct) instances of medical decision-making in a state of decisional impairment, discussions broaden to encompass preserving one's dignity throughout the course of the disease, including during everyday care that may be provided by family members and/or professional caregivers. Centering advance-planning discussions around the preservation of dignity also means focusing less on hypothetical and unknown scenarios (e.g., dialysis in the event of renal failure) and more on highly likely scenarios (e.g., loss of independence for performing self-hygiene). Regarding the latter, nurses may be particularly well suited to invite a conversation as follows:

> Often times as dementia progresses, there is a need for help with personal care tasks, like using the bathroom or showering. One way to help your family or other caregivers to protect your dignity is to think about what kind of help you'd be most comfortable receiving when it comes to personal hygiene. For example, some people feel strongly about receiving assistance from a person of a certain gender, whereas others are more concerned about whether the person helping them is a family member versus a professional caregiver.

It is important to emphasize that discussions of the ethical implications of pursuing AD biomarker testing are relatively new. Nurses who engage in pre-test counseling and post-disclosure support of AD biomarker test candidates will be positioned to identify additional dilemmas. In illuminating and playing a key role in addressing such issues, nurses may shift the prototypical dementia ethics case study from one of a patient like Margo to that of a mildly symptomatic individual who has just learned of their positive AD biomarker status. This individual is likely to be wrestling with a broad set of concerns, including many that will warrant attention in the dementia ethics literature.

Implications for Preserving Human Dignity in Dementia Care

The approach described above represents a conceptual pivot away from hypercognitivist approaches that prioritize the preservation of decisional autonomy in states of advanced dementia. In contrast, the above-described nursing-oriented approach prioritizes the preservation of human dignity. Within this framework, distinctions between critical and experiential interests are less crucial, as we assert that interest in the preservation of dignity would override both experiential and critical interests should a conflict occur. Let us take the hypothetical example of an individual who, in discussions of their preferences for everyday care in an advanced state of dementia, expressed concern about maintaining an overall appearance of comportment in social settings. At mealtime in an assisted living environment, this now demented individual is noted to request seemingly unending servings of bacon at breakfast time and has acquired a habit of wiping grease on the napkins and sleeves of themselves and sometimes their table mates. Perhaps this individual, in the pre-dementia state, held deep convictions (either religious or moral) against consuming pork. An argument for the preservation of critical interests would favor instructing the kitchen staff to refrain from serving pork to this individual, regardless of their pleas upon seeing it on the plates of other residents. An argument for experiential interests, framed as the pursuit of activities that bring enjoyment in the moment, would favor serving the bacon. Clearly, the individual is enjoying this treat and it seems to be enhancing their quality of life. A dignity-oriented approach might favor mitigating the sloppiness and intrusiveness to others that are resulting from the consumption of bacon in the common dining area. Such an approach would take into consideration not only the obvious risks to dignity that breakfast with heaping helpings of bacon is posing, but would acknowledge that such indignities are compounded by the individual's long-held convictions against the consumption of pork. A dignity-focused solution may potentially involve serving a standard portion of bacon upon request, then shifting to offer the individual another enjoyable, but less messy, food item. If bacon were insisted upon, the additional serving could be brought to the individual's room so as to preserve dignity while eating in the common area. Note that this example is an oversimplification and is not intended to suggest that either the critical interests of a lifelong vegetarian or (mere) experiential interests of a person living with dementia should be unilaterally discarded. We argue that both should be considered, but that the ultimate decision should maximize dignity. We acknowledge that nurses with expertise in dementia care may have other ethically acceptable, dignity-maximizing solutions to the problem at hand, including some which creatively work around the serving of pork to this resident.

While the implications of such an approach are clear for nursing care, the application of a dignity lens also has implication for how clinicians ought to approach medical decision-making. To the extent that patients can use AD biomarker testing as a starting point for discussing their preferences for maintaining dignity over the course of cognitive, functional, and behavioral changes, patients can also be invited to consider how dignity can be maximized in the face of acute or terminal medical events that may occur in time. For example, in advance planning discussions of preferences regarding the use of life-sustaining treatments, nurses or other clinicians might invite patients to consider whether their preferences would differ if the treatments would require the application of physical restraints (e.g., hand mitts to prevent removal of tubing for intravenous hydration). In doing so, clinicians may guide patients to (a) understand dementia as extending beyond cognitive symptoms that limit decisional capacity to include behavioral symptoms like physically resisting invasive medical care, and (b) consider how treatments might impact an individual's dignity. From this lens, one can imagine "leeway" provisions that focus on the maintenance of dignity during the provision of medical care.

Conclusion

The landscape of ethical issues in dementia care is shifting, and as the field transitions to an era of biologically defined AD, nurses will have a key role in identifying and responding to emerging ethical dilemmas, including those arising during pre-test counseling for biomarker tests of AD risk. In doing so, nurses have a unique opportunity to reject historical hypercognitive biases and to guide patients, families, and other clinicians toward giving equal consideration to the interpersonal and behavioral implications of AD and working to proactively identify plans for promoting dignity throughout the disease course.

Acknowledgment

Portions of this essay first appeared in the unpublished master's thesis, *Conceptualizing Dementia as a Relationship-Transforming Phenomenon*, written and defended by Jennifer Lingler in 2003 under the advisement of Lisa S. Parker, PhD, Director, University of Pittsburgh Center for Bioethics and Health Law.

References

Alzheimer's Association. (2016). *End of life decisions* [Brochure]. https://www.alz.org/natio nal/documents/brochure_endoflifedecisions.pdf.

Anderson, J. G., Bartmess, M., Hundt, E., & Jacelon, C. (2021). "A little bit of their souls": Investigating the concept of dignity for people living with dementia using caregivers' blogs. *Journal of Family Nursing, 27*(1), 43–54.

Buchanan, A., & Brock, D. W. (1989). *Deciding for others: The ethics of surrogate decision making.* Cambridge University Press.

Byers, P. (2020). Eudaimonia and well-being: Questioning the moral authority of advance directives in dementia. *Theoretical Medicine and Bioethics, 41*(1), 23–37.

Cowley, C. (2018). Dementia, identity and the role of friends. *Medicine, Health Care and Philosophy, 21*(2), 255–264.

De Sabbata, K. (2020). Dementia, treatment decisions, and the UN convention on the rights of persons with disabilities: A new framework for old problems. *Frontiers in Psychiatry, 11*, 1–16.

Dresser, R. (1986). Life, death, and incompetent patients: Conceptual infirmities and hidden values in the law. *Arizona Law Review, 28*, 373–405.

Dresser, R. (1994). Missing persons: Legal perceptions of incompetent patients. *Rutgers Law Review, 46*, 609–719.

Dresser, R. (1995). Dworkin on dementia: Elegant theory, questionable policy. *Hastings Center Report, 25*, (6), 32–38.

Dworkin, R. (1994). *Life's dominion: An argument about abortion, euthanasia, and individual freedom.* Vintage Books.

Firlik, A. D. (1991). Margo's logo. *Journal of the American Medical Association, 265*(2), 201–201.

Groves, K. (2006). Justified paternalism: The nature of beneficence in the care of dementia patients. *Penn Bioethics Journal, 2*(2), 17–20.

Jack, C. R., Jr., Bennett, D. A., Blennow, K., Carrillo, M. C., Dunn, B., Haeberlein, S. B., Holtzman, D. M., Jagust, W., Jessen, F., Karlawish, J., Liu, E., Molinuevo, J. L., Molineuvo, J. L., Montine, T., Phelps, C., Rankin, K. P., Rowe, C. C., Scheltens, P., Siemers, E., … Silverberg, N. (2018). NIA-AA research framework: Toward a biological definition of Alzheimer's disease. *Alzheimer's & Dementia, 14*(4), 535–562.

Jaworska, A. (1999). Respecting the margins of agency: Alzheimer's patients and the capacity to value. *Philosophy & Public Affairs, 28*(2), 105–138.

Kant, I. (2007). *Anthropology from a pragmatic point of view.* Cambridge University Press (Original work published 1798).

Kim, H., & Lingler, J. H. (2019). Disclosure of amyloid PET scan results: A systematic review. In J. T. Becker & A. Cohen (Eds.), *Progress in molecular biology and translational science*, vol. 165: *Brain imaging* (pp. 401–414). Elsevier.

Kitwood, T., & Bredin, K. (1992). Towards a theory of dementia care: Personhood and well-being. *Ageing and Society, 12*, 269–287.

Lingler, J. H., Butters, M. A., Gentry, A. L., Hu, L., Hunsaker, A. E., Klunk, W. E., Mattos, M. K., Parker, L. S., Roberts, J. S., & Schulz, R. (2016). Development of a standardized approach to disclosing amyloid imaging research results in mild cognitive impairment. *Journal of Alzheimer's Disease, 52*(1), 17–24.

Lingler, J. H., & Hu, L. (2016). Qualitative evidence in working with cognitively impaired older adults. In K. Olson, R. A. Young, & I. Z. Schultz (Eds.), *Handbook of qualitative health research for evidence-based practice* (pp. 277–289). Springer.

Lingler, J. H., Roberts, J. S., Kim, H., Morris, J. L., Hu, L., Mattos, M., McDade, E., & Lopez, O. L. (2018). Amyloid positron emission tomography candidates may focus more on benefits than risks of results disclosure. *Alzheimer's & Dementia: Diagnosis, Assessment & Disease Monitoring, 10,* 413–420.

Lingler, J. H., Sereika, S., Butters, M. A., Cohen, A. D., Klunk, W. E., Knox, M. L., McDade, E., Nadkarni, N. K., Roberts, J. S., Tamres, L. K., & Lopez, O. L. (2020). A randomized controlled trial (RCT) of amyloid positron emission tomography (PET) results disclosure in mild cognitive impairment (MCI). *Alzheimer's & Dementia, 16,* 1330–1337.

McKhann, G., Drachman, D., Folstein, M., Katzman, R., Price, D., & Stadlan, E. M. (1984). Clinical diagnosis of Alzheimer's disease: Report of the NINCDS-ADRDA Work Group under the auspices of Department of Health and Human Services Task Force on Alzheimer's Disease. *Neurology, 34*(7), 939–939.

McKhann, G. M., Knopman, D. S., Chertkow, H., Hyman, B. T., Jack, C. R., Jr., Kawas, C. H., Klunk, W. E., Koroshetz, W. J., Manly, J. J., Mayeux, R., Mohs, R. C., Morris, J. C., Rossor, M. N., Scheltens, P. S., Carrillo, M. C., Thies, B., Weintraub, S., & Phelps, C. H. (2011). The diagnosis of dementia due to Alzheimer's disease: Recommendations from the National Institute on Aging-Alzheimer's Association workgroups on diagnostic guidelines for Alzheimer's disease. *Alzheimer's & Dementia, 7*(3), 263–269.

Post, S. G. (1995). *The moral challenge of Alzheimer's disease.* Johns Hopkins University Press.

Post, S. G. (1998). The fear of forgetfulness: A grassroots approach to an ethics of Alzheimer's disease. *The Journal of Clinical Ethics, 9*(1), 71–79.

Schermer, M. H., & Richard, E. (2019). On the reconceptualization of Alzheimer's disease. *Bioethics, 33*(1), 138–145.

Stites, S. D., Rubright, J. D., & Karlawish, J. (2018). What features of stigma do the public most commonly attribute to Alzheimer's disease dementia? Results of a survey of the US general public. *Alzheimer's & Dementia, 14*(7), 925–932.

Tang, W., Kannaley, K., Friedman, D. B., Edwards, V. J., Wilcox, S., Levkoff, S. E., Hunter, R. H., Irmiter, C., & Belza, B. (2017). Concern about developing Alzheimer's disease or dementia and intention to be screened: An analysis of national survey data. *Archives of Gerontology & Geriatrics, 71,* 43–49.

Vanderschaeghe, G., Schaeverbeke, J., Bruffaerts, R., Vandenberghe, R., & Dierickx, K. (2017). Amnestic MCI patients' experiences after disclosure of their amyloid PET result in a research context. *Alzheimer's Research & Therapy, 9*(1), 1–16.

17

Relational Autonomy

A Critical Reading for Palliative and End-of-Life Care

Philip J. Larkin

The Case of Maneem

> Maneem is a 78-year-old man from an Indian Hindu tradition with advanced renal disease, receiving dialysis three times per week and on a waiting list for renal transplantation. His health is failing and the opportunity for a successful transplant increasingly unlikely. Maneem informs the clinical team of his decision to withdraw from the transplant list and stop dialysis to be able to spend some quality time with his family, conscious that to do so will mean eventual death. His clinical team are unhappy with his decision and seek ways to challenge his decision, arguing that life-sustaining interventions should be continued. His family find themselves in a dilemma; they do not want him to die, but neither do they want to see him suffer. They feel unsure of how to best support Maneem.

The case of Maneem is not unusual. Many decisions about treatments involve deliberation about the right course of action in a given situation and trying to find the best possible outcome. Often, the clinical outcome does not resolve all questions that complex care management evokes. Of all the main life transitions, death and dying provoke significant debate about rights, wishes, and choices. A recent paper by Parks and Howard (2021) on the experience of dying well in nursing homes during the COVID pandemic attests to this debate, much of which hinges on the interpretation of autonomy and the extent to which autonomous decisions can be made given the frailty of the person, the value and legality of "proxy" decision-making by family or close others, and who has the right to make decisions—the person, their family, or the clinical team. Historically, the use of principalist views on autonomy in ethical decision-making (Beauchamp & Childress, 2019) are most evident in how complex decisions around living and dying are made. Such discussion often rests on the primacy of the individual to make clear and decisive choices, being aware of and fully informed of the consequences of those decisions. The criteria for being considered competent, informed, and independent in decision-making are the topic of debate in both current literature and the media but, generally speaking, this approach has served clinical decision-making in palliative and end-of-life care quite well. Questions of the complexity of autonomy are linked to frailty, challenging symptom management and the process of death and dying (Fontalis et al., 2018; Gruenewald & Vandekieft, 2020; McNamara, 2004; Munro et al., 2020; Smith et al., 2020).

However, the practice of palliative care is evolving. The delivery of care has become increasingly complex. There has been a strategic shift from palliative care as a practice entirely devoted to the careful management of dying to one where earlier intervention and the inclusion of chronic life-limiting illness has redefined palliative and end-of-life care in terms of its overall scope. Public demand for greater involvement in their care decisions, the use of advance care planning, and the international debate on right to life and right to death mean that understanding the evolution of palliative and end-of-life care is critical to interpreting the place of autonomy and the continuing value of the biomedical approach as the *sine qua non* to complex decision-making. Maneem's case cited above questions how these rights and choices are determined and understood by all players: patient, family, and clinicians. Moreover, how can Maneem's decision be respected, valued, possibly challenged, and certainly enacted?

In this chapter, following a brief explanation of the changing dynamic of palliative and end-of-life care, a case will be proposed that our current focus on personal autonomy tailored to the individual may be erroneous and that a relational approach derived essentially from feminist philosophies, taking into account the wider personal and societal implications of clinical decisions, may be more valuable in providing optimal care for people living in the transition between living and dying. Based on Bergum and Dossetor's seminal work on relational ethics as the basis of respect (Bergum & Dossetor, 2005), this chapter will argue that although autonomy remains an essential and valued component of people's experience as their life closes, the application of a relational approach as goals of care change can lead to a richer and more meaningful experience for the person who is dying, their wider community, and the professional care team. To provide context, some hypothetical case studies will be presented. First, an understanding of palliative and end-of-life care and current international debate is needed.

Palliative and End-of-Life Care: An Evolving Dimension of Care

The use of the term "palliative *and* end-of-life care (PEOLC)" as a single phrase is itself a challenge. Historically, the modern construction of palliative care is derived from the UK hospice or "end-of-life" model of care postulated by Cecily Saunders (1918–2005) with its focus on the care of the dying through optimal symptom management (Clark, 2018). The term "palliative care" has its origins in French-speaking Canada, where the image of hospice related to charity warranted a shift toward more culturally appropriate language (Mount, 2005). Although both terms have been used interchangeably, palliative care has become the more globally acceptable term. The original World Health Organization (WHO) definition of palliative care in 1990 proposed palliative care as:

> the active, total care of patients with progressive, far advanced disease and limited life expectancy whose disease is not responsive to curative treatment. It refers to the control of pain and of other symptoms as well as the treatment of social, psychological, and spiritual problems. (WHO, 1990)

This supported the view of a clinical practice directed toward the terminally ill (a term avoided in current thought) at a point when curative options were no longer possible. It implied that care was multidimensional, albeit that pain management was seen as the primary predictor of good palliative care. Overall, the definition indicated that palliative care would be introduced at a time point following the cessation of active treatment, up to and including death and bereavement. This was criticized for its overt cancer-orientated focus, implication that clinicians could "control" symptoms, and focus on the last days and weeks of life. Counterarguments proposed that the holistic approach advocated in this definition was of equal benefit earlier in the disease trajectory and to a wider and more diverse range of chronic and life-limiting conditions beyond cancer (e.g., heart failure, chronic obstructive respiratory disease, and dementia care). Therefore, a revised WHO definition (2002, n.p.) proposed:

> Palliative care is an approach that improves the quality of life of patients and their families facing problems associated with life-threatening illness, through the prevention and relief of suffering by means of early identification and impeccable assessment and treatment of pain and other problems (physical, psychosocial, and spiritual).

A study by Temel et al. (2010) into early palliative care for people with lung cancer was a catalyst to seeing palliative care as more than a practice for the dying. The essential difference is an *approach* to care (rather than a specialist practice) delivered by all healthcare professionals in a variety of settings.

However, to some degree, both definitions retain the focus toward a medically led responsibility for clinical care, while the broader social determinants of health such as social networks, gender, and culture, which may impact how PEOLC decisions are made, receive limited attention, despite the fact that these determinants are known to have a significant impact on issues of access, resource allocation, and decision-making. Consequently, the International Association for Hospice and Palliative Care (IAHPC) has stated that the 2002 definition remains limited and reductionist in approach; it argues for a new definition which is more inclusive of the need to advocate for global political engagement to ensure equity of access to essential medicines and normalization within the standard of delivery of care to relieve serious health-related suffering:

> Palliative care is the active holistic care of individuals across all ages with serious health-related suffering due to severe illness, and especially of those near the end of life. It aims to improve the quality of life of patients, their families and their caregivers. (IAHPC, 2018, n.p.)

Confirming the need for optimal symptom management and adopting some of the language of preceding definitions, the IAHPC definition reflects the wider social determinants mentioned earlier, including effective communication strategies, and targets governments to take responsibility for integrating palliative care into health systems through ensuring equitable access.

The Impact of Changing Definitions for Practice

Historically, the focus on care in the last days of life meant that patients and families were largely dependent on clinicians to predict and plan the trajectory of care toward death. Engagement with patients and families was seen in terms of information and advice in the face of rapid deterioration. The changing perspective on palliative care has led to new considerations in terms of the meaning and interpretation of autonomy, how decisions are made, and by whom. Early intervention of palliative care has become a critical element of current service provision, and its benefits to patients and clinical services have been evidenced through both qualitative and quantitative studies (Bekelman et al., 2018; El-Jawahari et al., 2017; Hannon et al., 2017). With an approach to care which favors intervention at critical moments of complex symptom management and suspension of services if the clinical situation stabilizes, clinicians must now embrace the contextual elements of choices made by virtue of a much deeper engagement between the palliative care provider, patient, and family over a longer period of time than just in the last days of life. Wishes and choices can be discussed and debated, and of course changed, over time. It has also meant a closer proximity to the wider family perspectives on how decisions are made, and although the extent of family engagement in decision-making varies by legal jurisdiction and authority, the early introduction of palliative care clearly warrants a review of how complex care is managed.

Early palliative care has challenges. Despite the fact that it may be beneficial in terms of enabling patients to better understand their values and preferences when end of life occurs, prioritizing early intervention may inadvertently obscure the needs of those who are actively dying. Early intervention is an ideal; in practice, the main focus of many palliative care services is still end of life. Balance is needed in terms of how palliative care is delivered and that critical elements of end-of-life care are not forgotten.

Although calls for this third IAHPC definition have also gained traction within the global palliative community, the 2002 WHO definition remains in force. The global perspective proposed by the IAHPC is underpinned by a social justice argument that PEOLC differs according to access, availability, and culture, reflecting different worldviews. From a relational ethics perspective, the expectation that the autonomous individual only makes decisions based on their sole interpretation of their dilemma is erroneous and indeed may conflict with cultures where decisions are made in community. Therefore, a system of ethical decision-making based on the primacy of the individual to make their own individually expressed choices in terms of matters of living and dying may fail to heed "real-world" contextual issues for which the wider network would need to be involved. In PEOLC, these issues can include deeply challenging questions around care, provision for others after death, legacies (such as wills and testaments), and rites and rituals of remembrance which may need a range of views to help the person reach the most appropriate decision.

Therefore, it would appear that the IAHPC definition best reflects the basis of relational approaches to ethical decision-making in PEOLC, that is, placing decisions in the wider context of people's lives and connections, offering a richer and more responsive solution to complex and challenging PEOLC decisions. Examples of this will be considered later. For some, particularly clinicians, the risk of adopting this new definition is that palliative care would no longer be seen as a clinical discipline but rather as a social movement. For others, the latter cannot be ignored. Both present essential arguments for the future of palliative care. In the next section, this challenge will be considered further, unpacking one approach to relational ethics as proposed by Bergum and Dossetor and its benefit to better understanding of PEOLC.

Relational Ethics: The Work of Bergum and Dossetor

Although this chapter focuses on the application of one specific relational approach, theories of relational ethics have been the subject of contemporary debate within philosophy and health sciences (Christman, 2004, 2014; MacKenzie, 2019, 2021; MacKenzie & Stoljar, 2000; Westlund, 2009, 2012), including those working in palliative care (Abma, 2005; Heidenreich et al., 2018; Jennings, 2019; Olsman et al., 2016; Pergert & Lützén, 2012; Ramvi & Ueland, 2019; Weigand et al., 2015; Wright et al., 2018). The call for a relational ethics within feminist philosophy holds weight because of its challenge to social oppression, exclusion, and discrimination, emphasizing the multifaceted nature of autonomy, arguing that our individual identity is shaped by the intersection of our relationships across networks (MacKenzie, 2019). From this perspective, relational autonomy endorses normative individualism, that is, the importance of rights, freedom, and autonomy, but at the same time rejects the primacy of methodological individualism, which dictates that we only understand and interpret the world as an individual, with limited attention paid to the wider social world and relationship. In effect, relational autonomy argues that individual autonomy is best understood in relational terms (Westlund, 2012). There has been a critical position taken regarding these perspectives, but overall, the benefit of a relational ethic has been endorsed (Christman, 2004; Westlund, 2009). The strength of feminist perspectives reflecting issues of vulnerability, patriarchy, and exclusion speak particularly to the work of Vangie Bergum and John Dossetor and their 2005 publication, *Relational Ethics: The Full Meaning of Respect*. Reporting on a study funded by the Social Sciences and Humanities Research Council of Canada and based at the University of Alberta, Canada, this study, situated within feminist philosophy, sought to understand the nature of relationship and its impact on how ethical decisions are made. Through an interprofessional group, including palliative care practitioners, Bergum, a nurse scientist, and Dossetor, a physician and bioethicist, led a qualitative process of interactive engagement and discussion with clinicians, academics, teachers, and students to understand where a relational approach sat within the predominant bioethical paradigm of principle-based ethics (Beauchamp & Childress, 2019). They identified a number of specific clinical and ethical scenarios to demonstrate how a focus on relationship to ethical decision-making based on interdependence can lead to more informed and hopefully better decisions. The issue of relationality and critical appraisal of the application of principle-based biomedical ethics was already part of academic discourse, and the work of Bergum and Dossetor drew on a wide range of resources and evidence, but were particularly influenced by Sally Gadow (1999) and Edmund Pellegrino (2002) and their ethical discourse in nursing and medicine, respectively. Both served to explain how the focus on universal principles to address moral dilemmas was of increasingly limited value in a changing dynamic and pluralist society and were critical of the influence of principle-based ethics which were based on rational thought and removed from the reality of people's lives, their life story, and character. In particular, Gadow (1999) discussed the context of "layered" worldviews which inform choices and decisions. In this approach, true understanding of a given situation requires a combination of subjective, objective, and intersubjective knowledge. Past history is always included, developed, and shaped, so that how decisions have been made previously may influence the pattern of decision-making in a current dilemma.

Layering knowledge, rather than trying to "dissect" the problem and apply universal principles, means that, in real-world situations, "nothing is lost, everything is attended to, but changed and enhanced in a way that makes for greater usefulness" (Bergum & Dossetor, 2005, p. 48). Bergum and Dossetor describe their relational ethic through an analysis of four themes derived from their research: engagement, mutual respect, embodiment, and environment.

Engagement suggests the need to address not only rational decision-making (what is the right thing to do in this situation for all concerned) but also the "emotional aspects of others' lives" (Bergum & Dossetor, 2005, p. xii). In brief, both rational and emotional perspectives should be given equal status, reflecting not only the abstract complexity of an ethical dilemma, but also its personal impact on those who experience it. This requires a combination of approaches to gather both subjective and objective information through dialogue to understand the totality of a situation to aid better decision-making.

Mutual respect acknowledges our own limitations in understanding how others' cultural worldviews impact how information is sought and interpreted and how decisions are made at both individual and community levels. Reciprocity is key, respecting that contrasting positions are not necessarily wrong, and appreciating that the way to solution requires a respectful listening to each perspective proposed.

Embodiment seeks to evoke the reality of a lived experience through story. Listening to the story of a given situation, its impact on persons, the challenges and opportunities addressed, transforms an ethical dilemma from an abstract case to be adjudicated, to one that needs to be shaped and nurtured within the real-world existence of those who are experiencing it. Finally, *environment* encapsulates the three previous themes through challenging current notions of individual autonomy by arguing that some decisions (possibly most) cannot be made without reference to the wider network of relationship that situates the individual in their world.

There are some caveats. The first is that this approach to relational thought does not seek to reject the normative mainstream bioethics promoting autonomy as a core principle such as proposed by Beauchamp and Childress (2019). Rather, it argues that autonomy is equally valued within a relational ethical approach, but seeks to situate that within the wider context in which lives are lived and experienced. It respects the value of individual experience and difference. Second, the relational approach is less about seeking solutions and more about asking the right questions which may enable a solution to emerge. This is only possible through a deep commitment to the dialogue and the process, rather than the outcome of a problem solved.

To conclude, the metaphor of a tree in full bloom is used to explain the benefit and importance of a relational ethic. For example, the trunk of the tree cannot be separated from the branch or roots. It is integral to the flow of nutrients to enable the tree to flourish. Bergum and Dossetor propose that "if one only lives through the branches (the rational mind) one misses the wisdom of the roots (the lived body) and wholeness is lost" (2005, p. 51).

This interrelatedness responds to persons in the full complexity of their lives through the establishment of relationship and so permits the true expression of the ethical life to be nurtured.

Application of a Relational Ethic to PEOLC

It would seem that the prevailing discourse on autonomy, at least in Western healthcare, argues that people make important decisions through focusing on their individualized self-interest in a rational and logical manner (Dove et al., 2017). An important question to be addressed here is why a relational approach to our understanding of autonomy has specific resonance with PEOLC. The right to self-determination, mitigation against the risk of medical paternalism, based on a clear set of principles and enshrined in law, gives structure to situations which are often nebulous and fluid (Gilbar & Miola, 2015; King & Moulton, 2006). Given the deeply personal nature of the transition toward death and dying (insofar as death is an individual experience and only experienced once in a lifetime), the imperative on healthcare professionals to do all that is within their power to enable patients to voice their needs and desires and have those needs and desires enacted and respected as far as possible would seem to be without question. To do less than this, a clear underlying principle of PEOLC, would challenge what is meant by optimal care for dying people. However, dying as an individual experience is not necessarily a private one, and engagement with family and those close to the patient is usually encouraged and prioritized, supported by a multi-professional team (WHO, 2002). Clinical engagement is defined at the level of patient *and* family in tandem, ensuring that both are supported in the transition from living to dying in equal measure, albeit with different foci. Proponents of a more relational approach to ethical decision-making and certainly those engaged in PEOLC would argue that individuals rarely, if ever, make critical decisions based on their sole self-interest. In a relational context, our interrelatedness to others in society determines how we interface with the world around us and how that influences how and why we make certain decisions. Of course, this reflects complex understanding regarding the capacity of the patient to make autonomous decisions, the place and rights of family to be part of that decision, and the duties of the clinician (real or perceived) in terms of responsibility for how those decisions are made and how the consequences of those decisions are managed. People in receipt of palliative care are often frail, with variable levels of capacity and trajectories of illness which can be unpredictable and elusive in terms of prognosis. For clinical practice, this raises two important questions:

- Does a principle-based approach to ethical decision-making offer sufficient scope to appreciate the complexity of clinical decision-making at end of life?
- What value is placed on family or community in decision-making processes around end-of-life care? In effect, is autonomy essentially different when people are living with chronic life-limiting illness or life is ending?

Using three hypothetical case studies derived from practice, the final part of this chapter will present an argument that the use of a relational ethical framework can offer an alternative structure to address ethical questions in PEOLC in terms of their complexity and responsiveness to patient and family needs.

Case 1: Simon

Simon is a 75-year-old man with a diagnosis of congestive heart failure (CHF) and chronic obstructive pulmonary disease (COPD). He lives with his wife, Anne; they have been married for 50 years and they have five adult children. Their youngest daughter, Elaine, lives with them and is his main caregiver. He is frail, breathless, with moderate leg edema, and requires continual oxygen for comfort, although of minimal clinical value. He has been admitted to the hospital due to a possible chest infection.

Anxiety has been a lifelong problem for Simon, exacerbated by his current disease. He has had recurrent dreams about suffocating and choking to death. He wakes up distressed and shouting for help.

On admission, Simon is asked what he wishes to do with regard to resuscitation if it is required. Simon is clear that he wishes to be resuscitated in all circumstances. His wife supports his decision, although she is aware that any attempt at resuscitation is unlikely to be successful. Their children, especially Elaine, are of a different view; as a group, they feel very strongly that to even attempt resuscitation is cruel and inappropriate. They oppose their father's wishes.

Contrary to the idea that autonomy is exclusively determined at the level of the individual, Bergum and Dossetor, (2005) argue that a relational ethic is centered on persons and not the dilemma itself. A relational ethic acknowledges the deep impact of disease not only on the person, but also on those close to the sick individual. Further, it contends that the interests of the wider network who are directly impacted by the disease are morally relevant. It does not seek to deny the right of Simon to make autonomous decisions in principle, but rather seeks to set those decisions within the larger context of what is happening to all involved: his wife, his children, and the professionals. Second, whereas it may be argued that a principle-based approach seeks solutions, a relational dialogue with Simon and his family does not seek to resolve the problem, but to ask pertinent questions so that all perspectives are valued.

As a clinical practice, despite calls for early intervention noted earlier, palliative care is still often introduced later in the patient's journey through illness. The risk for a practitioner is to arrive at one point in time and to fail to address sufficiently the context in which the person currently lives now or has lived in the past; worse is to try to "fill the gap" in the absence of information or context. For Simon and Anne, their 50 years of marriage mean that they will have encountered other dilemmas and managed to find solutions. A question on how they have managed to resolve these earlier situations may give insight into how best to address this one. This speaks to an approach which values mutual respect, learning from Simon and Anne, rather than trying to educate them on the right decision. Further, it enables both groups (parents and children) to develop ways to listen to each other's perspective without having to argue for contrasting positions which may only lead to entrenchment and division. Setting this discussion within the life story of Simon and Anne may also speak to this situation, where the steps that have led to this decision can be explored and shared as a family. Through a process of engagement, with the clinician acting as a guide rather than a leader, it may be possible to blend the emotional nature of the situation with some of the "real-world" questions that need to be asked. For example, where is Elaine as the principal caregiver in this scenario, and why is she opposed to her parent's view? Who is "leading" the children's response and why? What fears and worries exist on both sides, and how can they be voiced? At the same time, how can rights and duties be made visible so that options and choices become clear. For example, the fact that Simon is asked his wishes on admission to hospital would suggest that choices are possible, and if so, how does Simon's choice resonate with the professional caregivers, as well as close family members? Datta-Barusa and Hauser (2018) apply four communication strategies from the domain of psychiatry to palliative care, all of which speak to communication with Simon and his family. These include being attentive to the impact of communication on the clinical caregiver; the need to develop skills in active listening; the appropriate use of silence to enable reflection; and having the capacity to sensitively bring the critical issues to the fore and "name" them to avoid ambiguity. Palliative care and psychiatry share a number of the same priorities, particularly related to complex communication. Application of these strategies may help solutions to emerge which would help avoid fragmentation within the family unit. Bergum and Dossetor describe this as enabling persons to experience "the self and the other more clearly through the honest effort to keep conversation open" (2005, p. 55).

Case 2: Clara

Clara is a 25-year-old woman, the victim of a road traffic accident. She has sustained severe head injuries and was admitted to the intensive care unit. Her prognosis is very poor, but at this time, her clinical situation has stabilized. Clara's family have traveled from another part of the country to be with her, aware that it is extremely unlikely that she will survive.

Clara does not have an advance care directive or organ donation card, although she has previously expressed a desire to donate her organs in a life-threatening situation. Clara may survive without respiratory support but would need continual care for the rest of her life. Her family express their view that Clara would not wish to live if this were the case. The clinical team and the family are divided as to the best action to take, given that she could survive for a number of years if respiratory support was stopped, but it would impact significantly on the quality of her life and her personal autonomy.

There are clearly some similarities between the cases of Clara and Simon. A key question here is the place of the family as a "proxy voice" for Clara, notably in the lack of evidence of any written or verbal instruction from Clara herself (Baran & Sanders, 2019). The case also addresses an issue of medical culture, insofar as the legitimacy of the family to make decisions may be medical or legislatively determined based on jurisdiction and practice. However, one would expect the family to be dealt with in a respectful way, welcoming their contribution and incorporating their perspective where possible. In this situation, there does not appear to be a contrast of views, but a genuine lack of certainty over the future. Gedge et al. (2007) present the limitations of the traditional "principalist" approaches to decisions of withdrawing or withholding treatment in the context of critical care, arguing that the practitioner often holds an ambiguous position, unclear what information should be shared and with whom, working to solve a clinical problem, rather than asking appropriate questions to better understand the complexities of the situation. Perhaps an opening question here would begin with "I wonder . . ." which opens the possibility to diverse outcomes, none of which can be predicted. Here, the flexibility of the relational approach comes to the fore, teasing out how people would live with a complex and challenging situation. Clara's death would require one set of ethical questions around the choices that she made around organ donation and voiced to others. Her life would evoke deeper questions about the challenge of care, responsibilities, and a vision for the future. A critical element here is time, making decisions now that impact the immediate and the unforeseen future. The timing of conversations is also critical, as a stable clinical condition as described here can deteriorate quickly. Questions related to respect for Clara's wishes should also ask about the environment of care and network willing to take responsibility for Clara's care. Clara's survival is predicated on the interdependence between those persons close to her, but the risks and challenges for all need to be clear and explicit, even though the future cannot be predicted. For Bergum and Dossetor (2005), they describe this as "letting go of sureness" (p. 57), where the approach is more about a gentle expectation of realities and perspectives toward living with the unknown.

Case 3: Maria

Maria is a 35-year-old woman with amyotrophic lateral sclerosis (ALS). Her disease has progressed rapidly. She is unable to walk without assistance and is using a wheelchair. Maria has been told that the prognosis of her illness is relatively short, possibly 6–8 months, and that she will need to be admitted to a hospital or hospice in the last months and weeks of life. It is not clear what Maria has understood about her illness.

Maria has a clinical history of alcohol and heroin dependency. She has also been a victim of domestic violence, and her last partner, André, is not allowed to be alone with her and the children. André is not believed to be the father of the children. Maria's children (Eliane, aged 4, and Rahul, aged 15 months) were placed in foster care because of her social problems and only have limited contact with their mother. Maria lives alone in a first-floor apartment, supported by community services. She has family who live locally and who visit, although they, too, have alcohol and drug dependency issues and are in a variety of rehabilitation programs. Her care at home has become increasingly difficult due to her physical care needs.

Maria's case is not atypical of those seen in PEOLC. It reflects the complex interplay between physical, psychosocial, and spiritual symptoms which underpin contemporary palliative care practice. Physical pain and suffering, which always need to be addressed, may be eclipsed by the enormity of the wider context in which people live their lives and which, in Maria's case, led to destructive health behaviors, isolation, and vulnerability. A principalist approach to this case might argue that the risks imposed by Maria's situation warrant an urgent intervention to ensure her safety and the onus (and power) rests with the clinician to make decisions for Maria in her current state of vulnerability. In effect, Maria's ability to make autonomous decisions is inhibited by the complexity of her health status and social situation. From a relational perspective, the context of environment is critical to understanding how best to respond. In Maria's situation, there are not only clinical and ethical decisions to be made, but legal implications that need to be addressed in relation to her and the care arrangements for her children. A multi-professional network, both within and outside the palliative care team, will be necessary to plan appropriately for Maria's place of care. Multiple voices will be needed to create realistic options and choices to support Maria.

Maria's story and situatedness in a challenging dynamic of relationship (André, her children, her own family with their own lived experiences) need to be acknowledged. For the professional caregiver, the layers of suffering in Maria's life cannot be ignored or glossed over. A blog debate by Selman and colleagues in the *British Medical Journal* in 2019 argued that palliative care could be accused at one time of adopting a "chronic niceness" label, where the desire to construct a "care-full" environment which is clean and neat, and where everyone is kind and caring, belies the reality of people's lives, and that relationships between caregivers and patients can be challenging and difficult. An opening question to the healthcare professional is an acknowledgment of one's personal views on issues such as addiction and domestic violence which may color judgment and influence the care response, albeit subconsciously. From a position of mutual respect, Maria may have entrenched views of authority and their negative influence on her life. This may influence her capacity to express her needs and to feel heard. Conversely, a professional approach that only sees Maria as a victim or responsible for her own circumstances may obscure the opportunity for open and frank discussion and for shared decisions to be made. Understanding Maria's priorities, which may be inherently different from those of the professional team, is critical. The goals of care need to be explicit and, through a process of dialogue, ensure that Maria clearly understands the ongoing implications of her progressive disease and the probable time frame. The capacity of her wider family to provide necessary support needs to be addressed without the risk of alienation. Bergum and Dossetor (2005) argue that "conversation requires openness, in which one must be willing and able to reveal oneself to others and also be willing and able to accept others' revelations" (p. 130). Such openness may enable the capacity to hear questions which are not overtly expressed and may reduce Maria's sense of alienation and separation. However, it requires authenticity on the part of the professional and a willingness to appear vulnerable. That in itself means that an approach to Maria's case diverts attention from goals to be achieved toward persons in the fullness of their lives.

Conclusions

The view of Hans-Georg Gadamer (1996) that the body and soul are inseparable means that every ethical question should begin with a deeper understanding of how we see each other as human persons. Arguing for the "absolute inseparability of the living body and life itself" (p. 71) fits well with the inclusive and tripartite nature of palliative care. Palliative care argues that our response to the needs exhibited by patients and families as they come to terms with life-limiting disease and end-of-life scenarios demands an approach that sees the treatment of physical symptoms in the wider context of the psycho-social and spiritual dimensions which make up the totality of the person. The deterioration of the body due to disease does not mean that life in all its richness and diversity has ended, and a relational ethic may assist in strengthening those elements of our human self when quality rather than quantity of life is the goal. The position of a relational ethic does not seek to overturn the given wisdom, and indeed, autonomy remains a key principle in how ethical decisions are made. However, the work of Bergum and Dossetor, as well as more contemporary authors, asks how approaches which seek generalizable principles, objectivity, and distance can really address the complex reality of living within community. In professions where hierarchy and structure are valued, "rules-based" approaches may fit well.

They argue that we need a call to relationship and an understanding that relationship in itself is an ethical responsibility. Relationship strengthens the need for collective responsibility which reflects our shared existence in humanity and asks us to situate autonomy in our interdependence, rather than an abstract construct to be upheld.

Reflecting on the three cases presented, the critical argument posed is that a relational ethic does not deny individual autonomy but situates it within a wider sociopolitical context and interdependent network which govern the reality of how people make real and meaningful decisions. The case of Maneem, which opened this chapter, offers a further example of the richness of a relational approach. Bergum and Dossetor (2005) argue that a relational ethic does not seek to solve a problem, but rather to ask the questions which enable ethical decisions to made which reflect a real-world situation. The clinical team see a problem that needs to be resolved and that Maneem's decision denies the potential for life if treatment continues. However, Maneem's culture also impacts his choices and decisions. Maneem's worldview as a practicing Hindu would favor the life cycle of birth and rebirth and so influence his understanding of living and dying. Focus on the clinical implications of the cessation of treatment may fail to incorporate his view of life as a continuum and death not as an endpoint. Engaging with Maneem, his family, and the clinical team on these important aspects of Maneem's view of the nature of human existence in a relational way can bring a perspective to find an equitable solution which is respectful of his wishes as well as the challenges faced by clinicians. Such an approach may help us to seek solutions to complex ethical dilemmas which are integral to the vision and scope of palliative and end-of-life care.

References

Abma, T. A. (2005). Struggling with the fragility of life: A relational-narrative approach to ethics in palliative nursing. *Nursing Ethics, 12*(4), 337–348.

Baran, C. N., & Sanders, J. J. (2019). Communication skills: Delivering bad news, conducting a goals of care family meeting, and advance care planning. *Primary Care: Clinics in Office Practice, 46*(3), 353–372.

Beauchamp, T. L., & Childress, J. F. (2019). Principles of biomedical ethics: Marking its fortieth anniversary. *The American Journal of Bioethics, 19*(11), 9–12.

Bekelman, D. B., Johnson-Koenke, R., Bowles, D. W., & Fischer, S. M. (2018). Improving early palliative care with a scalable, stepped peer navigator and social work intervention: A single-arm clinical trial. *Journal of Palliative Medicine, 21*(7), 1011–1016.

Bergum, V., & Dossetor, J. B. (2005). *Relational ethics: The full meaning of respect.* University Publishing Group.

Christman, J. (2004). Relational autonomy, liberal individualism, and the social constitution of selves. *Philosophical Studies, 117*(1–2), 143–164.

Christman, J. (2014). Relational autonomy and the social dynamics of paternalism. *Ethical Theory and Moral Practice, 17*(3), 369–382.

Clark, D. (2018). *Cicely Saunders: A life and legacy.* Oxford University Press.

Datta-Barua, I., & Hauser, J. (2018). Four communication skills from psychiatry useful in palliative care and how to teach them. *AMA Journal of Ethics, 20*(8), E717–E723.

Dove, E. S., Kelly, S. E., Lucivero, F., Machirori, M., Dheensa, S., & Prainsack, B. (2017). Beyond individualism: Is there a place for relational autonomy in clinical practice and research? *Clinical Ethics, 12*(3), 150–165.

El-Jawahri, A., Greer, J. A., Pirl, W. F., Park, E. R., Jackson, V. A., Back, A. L., Kamdar, M., Jacobsen, J., Chittenden, E. H., Rinaldi, S. P., Gallagher, E. R., Eusebio, J. R., Fishman, S., VanDusen, H., Li, Z., Muzikansky, A., & Temel, J. S. (2017). Effects of early integrated palliative care on caregivers of patients with lung and gastrointestinal cancer: A randomized clinical trial. *The Oncologist, 22*(12), 1528–1534.

Fontalis, A., Prousali, E., & Kulkarni, K. (2018). Euthanasia and assisted dying: What is the current position and what are the key arguments informing the debate? *Journal of the Royal Society of Medicine, 111*(11), 407–413.

Gadamer, H. G. (1996). *The enigma of health: The art of healing in a scientific age,* trans. Gaiger and N. Walker. Polity.

Gadow, S. (1999). Relational narrative: The postmodern turn in nursing ethics. *Scholarly Inquiry for Nursing Practice, 13*(1), 57–70.

Gedge, E., Giacomini, M., & Cook, D. (2007). Withholding and withdrawing life support in critical care settings: Ethical issues concerning consent. *Journal of Medical Ethics, 33*(4), 215–218.

Gilbar, R., & Miola, J. (2015). One size fits all? On patient autonomy, medical decision-making, and the impact of culture. *Medical Law Review, 23*(3), 375–399.

Gruenewald, D. A., & Vandekieft, G. (2020). Options of last resort: Palliative sedation, physician aid in dying, and voluntary cessation of eating and drinking. *Medical Clinics, 104*(3), 539–560.

Hannon, B., Swami, N., Rodin, G., Pope, A., & Zimmermann, C. (2017). Experiences of patients and caregivers with early palliative care: A qualitative study. *Palliative Medicine, 31*(1), 72–81.

Heidenreich, K., Bremer, A., Materstvedt, L. J., Tidefelt, U., & Svantesson, M. (2018). Relational autonomy in the care of the vulnerable: Health care professionals' reasoning in moral case deliberation (MCD). *Medicine, Health Care and Philosophy, 21*(4), 467–477.

International Association for Hospice and Palliative Care. (2018). *Global consensus based palliative care definition.* Retrieved January 1, 2021, from https://hospicecare.com/what-we-do/projects/consensus-based-definition-of-palliative-care/definition/.

Jennings, B. (2019). Relational ethics for public health: Interpreting solidarity and care. *Health Care Analysis, 27*(1), 4–12.

King, J. S., & Moulton, B. W. (2006). Rethinking informed consent: The case for shared medical decision-making. *American Journal of Law & Medicine, 32*(4), 429–501.

Mackenzie, C. (2019). Feminist innovation in philosophy: Relational autonomy and social justice. *Women's studies international forum 72,* 144–151). Pergamon.

Mackenzie, C. (2021). Relational equality and the debate between externalist and internalist theories of relational autonomy. In N. Stojar & K. Voigt (Eds.), *Autonomy and equality* (pp. 32–56). Routledge.

Mackenzie, C., & Stoljar, N. (Eds.). (2000). *Relational autonomy: Feminist perspectives on autonomy, agency, and the social self.* Oxford University Press.

McNamara, B. (2004). Good enough death: Autonomy and choice in Australian palliative care. *Social Science & Medicine, 58*(5), 929–938.

Mount, B. M. (2005). In memory of . . . snapshots of Cicely: Reflections at the end of an era. *Journal of Palliative Care, 21*(3), 133–135.

Munro, C., Romanova, A., Webber, C., Kekewich, M., Richard, R., & Tanuseputro, P. (2020). Involvement of palliative care in patients requesting medical assistance in dying. *Canadian Family Physician*, 66(11), 833–842.

Olsman, E., Willems, D., & Leget, C. (2016). Solicitude: Balancing compassion and empowerment in a relational ethics of hope—an empirical-ethical study in palliative care. *Medicine, Health Care and Philosophy*, 19(1), 11–20.

Parks, J. A., & Howard, M. (2021). Dying well in nursing homes during COVID-19 and beyond: The need for a relational and familial ethic. *Bioethics*, 35(6), 589–595.

Pellegrino, E. D. (2002). Medical evidence and virtue ethics: A commentary on Zarkovich and Upshur. *Theoretical Medicine and Bioethics*, 23(4–5), 397–402.

Pergert, P., & Lützén, K. (2012). Balancing truth-telling in the preservation of hope: A relational ethics approach. *Nursing Ethics*, 19(1), 21–29.

Ramvi, E., & Ueland, V. I. (2019). Between the patient and the next of kin in end-of-life care: A critical study based on feminist theory. *Nursing Ethics*, 26(1), 201–211.

Selman, L., Sallnow, L., Taylor, R., O'Mahony, S., & Smith, R. (2019). Is palliative care having an existential crisis? Retrieved January 21, 2021, from https://blogs.bmj.com/bmj/2019/11/12/is-palliative-care-having-an-existential-crisis/.

Smith, M. A., Torres, L., & Burton, T. C. (2020). Patient rights at the end of life: The ethics of aid-in-dying. *Professional Case Management*, 25(2), 77–84.

Temel, J. S., Greer, J. A., Muzikansky, A., Gallagher, E. R., Admane, S., Jackson, V. A., Dahlin, C. M., Blinderman, C. D., Jacobsen, J., Pirl, W. F., Billings, J. A., & Lynch, T. J. (2010). Early palliative care for patients with metastatic non–small-cell lung cancer. *New England Journal of Medicine*, 363(8), 733–742.

Westlund, A. C. (2009). Rethinking relational autonomy. *Hypatia*, 24(4), 26–49.

Westlund, A. (2012). Autonomy in relation. In S. L. Crasnow & A. M. Superson (Eds.), *Out from the shadows: Analytical feminist contributions to traditional philosophy* (pp. 59–82). Oxford University Press.

Wiegand, D. L., MacMillan, J., dos Santos, M. R., & Bousso, R. S. (2015). Palliative and end-of-life ethical dilemmas in the intensive care unit. *AACN Advanced Critical Care*, 26(2), 142–150.

World Health Organization. (1990/2002). Definition of palliative care. Retrieved January 21, 2021, from https://www.who.int/news-room/fact-sheets/detail/palliative-care.

Wright, D. K., Brajtman, S., & Macdonald, M. E. (2018). Relational ethics of delirium care: Findings from a hospice ethnography. *Nursing Inquiry*, 25(3), e12234.

18

Help Wanted

Technology, ICU Nurses, and Death

Helen Stanton Chapple and Megan Gillen

Nurses are experts in managing intensive care unit (ICU) rescue/life-saving technology. One of the satisfactions in being an ICU nurse is becoming highly skilled in operating particular kinds of machinery, such as the intra-aortic balloon pump (IABP), extracorporeal membrane oxygenation (ECMO), left ventricular assist device (LVAD), and/or continuous veno-venous hemofiltration (CVVH) after physicians have placed appropriate machine parts into the patient. Nurses manage all of this, along with an often-inert human hidden under lines, cords, dressings, masks, and tubes. Such expertise must be honed with practice. Nurses understand what a particular technology is meant to do to improve their patients' welfare, and one of the satisfactions of the role is for nurses to feel confident in their proficiency.

Yet nurses are also the ones who struggle regularly and intimately with technology's broken promises. As they assiduously manage this seeming cyborg, patient plus machines, they are acutely aware of three factors: the patient's age, her comorbidities, and the passage of time. An 85-year-old with diabetes and congestive heart failure whose acute problems fail to abate over time will activate the nurse's internal alarms faster than a healthy 60-year-old with a stubborn pneumonia. Acute-on-chronic illness in the setting of advanced age diminishes the chances that technology will restore the patient's future prospects. Experience advises the patient's nurses that hopes for limitless tomorrows will turn out to be misplaced, regardless of their meticulous care. When organ systems do not respond convincingly to extensive technological support, then presumed current suffering and alienation are irredeemable. The patient becomes "other," segregated from fellow humans who are delivering care and living into the illusion of their own unlimited futures (Chapple, 2015). On admission, the patient's right-now stability and prospects for future recovery seem fused to the application of specific technologies. But over time, her presumed immediate suffering becomes more compelling and fragile than a fantasized future resilience. For the nurse, convinced of the patient's ultimate death, patient/machine management is now blanketed by moral distress (Hamric & Blackhall, 2007) and emotional labor (Mauno et al., 2016).

Now nurses mumble—to themselves and each other. They feel a moral responsibility to make things different. They seek resolution to their distress by bringing the participants (team and family—the patient is typically too sick to participate) to acknowledge that the patient has entered "mortal time" (McQuellon & Cowan, 2010), but they may not feel powerful enough to make any difference, as the interview in this chapter shows. The failures of technology may come to form a pattern, weighing more heavily over time (Epstein & Hamric, 2009). Stress, burnout, and compassion fatigue among ICU nurses compromise their care of patients and of themselves, and can cause them to leave the profession.

These machines managed by nurses are part of the rescue project that has emerged in the U.S. healthcare system to express its rejection of human finitude. When the nurse-run technologies fail to live up to societal expectations, nurses are the ones who pick up the pieces. The work is physically, emotionally, intellectually, ethically, and spiritually taxing. How did this state of affairs come to be? What are its features? What keeps it in place? What does it mean for ICU nurses and for the wider culture as a whole? In this chapter we explore these questions using a case interview to show that ICU nurses shoulder a burden that society disdains: negotiating the transition to dying while making it as meaningful as possible. We explore the connection between the nurse and the machines used in the ICU as an unrecognized component of their stress. Along the way we notice an interaction between ICU nurses and their professional association that appears to be supportive but may complicate their problems. Finally, we suggest possible countermeasures that may prove efficacious.

The Phenomenon of the ICU as a Manifestation of Terror Management

Solomon, Greenberg, and Pyszczynski (2015) have asserted that being a mature human entails the knowledge of death. If death is imminent, terror (fight, flight, or freeze) is the biologic response. According to these authors' extensive research, humans shield themselves from both imminent death itself and any casual reminders of its ultimate inevitability. They use adaptive human responses to mitigate their awareness and fear of death, called "terror management," by deepening their involvement in cultural worldviews and striving to enhance self-esteem.

The ICU in the United States is a profound cultural expression of terror management in its origins, persistence, growth, and day-to-day operations. The U.S. healthcare delivery system is built around the project of rescue, central to its economics and its self-image. Since the discovery of successful cardiopulmonary resuscitation (CPR) in the mid-1960s, rescue and stabilization have emerged as the default mode of operation on the street, in the emergency department (ED), and especially in the ICU. They capitalize speed and technology in an idealized, egalitarian effort to defeat imminent death (Chapple, 2010). The ICU is the front lines in the crusade against mortality. Death is close here. Yet it is also far. The battlements are tall and strong, constantly reinforced by technological innovation and adoption (Callahan, 2009). This is the culmination of a profound societal response to the fear of dying, fully capitalized and ever-expanding.

The statistics of ICU care in the United States illustrate its central place in U.S. healthcare delivery. Prior to the pandemic, trends showed an increasing number of ICU beds even as the number of U.S. hospitals housing them declined (Wallace et al., 2017). When more beds are available, demand for them increases, proving its elasticity (Gooch & Khan, 2014). The role of ICU care became even more dramatic in the eyes of the U.S. public during the Covid-19 pandemic when real and potential shortages of ICU beds, ventilators, personal protective equipment, and staff gained media attention. Prior to Covid, ICU patients died most often from multisystem organ failure, cardiac and circulatory failure, and sepsis, with the rate of mortality ranging from 10% to 29% of ICU admissions (Society of Critical Care Medicine, 2016). By 2021, Covid-19 ranked as the third leading cause of death in the US overall, after heart disease and cancer (Xu et al., 2022).

ICU deaths prior to Covid had fallen overall by 35% from 1998 to 2012 (Zimmerman et al., 2013). This decline might surprise ICU clinicians, who are deeply aware of its inadequacies. Critical care is also an economic driver on many levels. ICU care comprised up 3% of healthcare costs and 1% of U.S. national GDP as of 2005 (Gooch & Kahn, 2014). Garrett (2015) notices that rescue seems an unimpeachable first priority because the direness of the need cancels other considerations. Yet an awareness of rescue's context warrant ethical attention due to its frequency, its demand on resources needed elsewhere, and what preventive measures enacted on the front end could mitigate the need for it.

What does this plethora of rescue mean to the general public? To be in the ICU is to be surrounded by high-tech interventions (see later discussion in this chapter) and improved nurse availability. Yet the true complexity of ICU care is opaque even to some clinicians. The media fails to do it justice; entry to and immersion in the ICU are shocking to the uninitiated. Longing and fear of even greater loss in the face of life-threatening illness can overwhelm patients' families, not to mention the impacts of stress and fatigue. And what of the patients? They become almost unrecognizable. Attaching biomechanical objects to the insides and outsides of patients creates mélanges of suffering that are difficult to witness, much less shepherd. But they are also creatures of hope, a priceless hodgepodge of rescue and dying. Patients' sequestration in ICUs maintains the public's obliviousness regarding their complexity—not to mention that the dazzle of activity, urgency, and drama in the ICU can be overpowering.

For ICU nurses, by contrast, the path is well-worn: using machines and monitors to stabilize fragile life forces within bodies. Just as they know the machines, they are attentive to the existential threat implied by their deployment and the emotional labor, for the participants but especially for the nurses, that they portend. No one else in the situation is more aware of that labor, because it is no one else's place to tend to the machines, the patient's body, and their nexus. Accommodating the existential reality of the human condition *in* extended *extremis* is their daily work. The ICU nurse plus the patient/machine are at the center of the rescue/dying praxis that allegedly justifies the unit's existence.

Case Interview

When neither the patient's living nor dying are clear to everyone in the situation, conflict can occur regarding the appropriate treatment plan. Physicians often play a significant role in family decision-making when the patient is unable to participate (Shapiro, 2019). In the case that follows, the treating physician plays a particularly dominant role. Regardless of who drives the plan, the ICU nurse may be caught in the middle. We argue that the dynamics encouraging aggressive care operate within the situation itself, often unchecked. The interview with the ICU nurse who cared for Ms. W occurred 14 months after her demise, but the details are still sharp in her memory.

So, Tell Me About Ms W. What Do You Remember About Taking Care of Her?

The patient's husband wanted to withdraw life support so badly and the doctors weren't letting him. Her last two nights, her husband would come and say that she never wanted any of this. Then they would talk him into more interventions, like more meds, chest tubes, and cardioversion. He had signed the universal consent at admission to the ICU, but I don't think he knew what he was signing. They would do interventions without discussing things with him because they were emergent. I'd ask, "Do you think the husband would have wanted that?" But they'd say she was still a full code so we would have to "do everything." They were being so awful.

Here the nurse is reacting to the argument that the goal of future survival justifies the means, which she sees perhaps as harming the patient in the present, and certainly disrespecting the patient's autonomy.

What Kinds of Interventions Were You Doing?

I never left the bedside [during my shift]. I was drawing labs and blood gases constantly. The respiratory therapist was making changes on the vent based on the gases. I was titrating multiple pressors and hanging antibiotics, sedatives, and antiarrhythmics. She had about 12 IV channels running through a central line, and multiple peripheral IVs with three IV poles. We were turning her and had to do baths because her fevers were so high, she was sweating. We had to change her IV and central line dressings too because of how diaphoretic she was. I had to chart her vital signs and her In's and Out's each time. Her vital signs were so out of whack. She was so uncomfortable. Her husband and daughter went home at night. I just stayed in there with her all night until they showed up in the morning.

How Did You Feel?

It made me feel terrible. At admission, she had been DNR/DNI.[1] The attending told the family to give him 5 days. It was just the flu. She was healthy otherwise and they'd be able to fix it. But 16-year-olds die from the flu. He started asking for withdrawal after the 5 days. Well, it had been 14 days and her husband felt like he had betrayed her. He felt defeated. I honestly wish I had done more. I was more focused on doing tasks at night and comforting him in the morning when he got there. I should've been there to give him more of a voice.

On the day they withdrew, her husband came in at 6 a.m. I could tell he hadn't slept. He said that he had been up all night going over her directives. He said to me, "Take the tube out now. I don't want to wait for the doctors. I want everything off now." I had to tell the resident. The resident cornered him and said, "We will not kill your wife." And the husband was crying. I was so defeated because I felt like the husband didn't know how wrong all of this was.

They pulled the tube finally, and she didn't even take a breath. I know it sounds cold, but her death brought me peace. Her family was afraid to touch her. There are so many alarms and machines. She should've been loved on. She didn't deserve to be in pain and be poked and prodded at. I felt like we were torturing her.

This interview shows the nurse's awkward position as she juggles the pressing and unpredictable needs of the patient and the patient record (diaphoresis, baths, documentation); adjusts IV drip rates to respond to vital sign fluctuation; and struggles with the patient's discomfort and her own through her night shifts. She is bereft of daytime resources like palliative care and ethics consultation, unavailable

---

[1] Do Not Resuscitate/Do Not Intubate.

in this hospital during off hours. Here, months later, she is second-guessing her care, wishing she had empowered the patient's husband (or herself) to speak up more forcefully, attesting to his powerlessness in the face of the medical team. The nurse takes on the emotional labor of (1) the unacknowledged but imminent death, (2) empathy for the spouse, and (3) misgivings about the treatment plan. She is juggling the power dynamics in the situation as she engages the minute-by-minute struggle to maintain the patient's stability. The wisdom of any intervention may be open to question in a seriously ill, possibly dying patient. But they pile on so quickly in the ICU (enabled, and perhaps seen as ethically justified, by the use of a universal consent form) that their sheer momentum can overwhelm the nurses' voiced concerns. The machines and the urgency of stabilization seem to be their own drivers. Obeying their demands can feel like hypocrisy to the nurse. And underneath it all is the constant fear of errors, exacerbated by the complexity of the required tasks.

While juggling these responsibilities, the ICU nurse caring for such a patient has both overt and covert roles in implementing a treatment plan oriented toward stabilization.

Overt Roles of the ICU Nurse

The visible work of the ICU nurse is not hidden, but even physicians may fail to appreciate its convolutions. In managing the machines, the patient's body, and the connections between the two, the nurse is enacting both care and hard science on the patient's behalf (Vilelas & Diogo, 2014), as the case illustrates. Besides operating and maintaining the machines, the nurse becomes their human face and hands (see Table 18.1 for a partial list of interventions and their connections). Apart from the ventilator, the nurse manages not only the machines but also all their connections: to the wall, the patient, and the bed (see Figure 18.1). The nurse's understanding is intimate; these technological breakthroughs are routine tools (Koenig, 1988). One must attend to their interconnections, plugs, infusion, and drainage bags; keep the lines untangled, labeled, and in-date; dressings clean, dry and intact, all while documenting the influence of machines and the body's response to their effects in minute detail.

The nurse watches the various displays, tweaking and adjusting how the machines affect the patient and each other. The nurse is noticing (and perhaps hand-recording) the data that indicate trends occurring in the internal and external environment of the patient. The nurse regularly obtains samples of blood and other body fluids. Continuous assessment is necessary to recognize difficulties immediately, make adjustments, and alert other clinicians. How can one travel for an off-unit procedure with all these attachments? How should

Table 18.1 Sample Interventions and Connectors

Machine or Action	Connector	Patient Contact
Ventilator	Ventilator tubing	Endotracheal tube
Cardiac monitor	One line splits into five	Five sticky patches on chest
BP monitor	One line to cuff	Sleeve that tightens on patient's arm
Oxygenation monitor	One line to probe	Sticky patch or finger clamp
Blood gas monitor	IV lines	Arterial line, radial or groin
Multiple IV infusion pumps	One line	Central and peripheral IV lines
Urine drainage	Tubing	Indwelling urethral catheter
Intra-aortic balloon pump	One line	Central line, groin
Ventricular assist device	Tubing	Abdominal insertion site
Continuous renal replacement therapy (dialysis)	Tubing	Fistula or central line
Extracorporeal membrane oxygenation	Tubing	Open chest
Blood transfusion	Blood tubing	Central or peripheral IV
Tube feeding	Tubing	Naso-gastric or gastric tube
Cardiac output monitor	One line, several ports	Central IV line, chest or groin

this patient be turned and bathed? Physiological changes like fever and sweating complicate the picture, as in the interview, often making it impossible to leave the room. The nurse also provides ongoing explanations and teaching to the family. It is not unlike spinning plates atop poles, racing from one to the other, making sure none shatters. "Ambiguity abounds . . . while caring for a patient . . . and monitoring a machine and trying to make the human technological and humanize technology . . . are mind-boggling and heart-rending chores" (Almerud et al., 2008, p. 135) As technical expertise increases, the nurse becomes a valuable resource for other clinicians, including physicians.

At the same time, the nurse's intimacy with the patient's body, unique among clinicians in its ongoing nature, can be a source of moral distress. The nurse may self-project and vow to avoid similar indignities for oneself. Alternatively, the nurse may minimize both the witnessed bodily suffering and one's complicity

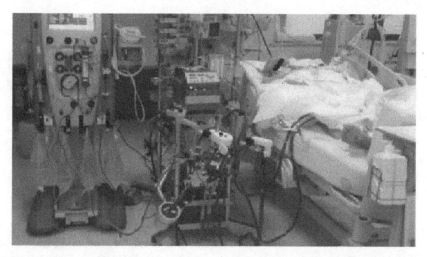

Figure 18.1 Patient under concurrent extracorporeal membrane oxygenation, plasmapheresis, and continuous renal replacement therapy (Savran et al., 2016).

in it as one enacts physicians' orders. The nurse hopes that achieving the goal of restoring the patient's future will justify the means. Certainly, the required attention to myriad details can serve as a distraction from the existential quandary the patient presents. Nurses' perception of patient suffering builds over time. Eventually they may lobby the team to reconsider the treatment plan, using the patient's suffering and the need to reinstate dignity as major motivators (Chapple, 2010; Kaufman, 2005).

This intense ICU work often confines the nurse to a small space, without consistent backup or witness. Non-nursing clinicians have greater mobility in their duties, able to refresh their eyes occasionally with sights other than the tethered patients in the ICU. While no other profession is trusted more highly by the public (Brenan & Jones, 2024) nurses see little recognition of their contribution, partly because of this isolating work model, and partly because the profession is not socialized to speak about its work (Buresh & Gordon, 2013).

To need such high-tech rescue is a crisis for the patient and family. Who in this situation can navigate the new perils? Who can interpret the meanings that apply as the dire situation persists without trajectory? Certainly not the patient. By now he or she is almost always too sick to offer or receive input about any care plan (Shapiro, 2019). The family also is compromised. Stressed and fatigued, in foreign territory, it is unlikely that they are prepared to absorb the implications of increasingly aggressive treatment. Neither are the ICU providers and physicians up to the task, engaged in responding to a deteriorating and fragmented rescue situation by directing the increased interventions needed to shore it up. "Medicine . . . has excluded from its view the possibility of the particularly embodied histories and particularly embodied projects of the patient, in order to gain power over the failing mechanism" (Bishop, 2011, p. 298). Bishop recommends humility in both what medicine purports to know and in the face of human finitude itself (Bishop, 2015). Dugdale (2015) notices that "it is recognition of finitude that helps bring into relief that which we most value" (p. 183). For the patient to flourish in the face of death, the physician must disclose that death is near, thereby acknowledging the finitude of medical prowess.

Yet even as many providers work hard to be realistic with themselves and with patients and families, flourishing in the face of death seems impossible once the patient is intubated and unable to direct care. Practiced in running the technology and in recognizing its painful shortcomings, the ICU nurses must also interpret the situations as best they can. Their perception of patient suffering mounts in concert with comorbidities and days of attempting rescue. Their emotional labor notices the patient's entry into "mortal time" (McQuellon & Cowan, 2010), makes it visible, and attempts to gain agreement for a care plan accommodating the new reality. The emotional labor and the moral distress of the nurse in the interview were plain as she struggled with how to navigate both.

Covert Role of the ICU Nurse: Describing the Emotions and the Labor of Emotional Labor

Anticipating death and managing its acknowledgment is a subtler role for the nurse than running the rescue technology. It garners less cache and legitimacy in the ICU environment, but many nurses are more than prepared to assume it. Certainly, they are more familiar with this unwelcome territory than the family may be. The nurse must mediate between the failing interventions of the machines and the family's and/or the team's resistance to the implications of a deteriorating body. Intimate on-the-job experience with dying and death inform the nurse, who has been foreseeing these inherent difficulties even as s/he has been spinning those technological plates so expertly. Epstein and Hamric (2009) call the repeated moral distress the nurse feels in these circumstances the "crescendo effect," meaning that the distress it causes can build with recurrence over time. If clinical rotations or other systemic factors delay provider attention to reorienting the care plan or meeting with the family, the nurse's frustration may increase.[2] Stress reducers such as mindfulness and reflection may or may not be effective in resolving nurses' distress as they witness and are complicit in preventable patient discomfort that they are powerless to mitigate (Schenck &

---

[2] Sarah Vittone, DBe, MSN, MA, RN, in a private conversation.

Neely, 2023). The nurse may feel that time is running out to prepare the family for the inevitability of their loved one's death.

These are the *emotions* of the emotional labor. What exactly is the *labor* here? What actions does the nurse take? The nurse joins a Greek chorus, in that the nurse cannot direct the patient's treatment plan. Meanwhile, nurses comment on the situation to peers, seeking validation and commiseration. Nurses speak in other ways as well, working to fill the void of meaning for other participants. They may urge the team to see "the big picture," to get them to acknowledge that a tipping point in the rescue effort has arrived (Chapple, 2010). Nurses interpret clinical comments about lab values and other indicators, telling the family, "I'm worried about your loved one," preparing them for bad news. Traditionally, nurses may not alter the care plan or overtly block it, so their actions must often be persuasive rather than determinative. In the case interview, the nurse wanted to give the husband "more of a voice." She felt that empowering him would enable him to speak with more force, galvanizing the medical team. If the family and the team decide that aggressive treatment is no longer appropriate, then by contrast, the nurse's compelled presence at the bedside may offer a new opportunity for leadership. Physicians often find other things to do while the nurse orchestrates the process of turning off the machines that no longer serve the patient's best interests, while ministering to the needs of both patient and family.

As we have seen, the one most involved in technological hands-on care is also the one most troubled by its use when it reneges on its promises, and who feels most responsible for enacting a technology-free transition. Healthcare workers embody society's concern for its ill members. As its agents, they enact a social contract. The position of the ICU nurse in navigating the territory of imminent death on behalf of society is both invisible and untenable. Who then understands and cares for the plight of the ICU nurse? From what quarters might support be found for the unacknowledged emotional labor that the job requires?

The Tenuous and Questionable Sources of Support for ICU Nurses

Considering the lack of social capital attributed to and claimed by nurses relative to physicians and similar healthcare providers, the list of prospects for assistance is short yet interesting: self-care, facility support, and professional resources. Certainly, the American Nurses Association (ANA) *Code of Ethics* (2015) prizes the nurse's own self-care, and "Resourceful" is every nurse's middle name. Yet self-care may be far down the list of personal priorities for the nurse, especially for ICU nurses (McElligott et al., 2009). The nurse's personal support networks become limited resources due to the confidentiality of patient care. The nurse cannot rely on society's empathy because the public's knowledge of the scope of nursing practice is woefully limited (Buresh & Gordon, 2013). But even the most enlightened self-care is a poor match for the system- and culture-wide imbalances endemic to the healthcare system (Hamric & Epstein, 2017). Daniel Chambliss (1996) noticed that bedside ethical quandaries faced especially by nurses were really systems issues in disguise. In the Ricou et al. (2018) study of burnout among ICU nurses, researchers state, "Although factors associated with burnout are known, they are part of the special environment of ICU" (p. 1). The very structure of the work is untenable for those who must perform it.

Can nurses find significant support from their employers? Hospitals may offer tangible assistance in terms of scheduling, enlightened staffing, support for professional development, and maintaining a "healthy work environment" (American Association of Critical Care Nurses, 2005, p. 189). But hospitals are the purveyors of the problem. Because they must be busy carrying out the wishes of the culture for full-bore rescue, their focus on ICU nurse welfare may not be robust.

The phenomenon of the ICU itself represents an ethical dilemma that is not well-articulated. Even though the problem of end-of-life decision-making has dominated the bioethics literature as the most likely topic of quandary ethics, the specific situatedness of the decision has rarely been tagged as the heart of the problem, with Chambliss (1996) and Shapiro (2019) being exceptions. And while moral distress, compassion fatigue, and burnout among ICU nurses is also widely discussed (see below), the connection between the machines populating the ICU and the nurses who manage them has rarely been identified as a specific contributor.

At least one entity has understood the connection between the ICU nurse, the place of work, and the machine. It has used this insight with a view toward supporting connections among all the entities involved. By reinforcing these entanglements, insight is not achieved. Instead, the human elements of emotional labor around the end of life become that much more difficult to parse.

The major professional association for ICU nurses is the American Association for Critical Care Nurses (AACN). Its annual conference, the National Teaching Institute (NTI), offers an intriguing mixture of support, education, exhortation, and entertainment tailored expressly for ICU nurses. Its messages are quite mixed, however, and the NTI experience may confuse as well as nurture its thousands of attendees. To the extent that NTI stands for and caters to ICU nurses by combining hundreds of educational offerings, revelry, and medical technology, its messages and experiences are worth exploring.

NTI: Support, but With Additional Agendas

Membership in the AACN is 130,000 strong in 200 chapters nationwide. The organization offers 15 types of professional certification, enabling nurses to challenge themselves to master specific domains of expertise. Its largest annual conference is the NTI, which attracted 9,000 worldwide attendees in 2018. That year, along with its hundreds of educational sessions and plenaries, its Critical Care Exposition sparkled with displays from 354 exhibitors.

The vital connection between the ICU nurse and the machine is weirdly reinforced and intensified at NTI. Here, in a carnival-like atmosphere, the plenary speakers lionize ICU nursing as heroic. Such recognition, so severely lacking in their grueling daily work, joins with celebration and display of the newest and shiniest versions of the technology that nurses work with every day, but *without the patients that make that relationship so fraught.* NTI delays the opening of the Exposition until the second day of the conference to build anticipation. Attendees crowd the gates at the appointed time, racing in when the doors open. The Expo atmosphere is festive and fun, encouraging unencumbered consumerism. The novelty of hands-on inspection of the newest versions of their rescue tools is hard for nurses to duplicate anywhere else. After all, they incur no emotional or financial risk in this giant space full of familiar devices and devoid of patients, family members, and shift work. The existential shadows cast by a cloud of expected death seem remote here in this place of brightly lit opportunity. Informational presentations in corporate display theaters offer drop-in opportunities to earn Continuing Education Unit credit as one browses the Expo and snags giveaways. Nurses fortunate enough to attend NTI soak up the vast amounts of information, to be sure. They network with each other and the vendors. They "play," literally and figuratively, with all the educational concepts and the tools of the ICU trade. They also revel in the attention, the praise, the gaiety, the dazzle and display, all of it justified by the goal of promoting excellence in ICU care. The tricky part is this: conference attendees become ambassadors and influencers for the Expo's corporate vendors to their home hospitals, sometimes by design, sometimes unwittingly. In the name of saving lives, nurses facilitate connections between buyer and seller. In doing so, they may be enabling the expansion and proliferation of the medical industrial project itself, along with over-treatment and unwanted care. Inadvertently, they may be cementing their own moral distress.

NTI's plenary sessions follow key points in terror management theory (Solomon et al., 2015). That is, they reinforce the importance of rescue in mainstream and ICU culture; they emphasize the significance of ICU nursing; and they celebrate the contributions that nurses make. But problems stow away in this message. Even as NTI encourages and feeds the recognition-starved nurse, it also ties that reward to excellence in promoting "hard science." It recruits nurses to advance the rescue project by bringing its latest iterations back home. And it defines professional success as ever more robust adherence to the rescue project in the form of scientific expertise, teamwork, and improving one's comfort level with the machines.

At the same time, attending NTI can increase the ICU nurse's fraught position. With saving lives as the major focus, the task of knitting patients and families together at the end of life receives only token attention. "Soft" issues, such as ethics, palliative care, and spiritual reflection support the nurse in the "trenches" of the ICU. They are indeed present at NTI. But lacking tangible flashy products, they can only whisper.

NTI's emphasis on empirical and operational knowledge is a one-sided message, insufficiently narrow for the ICU clinical experience. It implies that operational excellence alone (perhaps coupled with better staffing) will renew the ICU nurse's job satisfaction, because the machines are the means to an unquestioned good: saving lives. It is a partial truth, only. But the physical display of the Expo makes it powerful and difficult to abjure. In fact, the machines are the reason for the existence of the ICU—they become an end in themselves, even though they are advertised as a means to an end. The premier professional conference for ICU nurses may in fact undermine its attendees' well-being, if its messages transform the nurses into emissaries for their own job dissatisfaction. At home, the patients and their pain are added back in. Inadvertently, one's cognitive dissonance expands in an ever-increasing spiral as technology advances.

In some way that the U.S. public cannot articulate, these machines represent the promise of physical salvation that it requires from its healthcare system to manage its own mortal terror. Certainly, this promise is sometimes fulfilled, and machines along with their operators are successful in many cases as Zimmerman et al (2013) reported. ICU nurses' stress comes from pride in their operational expertise, combined with horror at their own and the machines' ruthlessness required to achieve the goal. What they may not realize is that they are also carrying the existential burden that society has pushed onto their shoulders because the reality of its own finitude is so unwelcome. ICU nurses ride the sharp edge of the knife, where the denial of death meets its foil: inexorable reality. It is hard to get comfortable. The outside world shields itself from deep knowledge of such a place.

Distress in the Difficult Position

While most may be unaware and therefore blissfully unconcerned about the plight of ICU clinicians, nursing and critical care research is replete with perplexity about it. The problem goes by many names: compassion fatigue, caregiver strain, survivor's guilt, burnout, moral injury, moral suffering, and post-traumatic stress, to name a few, along with moral distress. Each of them implies lowered "work engagement" (Mason et al., 2014). It is beyond the scope of this chapter to delve into this literature with the rigor it deserves. But the size of the discourse is impressive: more than 40,000 new listed in Google Scholar each year from 2018 to 2023, with the exception of the pandemic year of 2021, when the total was 35,000, regarding moral distress alone.

ICU nurses themselves have pointed to prolonged dying, inappropriateness of care, suffering, and undignified deaths as causes of distress (Wiegand & Funk, 2012). Other areas of pain are conflicts over palliative care (Curtis & Puntillo, 2007), communication failures (Moss et al., 2016), lack of involvement in decision-making (Azoulay et al., 2009; MacMillen, 2008), and concern over errors (Kaur et al., 2019). Covid-19 has added fear of contagion, bullying, stress, and anxiety (Falatah, 2021).

Regardless of the cause, the consequences are dire. If nurses retreat into themselves using protective tactics such as alienation and depersonalization, they and their patients suffer (Moss et al., 2016). Leaving becomes an attractive option (Lo et al., 2018). Beyond forsaking the ICU environment (Whittaker et al., 2018), they often relinquish the nursing profession altogether (22%, per Moss et al., 2016, p. 109), sometimes before the very research investigating their distress is complete (Ricou et al., 2018). If they stay, they may experience depression, anxiety, and physical stress responses at higher levels than the general population (Alderson et al., 2015; Davidson et al., 2019). Meanwhile, baby boomers—nurses and others—are aging into retirement. As they do, the supply of nurses declines just as the demand for them rises (American Association of Colleges of Nursing, 2019b).

Summarizing the Situation

Technological rescue from death is over-imagined in the public's mind as the expected remedy for chronic and acute conditions, manifesting itself in complex technologies that ICU nurses manage and that the general public has little hope of understanding. In many cases, nurses must dismantle them when they cannot make up for "the necessary fallibility of our knowledge of particulars" (Gorovitz & MacIntyre, 1975, p. 18); that is, the unfillable gaps in our understanding and ability to correct individual patient circumstances. As resilience disintegrates in dying, so the nurse removes its props. At the same time, the rescue project is overdetermined in the U.S. healthcare system due to reimbursement patterns focused on piecework (Chapple, 2010). The investment in ICU care represents a disproportionate share of the U.S. GDP (Gooch & Kahn, 2014). The result of this cultural approach to terror management is that death often comes as a terrible surprise. Managing its impact falls too heavily on the ICU nurse. Available sources of support for that nurse, including broad professional guidance, are inadequate and misleading. The major professional organization for ICU nurses encourages them to reinvest in their hard science expertise, a form of cultural re-immersion that Solomon and colleagues (2015) would deem inadequate for managing the reality of death. Further, this approach assists the technological imperative as much or more than it supports the nurses themselves, a yet unexamined ethical concern. Realistic tools for grappling with ICU nurses' difficult existential position are muted at the annual NTI gathering.

What can be done? Turning back the tide of healthcare technology is not a feasible or desired option. When it succeeds in stabilizing the patient and improving her chances for recovery, managing the complexities of patient care under its purview is a major source of satisfaction for nurses. Further, mortality in the ICU has decreased (Zimmerman et al., 2013). But when doubts about its benefits mount for individual patients, ICU nurses envision yet another bad outcome. They endure existential ordeals at the bedside that go almost entirely unnoticed and too often unrelieved.

If reliable support for the ICU nurses' position does not yet exist in the nurse's workplace, in its major professional association, or in society, then the role of the nurse needs to be reimagined as something more than the expert manager of the machines that define ICU territory. We know that empowerment and evidence of confidence in the nurse are factors that can decrease burnout and planned departure (Hauck et al., 2011). How can these remedies be implemented at the scale they are needed?

Support, Empowerment, and Ethical Tensions

Unfortunately, the crushing power dynamics in the ICU do not work in favor of creativity. The machines exert their inexorable energy, compelling routine deployment (Almerud et al., 2008). Unlike the situation in the interview, ethical norms usually grant hegemony to patient autonomy and by extension to surrogates such as family members over those of clinicians, even when those preferences may compromise prevailing standards of care (Wolpe, 1998). Workplace norms confer jurisdiction over the care plan to physicians and providers, as the case interview illustrated. Neither of these norms provides a routine opening for the nurse's view, nor seeks it as a matter of course. Shifting power to fully incorporate the nurse's perspective will require structural changes, uncomfortable but necessary. Failing to do so means that the system will not be able to make full use of the nurse's critical value as an expert and a stakeholder, not just in operating technology, but in the skills they develop in navigating the tension between life extension and death. The stakes for implementing a corrected vision of the ICU nurse are very high, both for nurses and for anyone who expects ICU care to be readily available now and in the future (Moss et al., 2016). How can appreciation and recognition for the crucial work these nurses do on behalf of society be turned into something that truly feeds them, repairs their tattered souls, and enables them to stay in their jobs?

Two domains require intervention. For the ICU nurse, support and empowerment may be more transformative than skill enhancement. At the same time, society must prepare itself to see the end of life not as aberrant and exceptional, but as a challenge to be met by the group as a whole. The responsibility for avoiding bad dying belongs to all of us, not just the ICU nurse, or even the hospice nurse. Rather than being a "private trouble," it is a civic responsibility (Jennings, 2014). We discuss these approaches separately, beginning with the ICU nurse.

Re-envisioning ICU Nursing Through Support and Empowerment

Garnering support for ICU nurses does not mean that their perspectives are always accurate or reliably predictive (Gwilliam et al., 2012). The crescendo effect (Epstein & Hamric, 2009) can darken their perception. Yet they almost always know important truths about the patient that no one else would know, such as how the patient reacts to stressors like turning and which family members visit most often. Their reflections regarding these truths and their own experiences deserve solicitation (Ben Moshe, 2019). As they work to humanize the technology we crave and to ease the transitions toward the finitude we abhor, they need support that is specific, clear, unquestioned, and unrelenting. Hospitals eager to undergird ICU clinicians can deploy interventions such as the following:

1. Ethics and palliative care consultation that is easily and routinely accessible 24/7;
2. Interventions aimed at defusing distress in the moment, such as "the art of pause" (Rushton, 2009); debriefing with chaplains and/or ethics consultants (Agency for Healthcare Research and Quality, 2019), or through Schwartz rounds (Goncalves, 2019); and mindfulness training (Said & Kheng, 2018; White, 2014);
3. Regular visits to ICU units by specialized staff such as moral distress consultation rounds (Hamric & Epstein, 2017) and bioethics rounds (Schmitz et al., 2018);

4. Hospital policies that limit overtime, provide safe staffing, and encourage self-care;

5. Non-high-tech professional development opportunities such as the End-of-Life Nursing Education Consortium (ELNEC) (American Association of Colleges of Nursing, 2019a), and Palliative Care in the ICU (IPAL ICU) (Nelson et al., 2010), funded and encouraged by the hospital.

Besides definitive supportive measures, nurses require specific arenas of empowerment (Traudt et al., 2016). Leadership in patient care planning is flawed without ICU nursing input. But communication is a fraught endeavor. Not only is it a well-known source of stress for nurses and other clinicians, but its failures also threaten patient safety (Maxfield et al., 2005). A commitment to solving these problems must be system-wide, from top management to the bedside. Nurses can benefit from accelerated training in communication skills that enable them to start from a non-defensive posture (Maxfield et al., 2005). Further, unspoken power differentials in meetings often silence less powerful colleagues. When those in charge rigorously solicit contributions from those of lesser rank, a more fruitful discussion is possible (Nembhard & Edmondson, 2006). Nursing eloquence directly contributes to patient safety, but it also indirectly enables the well-being of the nurses themselves (TeamSTEPPS) (Agency for Healthcare Research and Quality, 2014). Communication is listed first among six attributes of healthy work environments (American Association of Critical-Care Nurses, 2005, p. 189). With appropriate adjustments to staffing, the bedside ICU nurse can routinely lead daily rounds for the care team. The unit can similarly accommodate nurse-called and nurse-led family meetings. The nurse's experience and understanding of any tensions inherent in the patient's context are invaluable in care planning. Deliberately acknowledging and elevating the ICU nurse's role at the bedside enacts critical change in the institution's perspective on the practice of end-of-life care in the ICU and elsewhere. Covid-19 forced hospitals radically to reconfigure ICU leadership teams, proving that reimagining traditional roles is possible (Perlstein et al., 2021).

Cautions are needed here. As nurses become more empowered, an increase in ethical tensions can follow (Chambliss, 1996). Challenges to expanded roles can be expected. At the bedside, the nurse routinely reacts to shifts in the patient's clinical journey. How much influence should nurses have in shaping that journey? Resistance to such changes must be anticipated and countered. For example, it is a given that any clinician distress pales in comparison to the vital perspectives of the patient and the family. Yet nurses witness and inflict suffering on the patient—it seems necessary to define some moral standing for them that can coexist alongside the patient and the family. When the nurse seems overly pessimistic about the outcome for the patient, the team and/or the family may not endorse the nurses' perspective. But a nursing focus on big picture offers a necessary corrective to medicine's enmeshment in tweaking clinical details. In advocating for non-maleficence toward the patient, is it ethically appropriate for the nurse to elicit from the family a rationale for continuing aggressive rescue efforts? Nurses often want to give families an opportunity to prepare for a death that they see as inevitable. If families are not open to such an outcome, whether or not physicians have addressed it, what are the nurses' obligations in regard to laying such groundwork? How should the nurse or the team respond when families reject any suggestion of stepping back because they suspect that the team simply wants the bed for a more viable patient?

How Can Society Join With ICU Nurses and Share Their Struggle?

If the momentum of the rescue project sweeps dying aside, its aleatory prickliness remains. Supporting and empowering nurses, even on a societal level, is only one portion of the equation. A cultural shift is needed. We must sharpen our gaze about the realistic roles that technology can play when death is on the horizon, especially for patients with chronic illness. At the same time, society needs to take up a greater awareness of the position of those who, by default, must negotiate such liminal passages. Bruce Jennings (2014) calls for a population-based approach to palliative care, pointing out that "inadequate end-of-life care is neither a personal trouble nor a family failing primarily; it is a function of a failing civic system of health care and communal provision" (p. 273). Dying is appropriately a public health concern, one that calls for a multilayered demonstration of solidarity from the not yet dying (Chapple, 2018; Jennings, 2014). What roles might public health take up? Rao, Anderson, and Smith (2002) suggest surveying those with end-of-life experience to understand their needs; exploring cultural attitudes about death and dying as a frame for encouraging conversation; and partnering with healthcare facilities to extend discharge planning forward to advance care planning in the setting of chronic illness. Palliative care itself is moving quickly out of hospitals and into the community with a view toward seamless delivery across settings (Kamal et al., 2013). Ongoing efforts at healthcare reform can help incorporate palliative care into the healthcare system (Stjernsward et al., 2007).

Conclusion

Intensive care's complexity continues to expand with medical advances. Its opaque nature adds to its impressiveness, dazzle, and drama. Its nurses enact the social contract between society and its most seriously ill members, as they operate its technology to glean whatever physical survival might be available for each patient. Yet they recognize that meaning exists apart from the machines, even as the machines erase the personhood of their subjects. It is heavy work. Nurses need concentrated support and empowerment to alleviate the soul-stealing features of facing death through continuous and ever-expanding rescue. A vision of civic palliative care and interaction between hospitals and public health around end-of-life issues may chip away at the public's reliance on avoidance as its major terror-management strategy.

Solomon et al. (2015) encourage individuals to shift their customary habits (clinging to culture, personal contributions, and distraction) in managing their fears of death. They suggest adopting a more conscious approach that balances assurance with openness to ambivalence. Uncertainty about the future is the price we pay for being human—we feel it every day we draw breath. How can we get comfortable in that uncertain space? ICU nurses struggle mightily with uncertain futures—their own and their patients'. They are intimates with skepticism and doubt. How exactly can what ICU nurses live within transform them and us? How could a more supported, reflective, and mindful ICU practice (White, 2014) crystallize their understanding of the suffering, loss, and alienation that is part of a routine shift? Could they then convey their knife-edge wisdom to the rest of society? Perhaps they could help us transcend our fear of demonstrating solidarity with those drawing close to the veil.

Our love of the technology beast (Callahan, 2009) seems unquenchable. We need ICU nurses to continue in their crucial work of recognizing the advent of mortality and negotiating the patient's transition from belonging among the cohort of the living to that of the Other, that is, Dying. If nurses are sacrificed on the altar of technology because they can no longer both cater to the cyborg and restore humanity to the patient at the end of life, where does that leave us?

References

Agency for Healthcare Research and Quality. (2014). *Pocket guide: TeamSTEPPS*. Retrieved from https://www.ahrq.gov/teamstepps/instructor/essentials/pocketguide.html#cus.

Agency for Healthcare Research and Quality. (2019, September). *Debriefing for clinical learning*. Retrieved from https://psnet.ahrq.gov/primer/debriefing-clinical-learning.

Alderson, M., Parent-Rocheleau, X., & Mishara, B. (2015). Critical review on suicide among nurses: What about work related factors? *Crisis, 36*(2), 91–101.

Almerud, S., Alapack, R. J., Fridlund, B., & Ekebergh, M. (2008). Beleaguered by technology: Care in technologically intense environments. *Nursing Philosophy, 9*, 55–61.

American Association of Colleges of Nursing. (2019a). *ELNEC fact sheet* (p. 4). American Association of Colleges of Nursing. Retrieved from https://www.aacnnursing.org/ELNEC/About.

American Association of Colleges of Nursing. (2019b). *Fact sheet: Nursing shortage* (pp. 1–6). American Association of Colleges of Nursing. Retrieved from https://www.aacnnursing. org/Portals/42/News/Factsheets/Nursing-Shortage-Factsheet.pdf.

American Association of Critical-Care Nurses. (2005). AACN standards for establishing and sustaining healthy work environments: A journey to excellence. *American Journal of Critical Care, 14*(3), 187–197.

American Nurses Association. (2015). *Code of ethics for nurses with interpretive statements.* Nursebooks.org.

Azoulay, E., Timsit, J. F., Soares, M., & Conflicus Study Investigators. (2009). Prevalence and factors of intensive care unit conflicts: The Conflicus Study. *American Journal of Respiratory Critical Care Medicine, 180*(9), 853–860.

Ben Moshe, N. (2019). The truth behind conscientious objection in medicine. *Journal of Medical Ethics, 45*, 404–410.

Bishop, J. P. (2011). *The anticipatory corpse: Medicine, power, and the care of the dying.* University of Notre Dame Press.

Bishop, J. P. (2015). Finitude. In L. S. Dugdale (Ed.), *Dying in the 21st century: Towards a new ethical framework for the art of dying* (pp. 19–31). MIT Press.

Brenan, M., & Jones, J. M. (2024, January 22). Ethics Ratings of Nearly All Professions Down in U.S. Gallup. https://news.gallup.com/poll/608903/ethics-ratings-nearly-professions-down.aspx

Buresh, B., & Gordon, S. (2013). *From silence to voice: What nurses know and must communicate to the public* (3rd ed.). ILR Press.

Callahan, D. (2009). *Taming the beloved beast: How medical technology costs are destroying our health care system.* Princeton University Press.

Chambliss, D. F. (1996). *Beyond caring: Hospitals, nurses, and the social organization of ethics.* University of Chicago Press.

Chapple, H. S. (2010). *No place for dying: Hospitals and the ideology of rescue.* Left Coast Press.

Chapple, H. S. (2015). Rescue: Faith in the unlimited future. *Sociology, 52*, 424–429.

Chapple, H. S. (2018). The disappearance of dying and why it matters. In A. C. G. M. Robben (Ed.), *A companion to the anthropology of death* (pp. 429–443). John Wiley & Sons.

Curtis, J. R., & Puntillo, K. (2007). Is there an epidemic of burnout and post-traumatic stress in critical care clinicians? *American Journal of Respiratory and Critical Care Medicine, 75*, 634–636.

Davidson, J. E., Proudfoot, J., Lee, K., & Zisook, S. (2019). Nurse suicide in the United States: Analysis of the Center for Disease Control 2014 National Violent Death Reporting System dataset. *Archives of Psychiatric Nursing, 33*(2019), 16–21.

Dugdale, L. S. (2015). Conclusion: Toward a new ethical framework for the art of dying well. In L. S. Dugdale (Ed.), *Dying in the twenty-first century: Toward a new ethical framework for the art of dying well* (pp. 173–192). MIT Press.

Epstein, E. G., & Hamric, A. B. (2009). Moral distress, moral residue, and the crescendo effect. *Journal of Clinical Ethics, 20*(4), 330–342.

Falatah, R. (2021). The impact of the coronavirus disease (COVID-19) pandemic on nurses' turnover intention: An integrative review. *Nursing Reports, 11*, 787–810.

Garrett, J. R. (2015). Collectivizing rescue obligations in bioethics. *American Journal of Bioethics, 15*(2), 3–11.

Goncalves, S. A. (2019). *Schwartz rounds: Self-care at its finest.* Retrieved from https://www.americannursetoday.com/schwartz-rounds-self-care/.

Gooch, R. A., & Kahn, J. M. (2014). ICU bed supply, utilization, and health care spending: An example of demand elasticity. *JAMA, 311*(6), 567–568.

Gorovitz, S., & MacIntyre, A. (1975). Toward a theory of medical fallibility. *The Hastings Center Report, 5*(6), 13–23.

Gwilliam, B., Keeley, V., Todd, C., Roberts, C., Gittins, M., Kelly, L., Barcley, S., & Stone, P. (2012). Prognosticating in patients with advanced cancer: Observational study comparing the accuracy of clinicians' and patients' estimates of survival. *Annals of Oncology, 24*(2), 482–488.

Hamric, A. B., & Blackhall, L. J. (2007). Nurse-physician perspectives on the care of dying patients in intensive care units: Collaboration, moral distress, and ethical climate. *Critical Care Medicine, 35*(2), 422–429.

Hamric, A. B., & Epstein, E. G. (2017). A health system-wide moral distress consultation service: Development and evaluation. *Healthcare Ethics Committee Forum, 29*(2), 127–143.

Hauck, A., Quinn Griffin, M. T., & Fitzpatrick, J. J. (2011). Structural empowerment and anticipated turnover among critical care nurses. *Journal of Nursing Management, 19,* 269–276.

Jennings, B. (2014). Solidarity, mortality: The tolling bell of civic palliative care. In C. Staudt & J. H. Ellens (Eds.), *Our changing journey to the end*, Vol. 2: *Reshaping death, dying and grief in America* (pp. 271–288). Praeger.

Kamal, A. H., Currow, D. C., Ritchie, C. S., Bull, J. T., & Abernethy, A. P. (2013). Community-based palliative care: The natural evolution for palliative care. *Journal of Pain and Symptom Management, 46*(2), 254–264.

Kaufman, S. (2005). *And a time to die: How American hospitals shape the end of life.* Simon and Schuster.

Kaur, A. P., Levinson, A. T., Monteiro, J. F. G., & Carino, G. P. (2019). The impact of errors on healthcare professionals in the critical care setting. *Journal of Critical Care, 52*(2019), 16–21.

Koenig, B. (1988). The technological imperative in medical practice: The social creation of a "routine" treatment. In M. Lock & D. Gordon (Eds.), *Biomedicine examined* (pp. 465–495). Kluwer Academic Press.

Lo, W. Y., Chien, L. Y., Hwang, F. M., Huang, N., & Chiou, S. T. (2018). From job stress to intention to leave among hospital nurses: A structural equation modelling approach. *Journal of Advanced Nursing, 74,* 677–688.

MacMillen, R. E. (2008). End of life decisions: Nurses' perceptions, feelings and experiences. *Intensive and Critical Care Nursing, 24*(4), 251–259.

Mason, V. M., Leslie, G., Clark, K., Lyons, P., Walke, E., Butler, C., & Griffin, M. (2014). Compassion fatigue, moral distress, and work engagement in surgical intensive care unit trauma nurses: A pilot study. *Dimensions of Critical Care Nursing, 33*(4), 215–225.

Mauno, S., Ruokolainen, M., Kinnunen, U., & De Bloom, J. (2016). Emotional labor and work engagement among nurses: Examining perceived compassion, leadership, and work ethic as stress buffers. *Journal of Advanced Nursing, 72*(5), 1169–1181. Retrieved from https://onlinelibrary.wiley.com/doi/pdf/10.1111/jan.12906.

Maxfield, D., Grenny, J., McMillan, R., Patterson, K., & Switzler, A. (2005). Silence kills: The seven crucial conversations for healthcare (pp. 1–18). AACN. Retrieved from https://www.aacn.org/nursing-excellence/healthy-work-environments/~/media/aacn-website/nursing-excellence/healthy-work-environment/silencekills.pdf?la=en

McElligott, D., Siemers, S., Thomas, L., & Kohn, N. (2009). Health promotion in nurses: Is there a healthy nurse in the house? *Applied Nursing Research, 22*(2009), 211–215.

McQuellon, R. P., & Cowan, M. A. (2010). *The art of conversation through serious illness.* Oxford University Press.

Moss, M., Good, V. S., Gozal, D., Kleinpell, R., & Sessler, C. N. (2016). A critical care societies collaborative statement: Burnout syndrome in critical care health-care professionals. *American Journal of Respiratory and Critical Care Medicine, 194*(1), 106–113.

Nelson, J. E., Bassett, R., Boss, R. D., Brasel, K. J., Campbell, M. L., Cortez, T. B., Curtis, J. R., Lustbader, D. R., Mulkerin, C., Puntillo, K. A., Ray, D. E., & Weissman, D. E. (2010). Models for structuring a clinical initiative to enhance palliative care in the intensive care unit: A report from the IPAL-ICU Project (Improving Palliative Care in the ICU). *Society of Critical Care Medicine, 38*(9), 1765–1772.

Nembhard, I. M., & Edmondson, A. C. (2006). Making it safe: The effects of leader inclusiveness on psychological safety and improvement efforts in healthcare teams. *Journal of Organizational Behavior, 27*(7), 941–966.

Perlstein, L., Denison, K., Kleinschmidt, C., Swift, L., & Su, G. (2021). Implementation of a dynamic nursing care model during a global pandemic. *Nursing Management,* 51–54. https://doi.org/10.1097/01.NUMA.0000731964.86644.05

Rao, J. K., Anderson, L. A., & Smith, S. M. (2002). End of life is a public health issue. *American Journal of Preventive Medicine, 23*(3), 215–220.

Ricou, B., Gigon, F., Durand-Steiner, E., Liesenberg, M., Chemin-Renais, C., Merlani, P., & Delaloya, S. (2018). Initiative for burnout of ICU caregivers: Feasibility and preliminary results of a psychological support. *Journal of Intensive Care Medicine, 35*(6), 562–569.

Rushton, C. H. (2009). Ethical discernment and action: The art of pause. *AACN Advanced Critical Care, 20*(1), 108–111.

Said, Z., & Kheng, G. L. (2018). A review of mindfulness and nursing stress among nurses. *International Journal of Counseling and Education, 3*(1), 1–18.

Savran, Y., Aydin, K., Gencpinar, T., & Eroz, E. (2016). Concurrent extracorporeal membrane oxygenation, plasmapheresis and continuous renal replacement therapy in a case of Wegener's granulomatosis. ResearchGate. Retrieved from https://www.researchgate.net/publication/306914884_Concurrent_Extracorporeal_Membrane_Oxygenation_Plasmapheresis_and_Continuous_Renal_Replacement_Therapy_in_a_Case_of_Wegener%27s_Granulomatosis.

Schenck, D., & Neely, S. (2023). *Into the field of suffering: Finding the other side of burnout.* Oxford University Press.

Schmitz, D., Gross, D., Frierson, C., Schubert, G. A., Schulze-Steinen, H., & Kersten, A. (2018). Ethics rounds: Affecting ethics quality at all organizational levels. *Journal of Medical Ethics, 44*(12), 805–809.

Shapiro, S. P. (2019). *Speaking for the dying: Life-and-death decisions in intensive care.* University of Chicago Press.

Society of Critical Care Medicine. (2016). *SCCM critical care statistics.* Retrieved from https://www.sccm.org/Communications/Critical-Care-Statistics.

Solomon, S., Greenberg, J., & Pyszczynski, T. (2015). *The worm at the core: On the role of death in life.* Random House.

Stjernsward, J., Foley, K. M., & Ferris, F. D. (2007). The public health strategy for palliative care. *Journal of Pain and Symptom Management, 33*(5), 486–493.

Traudt, T., Liaschenko, J., & Peden-McAlpine, C. (2016). Moral agency, moral imagination, and moral community: Antidotes to moral distress. *Journal of Clinical Ethics, 27*(3), 201–213.

Vilelas, J. M. da S., & Diogo, P. M. J. (2014). Emotional labor in nursing praxis. *Revista Gaucha de Enfermagem, 35*(3), 145–149.

Wallace, D. J., Seymour, C. W., & Kahn, J. M. (2017). Hospital-level changes in adult bed supply changes in the United States. *Critical Care Medicine, 45*(1), e67–e76.

White, L. (2014). Mindfulness in nursing: An evolutionary concept analysis. *Journal of Advanced Nursing, 70*(2), 282–294.

Whittaker, B. A., Gillum, D. R., & Kelly, J. M. (2018). Burnout, moral distress, and job turnover in critical care nurses. *International Journal of Studies in Nursing, 3*(3), 108–121.

Wiegand, D. L., & Funk, M. (2012). Consequences of clinical situations that cause critical care nurses to experience moral distress. *Nursing Ethics, 19*(4), 479–487.

Wolpe, P. R. (1998). The triumph of autonomy in American bioethics: A sociological view. In R. DeVries & J. Subedi (Eds.), *Bioethics and society: Constructing the ethical enterprise* (pp. 38–59). Prentice Hall.

Zimmerman, J. E., Kramer, A. A., & Knaus, W. A. (2013). Changes in hospital mortality for United States intensive care unit admissions from 1988 to 2012. *Critical Care, 17*(R81), 1–9. Retrieved from https://ccforum.biomedcentral.com/track/pdf/10.1186/cc12695.

19

Teaching With Pictures

Respect for the Vulnerable

Daniel A. Wilkenfeld and Christa M. Johnson

Introduction

Nursing ethics educators (and educators more generally) frequently find value in presenting and discussing with students tragic historical events in clinical practice or medical research. For example, discussing medical experiments conducted by the physicians working for the Nazi Party can yield important insight into the subsequent Nuremberg Code (as discussed in Shuster, 1997) and the ethical importance of informed consent. It is sometimes common practice to use photographs of victims in these presentations or even—in the case of more recent events—videos depicting these events. Such images evince deep emotions and can be powerful educational tools, inspiring students to be vigilant against ethical malfeasance in care and research. Nevertheless, we will argue that the use of images of the victims in these cases is ethically problematic. Specifically, we argue that it is not acceptable in a classroom setting to use identifiable photographs of people in a heightened vulnerable state without at least their implied consent, even for otherwise laudable goals. We will focus our argument on photographs, but our conclusions will apply, *a fortiori*, to videos as well. We do not look at unidentifiable narratives, as the fact that they could in principle be fictional places them in a somewhat different category. We think many of our considerations will apply to dignitary harms done even with de-identified pictures, but for the sake of starting the conversation, for the moment we restrict our thesis to identifiable images(/videos). As will be discussed in final section of the chapter, we do not mean to argue that *any* use of an image of someone in a state of heightened vulnerability is problematic, but only that the use of such an image for the purpose of classroom education without at least implicit consent[1] is problematic.

---

[1] If people explicitly agree to have their images used, it is more likely (though not certain) that ethical concerns are minimal. It is also commonplace in healthcare ethics that people can implicitly consent to what might otherwise be a rights violation by taking an action that indicates their acceptance (e.g., reaching their arm out to receive a shot).

In the next section we give some classic examples of the sorts of photos of people with heightened vulnerability that students are likely to use during their nursing education. In the subsequent section we give our positive argument that there are serious ethical concerns with using photographs of individuals in vulnerable situations without at least their implied consent. We argue from a variety of interrelated positions, including Kantian grounds, respect for persons, contractualist and contractarian grounds, as well as an argument modified from Thomas Nagel (1970, 1987) that relies on intuitions about what we might want for ourselves in such circumstances. In the fourth section we respond to the most frequent objections to this position, including various consequentialist arguments in favor of using photographs, the argument from an "obligation to bear witness," and an argument from the need to achieve justice. The third and fourth sections jointly present the core argument of the chapter—there are a variety of reasons against using such photographs for pedagogical purposes and the contrary arguments cannot stand against them; thus, the weight of ethical reasons favors not doing so. We will then discuss in the final section to what extent our argument regarding classroom use generalizes to other uses, including museums, historical texts, and (especially) news footage.

One crucial assumption of this chapter is that, in general, ends do not justify means, and that infringing on rights for the sake of a more diffuse greater good is at minimum *prima facie* ethically impermissible—that is, infringing rights in such cases always stands in need of further—and compelling—justification. We will motivate this point a bit in the section "Arguments for Using Images," but for now we will note that aside from the obvious deontological validity assuming that the ends do not automatically justify the means, one gets the same results on most ethical systems other than act-consequentialism. Here are a few examples. First, it would likely be endorsed by most varieties of rule-consequentialism (e.g., Hooker, 1990). Second, while it is notoriously difficult to make general claims about virtue ethics, it strikes us as at least *prima facie* plausible that the virtuous person does not exploit the vulnerability of one person for the benefit of others. We grant that not all cases of an end justifying a mean will take this exploitative form. However, the case at issue in this chapter *does* take such a form, and so the point is instructive for our purposes. Third—and just as importantly in the context of nursing education—using the vulnerable for the sake of a greater good is at the very least in strong tension with having a caring relationship. (We do not yet claim to have established that this is what is happening in the present case, though that is what we intend to do.)

Classic Examples: Willowbrook State School and Nazi Party Experiments

It is common practice in courses on applied ethics generally—and nursing ethics in particular—to illustrate the importance of ethical principles by examination of cases where they are violated. This can be done by way of either faculty presentation or an assignment for students to find and present on cases. When these cases are from the last hundred or so years, there are frequently photographs available of the victims of experiments or failed interventions. Students are then frequently asked to explain precisely where the ethical breakdown takes place, and how adherence to edicts of nursing ethics would have headed off tragic results.

One common example is the unethical treatment of children at the Willowbrook State School. This treatment included a notorious experiment wherein children were intentionally infected with hepatitis as part of a process to develop a vaccine (e.g., Robinson & Doody, pp. 150–151), but even aside from that, the children lived in such desperate conditions that Robert Kennedy famously referred to the facility as a "snake pit."[2] Students are led to explore whether adequate disclosure was given to the parents before experiments were run and to what extent the limited options available to parents of mentally disabled children eroded the validity of their consent.

This case exemplifies many of the features that we will argue are most problematic about using images for educational purposes. First, images from Willowbrook are widely available, including from (at least otherwise) respectable news outlets. (For reasons that will become obvious, we do not include any here.) Second, the images display children at their most vulnerable—indeed, it is for that very reason that these images are often employed in ethics classes. Third, not only are many of the victims still alive, but many of them are still suffering from abuse that might possibly be traced back in part to their mistreatment as children (Weiser, 2020).[3]

Perhaps the most interesting aspect of this case, though, is how often it is used to demonstrate and discuss questions surrounding informed consent and autonomy. While workers at the school clearly also violated the principle of nonmaleficence (doing no harm), the more interesting discussions generally arise regarding whether the parents (as surrogates for the patients) had full autonomy or gave valid consent for their children's treatment. We will argue that these very

---

[2] https://mn.gov/mnddc/parallels/five/5b/bobby-kennedy-snakepits.html.
[3] As a word of warning, the linked article contains images; the citation was needed to establish the continuing harm to the victims in question.

same considerations should also motivate educators to avoid the use of such images by either themselves or their students in ethics classes.

Another example invariably brought up in classrooms is the use of prisoners by the physicians working for the Nazi Party to conduct radically inhumane experiments (e.g., Robinson & Doody, pp. 151–152). On one hand, one might find the arguments against using images of these experiments to be less compelling than the case for Willowbrook, since some (though not all) of the victims will have already (as of this writing) passed away. Nevertheless, there are several aspects of the case that bring into relief the points we are making. First, ethical condemnation of those experiments is fairly universal. Second, it was precisely the respect for those individual victims that motivated the development of the Nuremburg Code and subsequent Belmont Report (National Commission for the Protection of Human Subjects of Biomedical & Behavioral Research, 1978) as the bases for responsible research (for a clear history of the development of such codes, see Karigan, 2001). Thus, the very same people who inspired the development of ethical codes for research, we will argue, are harmed by efforts to exhibit the importance of those codes through the display and pedagogical use of images depicting them.

Arguments Against Using Photographs of Vulnerable People in Classroom Settings

In this section we provide as many as five (depending on how one individuates) arguments against using photographs of people in vulnerable situations in classroom settings without at least their implied consent. For much of the remainder of the chapter we leave the "without their implied consent" implicit—if people want you to use their images, there is significantly less ethical reason against doing so. While these arguments are all thematically related by respecting individuals, they all rely on slightly different justifications and so can in principle be accepted or rejected independently. The critical point is that each of them provides a strong deontological constraint against using people's images, which we will go on to argue is sufficient to swamp any countervailing reasons. If one accepts the full battery of arguments, then the conclusion becomes simply that much stronger.

Kantian Considerations

Considered one of the predominant voices in deontological ethics, Immanuel Kant argued that (one version of) the fundamental rule of morality is that we should never treat other people as mere means to accomplish an end. (Alexander & Moore, 2021). At its most basic level, this is our main objection to using photographs of people in vulnerable situations for educational ends. The goal in using the images is clearly not to help the depicted individuals—the harm to them has already been done. (For objections to this claim pertaining to, e.g., the need for justice, see the section "Arguments in Favor of Using Images" below.) Showing the victims of experiments done by the Nazi Party or those at the Willowbrook School in a classroom setting certainly does nothing to benefit *them*—if anyone is in a position to help them, they are unlikely to be in a classroom full of students.

Of course, showing such images does have the potential to do good for other people. It can teach students to be morally vigilant, or even to shut down specific programs in the future. But that is precisely the sort of action that Kant says is what we should not do—using person A as a mere means for the benefit of person B.

It could be objected that we are not actually using the person, but rather something else. There are two versions of this objection—on the first, the key is that while one's image is something one has, it is not oneself, and therefore we can use it. The second is that we are not even using the subject or their image at all, but rather the scene in which they happen to be a part. However, both variants would make it too easy to get around Kantian concerns by merely tweaking the direct target of one's actions. Regarding the fact that it is just an image one possesses, it is generally recognized that one's image is vital to one's identity—anyone who has dealt with an Internal Review Board knows the emphasis placed on respecting people's images (albeit with a bit of nuance regarding precisely how the images could be identified). More importantly, by this logic we are not treating a person as a mere means when we simply steal all of their belongings—after all, what we are using are the belongings, not the person. A Kantian prohibition on theft would not be so easily circumvented. Of course, one might simply say, so much the worse for Kant's prohibition on theft. Yet, we take Kant's idea to be that to steal someone's belongings is to treat the person as a free goods dispenser whose own interests and values need not be taken into account—not as a person with their own ends associated with those goods. Similarly, to use someone's image is to treat the person as an open-source image hub, not as a person with their own ends and interests associated with their own image. Regarding the fact that it is not the person but the scene in which the person appears, the fact remains that the vulnerable person is in the scene. Importantly, the individual is not merely an incidental or replaceable part of the scene, but what makes the scene so allegedly instructive and moving. If the vulnerable person ceased to be in the image, then the image could not play the intended role. Thus, even if one wants to argue that it is "the scene" being used, insofar as the vulnerable individual is a necessary part of what makes the scene worth showing, one cannot get around considerations of harm to the individual. Of course, one could object that the individual is not a part of the scene—but rather only their image is—but then this second variant of the objection collapses into the first.

This is really the central line of this chapter—by using these images, we are *de facto* using some people for the benefit of others without benefit to themselves or respect for their own ends, which is the epitome of a Kantian moral transgression.

Respect for Persons/Autonomy

Perhaps the most basic reason not to use people's images is that it violates the ethical principle of respect for persons. This principle can derive from a variety of places. It is central to the Nuremberg Code in the form of "voluntary consent" (Moreno et al., 2017) and the Belmont Report in the form of "respect for persons" (Sims, 2010), which is (as noted above) somewhat ironic given how many of these images are used in the context of illustrating dangers of violating ethical prohibitions such as the very same Nuremberg Code and Belmont Report. They have also been incorporated into more recent professional ethics, very typically under the heading of a respect for "autonomy." While there is no univocal understanding of what autonomy amounts to (for a review, see Buss & Westlund, 2013), it presumably has something to do with the ability to decide what's important for oneself with respect to matters that are central to one's life or values.

The critical fact for present purposes is that—more or less by definition—the images of people in vulnerable situations are taken when they are vulnerable. Vulnerability is frequently something people might not want to project or advertise. If the pictures are identifiable, there is a potential real harm in others knowing about vulnerable past situations in which individuals have been. (Even if the pictures are not identifiable, there is a potential dignitary harm in being exposed in one's vulnerable moments, though for present purposes we mainly put those considerations aside.)

Note that while these harms might be lessened after the subject's death, it is not at all clear that they are eliminated. First, there is a very real possibility that the subjects have loved ones and/or descendants who are alive and who might not want the dignity of their loved one impeached. (Granted, if the descendants actively did want the images used, then it should be possible to obtain a form of consent by proxy.) Second, there is a strong presumption in human societies the world over that it is wrong to do something that would harm even a person who has died, as evidenced by the near universal condemnation of grave desecration (e.g., Staff & agencies, 2003).[4]

The Golden Rule and the Platinum Rule

A different approach to showing why it is wrong to use images of people in vulnerable situations without at least their implicit consent is simply that we would not want anyone to do so to us. If we were in a vulnerable situation, we can imagine scenarios where we would want the image presented in a classroom, but very few where we would be thrilled to discover this happening without our consent. This is potentially even more true in the case of the photo of a loved one. We (the authors—see below for discussion of people with different preferences) would not be thrilled to find even non-vulnerable images used for the sake of furthering someone else's goals—*a fortiori*, while reactions to a picture in a state of vulnerability could conceivably be positive, they could also range from frustration to humiliation to outright fury. It is not the place of students or educators to decide what the reaction would be. If we would not want it done to us, we should not be doing it to other people. Even if we didn't mind it done to us, we should acknowledge the real possibilities of those with different views. Note that one might object to an image being used without consent even in the case where one would have consented had one been asked—there is a harm in not being asked even in cases where one would have agreed.

Doing unto others as one would want done unto oneself might be among the oldest ethical principles in the world, but if one wants a more modern source, we could consult Nagel's *The Possibility of Altruism*. A central tenet of this work is that there is nothing ethically special about oneself or one's position (Nagel, 1970). One corollary of this is that we can generally figure out what's ethical by figuring out what we would want for ourselves or our loved ones (see also Nagel, 1987). The authors at least would not want pictures of our children in vulnerable situations used to educate classrooms, and so we should not do so with pictures of other people's children. One advantage of this approach is that it lets one reach an ethical conclusion without even necessarily being able to cite a specific normative foundational principle for it—it suffices that we know that it would wrong us to be confident that it also wrongs other people. (See below for a discussion of people with different preferences.)

One concern someone might have to this approach is that the requirement to treat others as you want to be treated seems to only work if you want to be

---

[4] "The desecration of any body will be condemned by everyone, there is not a sane person who would not be offended by this" (Staff & agencies, 2003).

treated especially well. For our purposes, if *I* would not mind my picture or a picture of a loved one in a vulnerable situation being used in this way, there seems to be no reason that I should refrain from sharing the images of others after all. This has led some to turn from the Golden Rule to what has been dubbed the "Platinum Rule": one ought to treat others as *they* want to be treated (Alessandra & O'Connor, 1996). The problem with the Platinum Rule is that one might not always know how someone wants to be treated. Moreover, we might find that in some situations it may be best to treat someone *better* than they want to be treated, or else that we need not treat someone as well, if their standards are too high.

Not wanting to take on board the Golden or the Platinum Rule, we turn back to Nagel. Nagel, for his part, mostly focuses on the general idea that we indeed have reasons to concern ourselves with the interests of others. What he does not focus on is the exact content of those reasons. For example, if I think you have a reason not to steal my umbrella, then consistency dictates that I accept that I have that same reason not to steal your umbrella (Nagel, 1987). And, as noted above, if I believe you have a reason not to share my images, then I must accept that I have that same reason. In making this argument, Nagel does consider the possibility that someone, upon being asked "How would you like it?" simply responds that they would not mind at all if someone, for instance, stole their umbrella. Nagel's response is incomplete, but instructive. His first instinct, and ours, is to point out that there do not seem to be many people who would respond that way. Perhaps the objection is empty, insofar as no one *really* does not care if someone steals their umbrella (or shares their images). Here, though, Nagel does go a bit further than the specific examples because perhaps someone really does not care about an umbrella. He states, "I think most people . . . would think that their own interests or harms matter, not only to themselves, but in a way that gives other people a reason to care about them, too" (1987, p. 67). The important move for our purposes is the shift from the specific case of the umbrella to a more general statement of one's own interests or harms. Nagel's view is not grounded in the very specific details of each case and whether an individual would want it to happen to them. Rather, it is grounded in moving from thinking that other people have a reason to care about our interests to recognizing that we have a reason to care about the interests and harms of others. So, the response to the concern is twofold. First, we are comfortable making the assumption that most people would not want their own vulnerable images or the vulnerable images of their loved ones used as a mere teaching tool in the classroom. Second, if we are wrong about that for some individuals, it is enough to note that others do care about such matters, and that such sharing of vulnerable images may constitute a harm to someone, such that we have reason to refrain from so doing, at least without inquiring about whether they mind (i.e., without receiving consent).

Perhaps this just is a justification of the Platinum Rule in the end. Yet, we contend that Nagel adds a stronger justification of and motivation for the move.

Contractarian and Contractualist Approaches

One final approach, or perhaps set of approaches, to showing that we ought not use images of people in vulnerable position without consent moves from what we would want individually to what we would agree to in setting up a social contract. There are more or less two ways that people conceive of the social contract. We begin with a Rawlsian approach. In developing his social contract approach to a theory of justice, Rawls (1971) has us imagine that a group of individuals are creating a new society from scratch. From this "Original Position," the contractors are given the task of setting the rules for the new society, including provisions for the allocation of primary goods, which include for our purposes the allocation of rights. The catch is that the contractors are said to be behind a "Veil of Ignorance"; that is, they do not know any identifying information about themselves. Each contractor is unaware of their race, gender, economic status, and so on. The idea is that, insofar as they might turn out to have any combination of cultural, ethnic, national, religious, gender, or disability identities, among others, they will select principles of justice that fairly represent everyone. Our interest here is not in what lessons Rawls gleans from this setup, but to consider what lessons might be learned for our particular case.

One of the upshots of the Veil of Ignorance often pointed to is that in the Original Position, the contractors are likely to play it safe, ensuring that the worst off in a society are well protected. After all, one of the contractors may turn out to be one of the worst off. With that general idea in mind, turn to the individuals at issue in our case. The images we are discussing are of people in vulnerable moments, images of people worse off in society than those in the classroom they are meant to help (and likely than many of those who might eventually be helped indirectly). Intuitively, then, we argue that the contractors would want to protect the victims of these medical atrocities (in case they happen to be one). In our view, protecting these victims entails protecting their images, as well. Specifically, the best way to protect them is to prevent the use of these images/ videos without their consent (see also note 5).

Of course, one might always push back on the content of a particular position that comes out of the Rawlsian setup. Perhaps the contractors are not that risk-averse. Perhaps contractors would sacrifice the interests of the victims for the benefits of sharing the images (benefits to which we will consider shortly in our objections). To argue that any set of contractors would actively choose one position over another is inevitably contentious. As such, though we do think the contractors would go this way, we turn to a second approach to a contract basis of morality.

Scanlon's contractualism shares with Rawlsian contractarianism the idea of an agreement. However, instead of focusing on what contractors would actively choose, Scanlon (1998) focuses instead on the negative position of what might be reasonably rejected. The idea here is that we ought only follow principles which no person could reasonably reject. Running the test for using vulnerable images, we contend that one could reasonably reject the use of their image in a classroom setting. Indeed, the authors are two such people who would reject that use. For reasons already mentioned and further defended below, we believe such a rejection to indeed be reasonable.

Arguments in Favor of Using Images

In the previous section we provided what we take to be strong *pro tanto* (i.e., strong but defeasible) reasons for thinking that it is wrong to use images of vulnerable people in a classroom setting without at least their implicit consent. However, that is of course only half the battle—in this section we argue that it is wrong to do so all-things-considered. This requires consideration of the main arguments in favor of using these sorts of images. In general, these arguments fall into one of two camps. Either they are fundamentally consequentialist, in which case they are (outside of extreme circumstances) insufficient to justify doing a strict moral harm, or they are deontological, in which case we argue they are ultimately under-motivated.

Consequentialist Arguments

Perhaps the main argument for using images of people in vulnerable situations is that they are necessary for students' education. Students need to know these sorts of things happened in order to have a full and well-rounded education, as well as to be in a position to help prevent them in the future. Relatedly, propagation of such images could deter future wrongdoers from exploiting people in vulnerable situations.

The problem with both lines of reasoning is that they run afoul of our assumption from the first section against ends justifying means—granting in essence that there might be a wrong being done in using the photographs (independent of any possible other wrong having been done in taking them), but asserting that since it is for a good end it is ethically acceptable. This view has well-known problems in that it can justify virtually anything. To pick a common example (Thomson, 1985), one would be justified by this logic in murdering and harvesting someone's organs if those same organs can be used to save the lives of five patients suffering from failures of different organs. While perhaps some die-hard consequentialists would dispute the following claim, most everyone else would acknowledge that there must be some constraints on what is allowable behavior that go beyond merely saying that it is ultimately done to bring about some good result.

Is it possible that the weight of consequentialist reasons can ultimately override any moral prohibition? Perhaps to save 10,000 or 100,000 people, a murder would be permissible, or even what one *ought to do* in that situation (Brennan, 1995; Cook, 2018; Johnson, 2020). Still, there would continue to be an active burden on the part of the murderer to justify that the case in question is *so* extreme that a meaningful threshold has been met. Of course, different moral prohibitions may not require so much at stake. Perhaps, we can permissibly lie to simply spare someone added hurt when the lie has low stakes and the pain is great. The point stands, however, that there is a burden to show that some threshold has been met, and we see no evidence that such a burden has or even can be met in the case of using vulnerable images in the classroom.

It's also worth noting that this whole line of reasoning is premised on the claim that those viewing images of the vulnerable are doing so toward the ultimate goal of some societal good. There are, however, both conceptual (Grue, 2016; Nguyen & Williams, 2020; Sontag, 2003) and empirical (Shelton & Waddell, 2020; Vaish et al., 2008) concerns that some people simply enjoy seeing pictures of the vulnerable. Examples of this have been referred to as tragedy porn, poverty porn, inspiration porn, moral outrage porn, and disaster porn. On Nguyen and Williams's account, "a representation is used as generic porn when it is engaged with for the sake of a gratifying reaction, freed from the usual costs and consequences of engaging with the represented content" (2020, p. 148). There is nothing *inherently* psychologically perverse about people enjoying sad or scary movies, but the possibility that those viewing the images are not doing so for solely noble purposes does call into question whether the net good being done would be justified even on purely consequentialist grounds.

Deontological Arguments

Granting that it would be difficult for all but the most extreme consequentialist arguments to justify using images of the vulnerable in a classroom setting, are there deontological reasons why it might make sense to do so? We look at some plausible candidates and argue that they do not apply in the present circumstance.

One argument (e.g., Cornish, 2017) is that at least some are under an obliga-tion to "witness" others' suffering and not turn away. This seems plausible, but also only of passing relevance to the present case. We can witness suffering—and even discuss it—without actively utilizing images of it. People likely have a right to have their suffering noticed, but that does not translate into a requirement that their suffering be publicized. Note that in order to fall under the present argument it really would have to be a requirement—even if there were a right to have one's suffering publicized, in the absence of even implicit consent that does not generate a right for other people to do the publicizing. Perhaps one might worry that our arguments against the use of images overgeneralize and would make it impossible even to discuss the relevant kinds of wrongs. However, mere discussions/texts avoid several pitfalls of images. First, they are easier to make unidentifiable. Second—for purposes of presenting ethical dilemmas—their reality is not an essential component of their pedagogical value. Discussing a case to exhibit a principle could be done just as readily with a hypothetical case as a real one. Since discussion of events like the ones described would poten-tially work, we are not taking advantage of the fact that they actually happened to some individuals.

Another way to approach the issue is to say that perhaps having their suffering publicized in a classroom somehow directly benefits the people being pictured, in which case it would not run afoul of Kantian or other constraints. We find it hard to see how this argument would go in the case of vulnerable images—the harm has already been done, and teaching about it at all (much less using images of it) does nothing to undo it. One might be tempted to say that if their suffering is not used for positive change then it was in vain, but a corollary of that argu-ment would seem to be that if it is used for positive change then it was *not* in vain, which seems wrong. Those who suffered from Nazi experiments did so need-lessly, and nothing we can do now can retroactively change that fact. Arguably it does a disservice to their suffering to imply that it might have had a (retroac-tive) purpose, as that detracts from the needlessness of it in the first place. (It is beyond the scope of this chapter to discuss the question of what we do with any knowledge gained from this suffering.)

One final deontological justification for using images might be that it helps the victimized achieve justice. This might apply in some settings (see the following section), but it is unclear how it would justify the use of images in a classroom. The dissemination of the video of George Floyd[5] being murdered *arguably* did him good by helping bring his murderer to justice, but it is not clear how showing

---

[5] Using his name does not conflict with our thesis, as (a) we restricted our thesis to images/videos, and (b) it is fairly clear that his family approved of the use of the video and its resultant production of justice.

the video of his murder after a nontrivial time lapse would be likely to do so. While it is perhaps possible that something shown in a classroom could lead to action being taken against the perpetrators of those very actions, that possibility seems sufficiently rare and remote as not to justify the general practice. One could contend that it is not just the victims themselves who are entitled to justice, but rather potentially a whole class of which the victim is a part. Perhaps there is deontological justification to seek justice for all Jews in response to Nazi atrocities. While we accept that Jews generally might be entitled to justice, doing so at a cost to individual victims would still seem a variant of using individuals for some other individuals' ends (even if those other individuals form a group of which the victim is a part). In any event it still would not seem relevant to classroom settings, where people are unlikely to be in a position to hold Nazi war criminals responsible for their actions.

Other Uses of Images

Granting that images of the vulnerable should not be used in classrooms without at least their implicit consent,[6] for what may or should they be used? In general, this question will turn on whether the proposed medium does good for the victims themselves (perhaps via good for a class of which the victim is a part). The question is not really whether such records should be maintained (the mere existence of documents in a vacuum does not much affect anyone) but on an ethical analysis for any particular use. Archives might make sense, but open museums and textbooks would remain problematic. (See Sontag [2003] for a similar argument that perhaps use of photographs is permissible if something can be done, but the stakes differ for "horrors long past.")

News sources and (oddly) social media might function differently. As mentioned in the previous section, the victim (or class of victims—see above) might in some sense benefit from justice being done to the perpetrator, in which case publicizing an atrocity in real time might be to the benefit (in some sense) of the vulnerable. Note, however, that even here we have at best a deontological standoff—a duty to provide justice and a duty to respect autonomy are at odds with each other, so it is not clear what the right thing to do is. Perhaps in such a case, consequentialist considerations should bear weight (though someone strongly committed to deontology would likely continue to base their arguments on other grounds). Our argument above was that in the case of classroom use

---

[6] Note that our arguments (particularly the Rawlsian variant) relied on both the vulnerability of the subject and the lack of consent—the two are not separable harms. We don't really see this as an either/or situation—using pictures of those in heightened vulnerability is *pro tanto* bad, but can be made acceptable by express or implicit consent.

there is no countervailing deontological consideration, which might not apply in the case of real-time accounts.

Conclusion and Connection to Nursing

There are clear pedagogical advantages to using images in classroom presentations—they tap into emotional resources and learning modalities that might otherwise remain latent. However, the fact that there are advantages to doing something does not entail that it is all-things-considered the right thing to do. In this chapter we have argued that there are deontological constraints against using images of the vulnerable in a classroom setting without at least their implicit consent. We could also not locate any countervailing deontological reason for doing so that withstood scrutiny. Assuming that we should not violate moral rules even for the sake of positive ends (which assumption we have hopefully at least rendered plausible), that speaks against using such images in classrooms. This has profound implications for how many of us go about running our classes, and so we encourage people to consider carefully just what they are doing in their daily education. At a minimum, we argue that those who disagree with our conclusions owe it to the victims of unethical behavior to invite their students to reflect on the potential costs of using their images. Even if the images are ultimately used, inviting students to consider the cost of their use should prompt ethically valuable conversation.

While most of the arguments (e.g., Kantian, contractualist) could apply to any classroom, and some (those based on a tension with the Nuremberg Code or the Belmont Report) would apply equally well to medicine, we do think there is a special obligation for nursing educators to be sensitive to these issues. Nursing ethics—even more than medicine—centers on knowledge of and advocacy for individuals. While it might be impossible to satisfy all the criteria for a caring relationship with distant individuals in photographs (see, e.g., Carper, 1979, for a classical statement), one of the most important aspects behind the logic of the need for caring "is the tendency to devalue the individual" (Carper, 1979, p. 12); this is precisely the value that we maintain is at issue here. And while nurses serve vital roles in discussions of policy and public health, on at least some conceptions the major defining factor of nursing is the emphasis on caregiving for individuals (Chinn, 2019). If nurses are not trained to be especially sensitive to respect for vulnerable individuals—even at the potential expense of some broader good—it is unlikely that anyone else will step in to fill that role.

References

Alessandra, T., & O'Connor, M. J. (1996). *The platinum rule.* Grand Central.

Alexander, L., & Moore, M. (2021). Deontological Ethics. In E. N. Zalta (Ed.), *The Stanford encyclopedia of philosophy.* Metaphysics Research Lab, Stanford University. https://plato.stanford.edu/archives/win2021/entries/ethics-deontological/.

National Commission for the Protection of Human Subjects of Biomedical, & Behavioral Research. (1978). *The Belmont report: Ethical principles and guidelines for the protection of human subjects of research* (Vol. 2). Department of Health, Education, and Welfare.

Brennan, S. (1995). Thresholds for rights. *The Southern Journal of Philosophy, 33*(2), 143–168.

Buss, S., & Westlund, A. (2013). Personal autonomy. In E. N. Zalta (Ed.), *Stanford encyclopedia of philosophy* (Summer 2013 ed.). https://plato.stanford.edu/archives/sum2013/entries/personal-autonomy/.

Carper, B. A. (1979). The ethics of caring. *Advances in Nursing Science, 1*(3), 11–20.

Chinn, P. L. (2019). *The discipline of nursing: Moving forward boldly.* Nursing Theory: A 50 Year Perspective, Past and Future, Case Western Reserve University Frances Payne Bolton School of Medicine.

Cook, T. (2018). Deontologists can be moderate. *Journal of Value Inquiry, 52*(2), 199–212.

Cornish, S. (2017). The responsibility to bear witness: Stephen Cornish on why MSF speaks out about what we see on the front lines of crisis. *Doctors Without Borders.* https://www.doctorswithoutborders.ca/article/responsibility-bear-witness-stephen-cornish-why-msf-speaks-out-about-what-we-see-front-lines.

Grue, J. (2016). The problem with inspiration porn: A tentative definition and a provisional critique. *Disability and Society, 31*(6), 838–849.

Hooker, B. (1990). Rule-consequentialism. *Mind, 99*(393), 67–77.

Johnson, C. M. (2020). How deontologists can be moderate. *Journal of Value Inquiry, 54*(2), 227–243.

Karigan, M. (2001). Ethics in clinical research: The nursing perspective. *The American Journal of Nursing, 101*(9), 26–31.

Moreno, J. D., Schmidt, U., & Joffe, S. (2017). The Nuremberg code 70 years later. *JAMA, 318*(9), 795–796.

Nagel, T. (1970). *The possibility of altruism.* Oxford University Press.

Nagel, T. (1987). *What does it all mean? A very short introduction to philosophy.* Oxford University Press.

Nguyen, C. T., & Williams, B. (2020). Moral outrage porn. *Journal of Ethics and Social Philosophy, 18*(2), 147–172.

Rawls, J. (1971). *A theory of justice.* Harvard University Press.

Robinson, S., & Doody, O. (2021). *Nursing and healthcare ethics* (6th ed.). Elsevier.

Scanlon, T. M. (1998). *What we owe to each other.* Harvard University Press.

Shelton, S., & Waddell, T. F. (2020). Does "inspiration porn" inspire? How disability and challenge impact attitudinal evaluations of advertising. *Journal of Current Issues & Research in Advertising, 42*(3), 258–276.

Shuster, E. (1997). Fifty years later: The significance of the Nuremberg Code. *New England Journal of Medicine, 337*(20), 1436–1440.

Sims, J. M. (2010). A brief review of the Belmont report. *Dimensions of Critical Care Nursing, 29*(4), 173–174.

Sontag, S. (2003). *Regarding the pain of others.* Farrar, Straus, and Giroux.

Staff & agencies. (2003, April 18). Horror at desecration of woman's body. *The Guardian.* https://www.theguardian.com/world/2003/apr/18/religion.uk.

Thomson, J. J. (1985). The trolley problem. *The Yale Law Journal, 94*(6), 1395–1415.

Vaish, A., Grossmann, T., & Woodward, A. (2008). Not all emotions are created equal: The negativity bias in social-emotional development. *Psychological Bulletin, 134*(3), 383–403.

Weiser, B. (2020, February 21). Beatings, burns and betrayal: The Willowbrook Scandal's legacy. *New York Times.* https://www.nytimes.com/2020/02/21/nyregion/willowbrook-state-school-staten-island.html?smid=url-share.

Index

For the benefit of digital users, indexed terms that span two pages (e.g., 52–53) may, on occasion, appear on only one of those pages.

Note: Tables and figures are indicated by an italic *t* and *f* following the page number.